THE HISTORY OF SURGICAL ANESTHESIA

☙ TO ❧

JOHN SILAS LUNDY

WHOSE COUNSEL AND
ENCOURAGEMENT
MADE THIS BOOK POSSIBLE

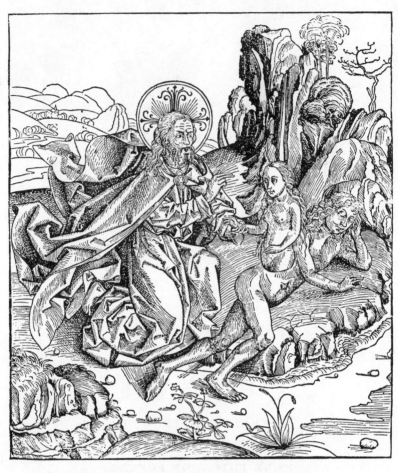

*"And the Lord God caused a deep sleep
to fall upon Adam, and he slept."*

Wood engraving attributed to Michael Wohlgemuth from
the *Nuremberg Chronicle*, 1493.

THE HISTORY OF SURGICAL ANESTHESIA

by

Thomas E. Keys, M.A., Sc.D. (h.c.)

Medical Library Consultant

formerly
Librarian of the Mayo Clinic

Honorary Member
American Society of Anesthesiologists

Foreword to the 1978
Reprint Edition
by K. Garth Huston, M.D.

With an Introductory Essay
by Chauncey D. Leake

A Concluding Chapter
"The Future of Anaesthesia"
by Noel A. Gillespie

And an Appendix
by John F. Fulton

ROBERT E. KRIEGER PUBLISHING COMPANY
HUNTINGTON, NEW YORK
1978

Original Edition 1945
Reprint 1978

617.9609

K44

Printed and Published by
ROBERT E. KRIEGER PUBLISHING CO., INC.
645 NEW YORK AVENUE
HUNTINGTON, NEW YORK 11743

Printed in the United States of America

Library of Congress Cataloging in Publication Data

Keys, Thomas Edward, 1908-
    The history of surgical anesthesia.

    Reprint of the 1963 edition published by Dover Publications,
New York.
    Bibliography: p.
    1. Anesthesiology—History.   I. Title.
[DNLM: 1. Anesthesiology—History.   WO211 K44h 1963a]
RD79.K4 1978   617'.96'09   77-14935
ISBN 0-88275-570-6

FOREWORD TO THE 1978 REPRINT EDITION

Few medical histories survive for thirty years. Dr. Keys' *The History of Surgical Anesthesia* has achieved this distinction, and deservedly so. Originally elegantly published by Henry Schuman in 1945, it was a compilation, distillation and synthesis of several earlier chronologies and histories by Dr. Keys. And it came at a proper time for the needed audience, just prior to the anesthesia centennial in 1946 and after the flourishing and development of anesthesia as a specialty during World War II. There was a flood of new residents in the field of anesthesiology, and it was correctly rumored that the answers to the historical questions on the Board examination could be found in this book.

The book was consequently soon out of print. Dover Publications, Inc. came out with a new edition, revised, with new photographs, bringing the history to 1963. There were two Dover editions. The History was translated into Japanese in 1966 and German in 1968, showing the international interest in what was the first great American medical discovery.

Now in 1978 Robert Krieger is reprinting what has become a classic, what antiquarian booksellers describe as "out-of-print, scarce" (translated "expensive"). This reprinting will bring the book back in the price range of students and residents, as it should be.

This is a reprinting, not a revision, and I think rightly so. In 1945 it was possible to synthesize and summarize the anesthesia achievements of a hundred years, including anesthesia pre-history. And in 1963 it was again possible to chronicle the changes that had occurred since 1945. In the last twenty years, however, the discoveries on all fronts have been so numerous and the state of the art in such a degree of flux that wisely, I think, Dr. Keys has elected to let someone else in the future bring order out of the present chaos. To cite a few examples:

1. Introduction of non-explosive, halogenated anesthetics with the subsequent problems related to liver, kidney and possible carcinogenesis. And the concomitant use of cautery by surgeons which has led to the almost total disuse of older (and excellent) explosive anesthetics (ether, cyclopropane, etc.).
2. The discovery of dissociative anesthetics (Ketamine) and anesthesia adjuvants (neuroleptanalgesia).
3. The discovery of long-acting local anesthetics, as well as local anesthetics that diffuse better through tissue planes, leading to an increased interest in regional anesthetic techniques for surgery and for diagnostic and therapeutic pain problems.

4. An increased interest in obstetric anesthesia and analgesia, with the qualification of excellent men in the combined specialties. This has been responsible for increased research leading to safer parturition for mother and babe.
5. Advances in the development of new muscle relaxants and to better knowledge of the physiology of the myoneural junction.
6. Advances in anesthesia techniques for cardiovascular and transplant surgery.
7. Worries about the effects of trace anesthesia gases on operating room personnel.
8. Increases in basic technology—invasive and non-invasive monitoring; ventilator technology, ready availability of blood-gas determinations; disposable anesthesia products, micropore blood filters, etc.
9. The active involvement of anesthesia personnel in various intensive care facilities outside the O.R.
10. Re-discovery and amplification of forgotten 18th century cardiopulmonary resuscitation techniques, with all of the current successful CPR advances.

Many other changes could be mentioned. One sign (or perhaps symptom) of the multitudinous changes is in the mass of anesthesia literature—in 1945 every important book on anesthesia could be contained on one (short) bookshelf and anesthesia journals could be counted on one hand. With the founding of independent anesthesia departments (and perhaps with what is popularly known as the publish-or-perish syndrome), no one person can keep track of anesthesia-related items and there are survey journals, abstracting journals, recorded tapes of meetings, computer print outs, and other aids, to keep those in active practice abreast of current developments in anesthesia and related fields.

In conclusion, Dr. Keys' book covers the development of anesthesia until 1963. And wisely, I think, he has left to another the shakedown of the chaff from the wheat in the current anesthesia scene.

K. Garth Huston, M.D.

Contents

		PAGE
List of Illustrations	. . . .	ii
Preface to the 1963 Edition	. . . .	iii
Preface	. . . .	ix
Introductory Essay by Chauncey D. Leake	. . . .	xiii

I. The Development of Anesthesia 3
  A—The Beginnings 3
  B—From Priestley to Morton 14
  C—The Acceptance of Anesthesia 31
  D—Local, Regional and Spinal Anesthesia 37
  E—Anoci-association; Refrigeration Anesthesia . . . 44
  F—Rectal Anesthesia 45
  G—"Twilight" Sleep 48
  H—Ethylene, Divinyl Oxide, Cyclopropane and Cyprome
      Ether 49
  I—Intravenous Anesthesia and Related Procedures . . 53
  J—Endotracheal Anesthesia 63
  K—Carbon Dioxide Absorption 69
  L—Physiologic Factors 71
  M—Pharmacologic Factors 80
  N—Anesthetic Apparatus 83
  O—Records and Statistics 86
  P—Concluding Comments 89
  References for Section I 93

II. A Chronology of Events Relating to Anesthesiology and Allied
    Subjects 103

III. Selected References by Subject 126

IV. Selected References by Author 150

The Future of Anæsthesia, by Noel A. Gillespie . . . 171

Appendix by John F. Fulton 177

Index 185

List of Illustrations

FRONTISPIECE: Wood engraving from the *Nuremberg Chronicle*, 1493

FIGURE   ON OR FACING PAGE

1. Early use of alcohol for anesthetic purposes 4
2. Title page to the first edition of Bullein's *Bulwarke of Defence* 5
3. Mesmer practicing animal magnetism 12
4. Hickman experimenting with anesthesia on animals . . 13
5. Title page to Humphry Davy's book 16
6. Humphry Davy's "gas machine" 17
7. Title page to Hickman's pamphlet 20
8. Crawford W. Long 20
9. Holograph letter by Crawford W. Long 21
10. Horace Wells 22
11. William T. G. Morton 23
12. John C. Warren 26
13. The first public demonstration of anesthesia with ether . 27
14. John Snow 28
15. Sir James Young Simpson 29
16. Title page of transactions of first meeting of the A. M. A. . 34
17. Queen Victoria in 1855 36
18. Friedrich Wilhelm Sertürner 37
19. Carl Koller 44
20. J. Leonard Corning 45
21. Title page of Pirogoff's book 46
22. Rudolph Matas 52
23. George W. Crile 53
24. James T. Gwathmey 54
25. Arno B. Luckhardt 55
26. Title page to first monograph on intravenous anesthesia . 57
27. Chauncey D. Leake 58
28. Ralph M. Waters 59
29. Sir Christopher Wren 60
30. Richard Lower 61
31. Initial Q from Vesalius's *Fabrica*, 1543 62
32. Emil Fischer 64
33. John S. Lundy 65
34. Original Fell-O'Dwyer apparatus 66
35. The Matas modification of O'Dwyer's intubating apparatus 67
36. Dennis E. Jackson 70
37. Model of Dennis Jackson's first anesthetic apparatus . . 71
38. Paul Bert 74
39. Paul Bert's anesthetic apparatus 75
40. Arthur E. Guedel 78
41. Wesley Bourne 79
42a and b. Letters from Royal Society of Medicine to Dr. Bourne 80,81
43a and b. W.T.G. Morton's Notice "To Surgeons and
   Physicians" 177,178

Preface to the 1963 Edition

THE ORIGINAL edition of this work appeared shortly before the end of World War II. Since that time my interest in the history of anesthesia has continued. In 1954 I was asked by Dr. Rudolf Frey, editor of *Der Anaesthesist*, to prepare an article[1] on historical anesthesia. This gave me an opportunity to review my book, epitomize the subject and rework the field. It also brought to light some minor inaccuracies, which have been corrected along with those mentioned earlier in some of the reviews of my book. In addition, the chronology of events and the sources for the chronology have been extended to 1953, and there have been brief additions to the text, references, and bibliography. A few of the portraits have been replaced with better or more recent likenesses.

In the fall of 1961 I was invited to read a paper on historical anesthesia[2] at the annual meeting of the Japan Pharmaceutical Library Association in Tokyo. In preparing for this lecture I found evidence that a Japanese surgeon, Seishu Hanaoka[3] introduced painless operations under narcosis some time prior to 1835. It does seem reasonable to believe that more facts have been and will be uncovered concerning the history of anesthesia as the older books and manuscripts are read and reread by the scholars interested in the subject. A recent paper by N. H. Keswani[4] suggests that the ancient Hindu literature is replete with references to pain-relieving plants and that concoctions from such plants were administered before painless surgery.

In the original edition of my book (pp. 21-22) it was reported that William Clarke administered ether to a patient prior to a dental extraction by Dr. Elijah Pope in January, 1842. I said that "This would appear to be the first use of ether anesthesia on record." My source was in a book by Lyman (ref. 23, p. 93). Since then I have found another source for this statement in a book by Hubbell.[5] This author also suggests why Clarke did not continue to use ether as an anesthetic agent:

> Another claimant for the early administration of sulphuric ether as an anesthetic, according to Professor Lyman . . . was the late Dr. W. E. Clark, [sic] of Chicago, Ill., who, while a student in Dr. E. M. Moore's office, Rochester, N.Y., in the winter of 1842, administered ether to a young woman for the extraction of a diseased tooth, which was done with the patient in an unconscious state. Dr. Moore believed, however, that the unconsciousness was hysterical, and advised his pupil to make no more experiments in that direction, and the advice was unfortunately followed.

As my readers are aware, I have always thought, from the study of the evidence, that Morton's contribution was the most important, and recently, in delving into the literature, I came across a letter from Oliver Wendell Holmes[6] to E. L. Snell giving support to this contention:

Boston, April 2, 1893.

My Dear Sir,—Few persons have or had better reason than myself to assert the claim of Dr. Morton to the introduction of artificial anaesthesia into surgical practice. The discovery was formally introduced to the scientific world in a paper read before the American Academy of Arts and Sciences by Dr. Henry J. Bigelow, one of the first, if not the first, of American surgeons.

On the evening before the reading of the paper containing the announcement of the discovery, Dr. Bigelow called at my office to recite this paper to me. He prefaced it in a few words which could never be forgotten.

He told me that a great discovery had been made, and its genuineness demonstrated at the Massachusetts General Hospital, of which he was one of the surgeons. This was the production of insensibility to pain during surgical operations by the inhalation of a certain vapor (the same afterward shown to be that of sulphuric ether). In a very short time, he said, this discovery will be all over Europe. He had taken a great interest in the alleged discovery, had been present at the first capital operation performed under its influence, and was from the first the adviser and supporter of Dr. W. T. G. Morton, who had induced the surgeons of the hospital to make trial of the means by which he proposed to work this new miracle. The discovery went all over the world like a conflagration.

The only question was whether Morton got advice from Dr. Charles T. Jackson, the chemist, which entitled that gentleman to a share, greater or less, in the merit of the discovery.

Later it was questioned whether he did not owe his first hint to Dr. Horace Wells, of Hartford, which need not be disputed. Both these gentlemen deserve "honourable mention" in connection with the discovery, but I have never a moment hesitated in awarding the essential credit of the great achievement to Dr. Morton.

[iv]

Preface to the 1963 Edition

This priceless gift to humanity went forth from the operating-theater of the Massachusetts General Hospital, and the man to whom the world owes it is Dr. William Thomas Green Morton.

Experiments have been made with other substances besides sulphuric ether for the production of anaesthesia. Among them, by far the most important is chloroform, the use of which was introduced by Sir James Y. Simpson. For this and for the employment of anaesthetics in midwifery he should have all due credit; but his attempt to appropriate the glory of making the great and immortal discovery, as revealed in his contribution to the eighth edition of the "Encyclopaedia Britannica," is unworthy of a man in his highly respectable position. In the ninth edition of the same work his article "Chloroform" is omitted and a fair enough account of the discovery is given under the title "Anaesthesia."

Yours very truly,

O. W. HOLMES

A sympathetic insight into Morton's[7] high professional attitude toward anesthesia is provided by his *Remarks on the Proper Mode of Administering Sulphuric Ether by Inhalation.* In this remarkable pamphlet Morton considers (1) the mode of administration, (2) the effects produced, (3) the symptoms of insensibility, (4) the difficulties and dangers, and (5) the best means of obviating and removing these.

As mentioned in the original text (p. 29), the early use of anesthesia developed rapidly in Europe. Ether was given a clinical trial in Paris on December 15, 1846, when Dr. Jobert invited the young American surgeon, F. Willis Fisher,[8] to act as his anesthetist. Fisher had heard about the introduction of anesthesia at the Massachusetts General Hospital in a letter he had received from a medical friend from Boston. This demonstration was unsuccessful. Nothing more was attempted by way of experiments until letters from Drs. Ware and Warren of Boston were published in the French medical journals. This revived interest in ether anesthesia, and on January 12, 1847, Dr. Malgaine reported before the French Academy of Medicine four successful operations performed on patients at the Hôpital St. Louis while they were under the influence of ether. This aroused considerable discussion and the general opinion was expressed that the new discovery was one of great importance.

After many more trials and experiments had been made, some failures and some successes, inhalation anesthesia was gradually adopted in France.

Meanwhile, in England, Dr. Francis Boott[9] had heard about ether anesthesia from his American colleague Dr. Jacob Bigelow, in a letter from Boston dated November 28, 1846. It was Dr. Bigelow's son, Dr. Henry Jacob Bigelow, who publicized the first public demonstration of anesthesia by reading a paper on this subject before the Boston Society of Medical Improvement on November 9, 1846. Interestingly enough, he previously had read an abstract of this paper before the American Academy of Arts and Sciences on November 3, 1846.

Dr. Boott, wishing to bring about the successful use of anesthesia in London, organized a demonstration. On December 19, 1846, he arranged for a tooth extraction in his own study while the patient was anesthetized. The patient was a Miss Dondale and the dentist-anesthetist was a Mr. Robinson. The dental surgery, accomplished without the least sense of pain, was highly successful.

As suggested in the first edition of my book, modern rectal anesthesia was attempted shortly after sulfuric ether became available as an anesthetic agent. It is interesting to learn in a recent article by Horine[10] that in the first century A.D., Dioscorides described the anesthetic effects of mandragora by its use in the form of a suppository or rectal injection. The sedative enema is also mentioned in Gerard's[11] *Herball*, published in 1633.

The development of trichlorethylene as an anesthetic agent should be discussed. In 1935 Cecil Striker,[12] Samuel Goldblatt, I. S. Warm and D. E. Jackson reported on its anesthetic value for operations of short duration in over 300 cases. This agent seems to have been neglected until 1939 when C. Langton Hewer[13-16] anesthetist at St. Bartholomew's Hospital, made his careful investigation. He concluded that purified trichlorethylene was an excellent inhalant drug for producing general analgesia. It was also found to be satisfactory if given in combination with nitrous oxide and oxygen, especially if sparks were present.

He discovered that it should not be used for a profound narcosis and not in a closed circuit apparatus with soda lime.

Joseph T. Clover,[17] the English anesthetist, became interested in nitrous oxide anesthesia in 1868. He discovered that chloroform apparatus was equally well adapted to the administration of nitrous oxide. He noticed in a few cases, however, some unsatisfactory results. Reasoning that this was due to the gas not being able to travel quickly enough along the tube during the forced motions of respiration, Clover invented a supplementary re-breathing bag which allowed for the re-breathing of a portion of the gas.

Another British pioneer in the development of nitrous oxide anesthesia was Alfred Coleman[18] (1828-1902), a dental surgeon. Apparently he was the first to devise a carbon dioxide absorber to be used clinically. The expired gas was passed over slaked lime contained in a gas tube before returning to the bag again.

Since the appearance of the original edition two of the contributors have died, Dr. Noel Gillespie (1904-1955), who wrote the concluding chapter, and Dr. John F. Fulton (1899-1960), who prepared the appendix. Many others mentioned in the text have also died. These include: Dr. Richard C. Adams (1906-1956), Dr. Walter M. Boothby (1880-1953), Dr. Howard Dittrick (1877-1954), Dr. Arthur E. Guedel (1883-1956), Dr. Arno B. Luckhardt (1885-1957), Dr. Rudolph Matas (1860-1957), Dr. Albert H. Miller (1872-1959), Dr. Emery A. Rovenstine (1895-1960), Dr. Henry S. Ruth (1899-1956), Dr. Brian C. Sword (1899-1956), and Dr. Edward B. Tuohy (1908-1959). There are probably many others that I have not heard about.

I consider it a great compliment that this book now appears in a paperback edition and I wish to thank Mr. Hayward Cirker, President of Dover Publications, for making this possible.

THOMAS E. KEYS

Rochester, Minnesota
November, 1962

[vii]

References for Preface to the 1963 Edition

1. KEYS, T. E.: An Epitome of the History of Surgical Anesthesia. Anaesthesist. 3:273-283 (Dec.) 1954.

2. ——: "An Epitome of the History of Western Surgical Anesthesia." (Read at the meeting of the Japan Pharmaceutical Library Association, Tokyo, Japan, November 11, 1961.) 25 pp. Mimeo. including trans. into Japanese.

3. HANAOKA, SEISHU: Quoted in Fujikawa, Yu: Japanese Medicine. New York, Paul B. Hoeber, Inc., 1934. pp. 57-58.

4. KESWANI, N. H.: Anæsthesia and Analgesia among the Ancients. Part I. Indian J. Anæsthesia. 9:231-242 (Nov.) 1961.

5. HUBBELL, A. A.: The Development of Ophthalmology in America, 1800 to 1870 . . . . Chicago, W. T. Keener & Co., 1907. p. 132.

6. HOLMES, O. W.: Letter to Mr. E. L. Snell, dated April 2, 1893. Reprinted in Practitioner 57:340-341 (Oct.) 1896.

7. MORTON, W. T. G.: Remarks on the Proper Mode of Administering Sulphuric Ether by Inhalation. Boston, Dalton & Wentworth, Printers, 1847. 44 pp.

8. FISHER, F. W.: The Ether Inhalation in Paris. Boston M. S. J. 36:109-113 (March 10) 1847.

9. BOOTT, FRANCIS: Surgical Operations Performed During Insensibility. Lancet 1:5-8 (Jan. 2) 1847.

10. HORINE, E. F.: Episodes in the History of Anesthesia. J. Hist. Med. 1:521-526 (Oct.) 1946.

11. GERARD, JOHN: The Herball, or General History of Plants (ed. by Thomas Johnson). London, Adam Islip, Joyce Norton and Richard Whitakers, 1633.

12. STRIKER, CECIL, and OTHERS: Clinical Experiences with the Use of Trichlorethylene in the Production of over 300 Analgesias and Anesthesias. Anesth. & Analg. 14:68-71 (March-April) 1935.

13. HEWER, C. L.: Trichlorethylene as an Inhalation Agent. Brit. M. J. 1:924-927 (June 21) 1941.

14. ——: Trichlorethylene as a General Analgesic and Anæsthetic. Proc. Roy. Soc. Med., Section on Anæsthetics. 35:463-468 (March 6) 1942.

15. ——: Further Observations on Trichlorethylene. Proc. Roy. Soc. Med., Section on Anæsthetics 36:463-465 (March 5) 1943.

16. ——: Trichlorethylene as an Anæsthetic Agent. Brit. M. Bull. 4, no. 2:108-110, 1946.

17. CLOVER, J. T.: in Duncum, Barbara: The Development of Inhalation Anesthesia. London, Oxford University Press, 1947. pp. 286-287.

18. COLEMAN, ALFRED: Economical Processes of Preparing and Administering Nitrous Oxide. Brit. M. J. 2:1056 (Dec. 31) 1881.

Preface

THIS BOOK had its beginning by way of a chance conversation with Dr. John S. Lundy, Chief of the Section on Anesthesia, Mayo Clinic. I asked Dr. Lundy if he was planning to include any historical material in his new book on anesthesia. Dr. Lundy said that he was and asked for my advice. We decided after considering different proposals that the most practical thing to do was to make a chronologic table. This was done and the table appeared in Lundy's *Clinical Anesthesia* (Saunders, 1942) as chapter 29, pp. 705-717.

In the preparation of the chronology, I had gathered together a considerable number of notes. On the invitation of Dr. Henry Ruth, the editor of *Anesthesiology*, I rewrote my notes into a series of five papers, which were published in *Anesthesiology* under the title "The Development of Anesthesia" as follows: 2:552-574 (Sept.) 1941; 3:11-23 (Jan.), 282-294 (May), 650-658 (Nov.) 1942 and 4:409-429 (July) 1943. A collected reprint was made incorporating these five articles and distributed to those interested. My bibliographic friends chided me a bit, for the source of the collected reprint was not given on either the cover or the title page. This was, to be sure, an oversight but had these same bibliographic friends bothered to read this reprint, they could have found in the first line of my "concluding comments" the sources given as numbered bibliographic references.

Before I had a chance to finish these papers the war broke out. I wrote the final two articles in spare evenings as a member of the Armed Forces, first in Washington, D. C., where I was assigned as assistant to the Librarian, Army Medical Library, and secondly in Cleveland, Ohio, where I was appointed Officer in Charge of the Cleveland Branch, Army Medical Library.

In Cleveland it was my good fortune to meet Dr. Howard Dittrick, the editor of *Current Researches in Anesthesia and Analgesia*. Dr. Dittrick asked me for a contribution to *Current Researches*.

I decided that a selected list of important references arranged by subject might be desired. This met with his approval and was published in two installments.

Meanwhile I had been urged by a few of my friends to make this contribution of a more permanent character; especially my good friend Chauncey Leake urged me to build it into a book. He wrote a letter to Henry Schuman advising this. Mr. Schuman offered publication. This offer was accepted and it was decided to include a revision of the five essays, a revision of the chronology and a selected list of references arranged by author and subject. Acknowledgment is hereby made to the W. B. Saunders Co., *Anesthesiology* and *Current Researches in Anesthesia and Analgesia* for permission to use the material referred to previously. I am indebted again to *Anesthesiology* for the use of the cuts which appeared in the original essays.

I am indebted to a considerable number of persons for their help and encouragement in this project. I especially wish to thank Dr. Lundy and his staff for their complete co-operation and for their many helpful suggestions. To my other friends in the field of anesthesiology and especially to Dr. Leake for his unfailing generosity in writing the introduction and for his boundless enthusiasm, to Drs. Ralph Waters and Noel Gillespie for their critical analysis of the book in its early stages and again to Dr. Gillespie for the concluding chapter I express my appreciation. It will be noted that Dr. Gillespie prefers the spelling "anæsthesia" which has therefore been used in his chapter. Dr. John F. Fulton has kindly consented to publish his bibliographic study of the *Letheon* tracts as an appendix. To Dr. Fulton and to Madeline Stanton, who assisted him, I wish to convey my appreciation.

Since the publication of the original essays it is with saddened heart that I bring to the attention of my readers the deaths of some of anesthesia's most profound contributors: Karl Albert Connell on October 18, 1941, at the age of sixty-three years; George Washington Crile on January 7, 1943, at the age of seventy-eight; James Tayloe Gwathmey on February 11, 1944, at the age of eighty; and Carl Koller on March 22, 1944, at the age of eighty-six. It is hoped that their contributions have received adequate attention within these pages.

A book of this nature necessitates a good deal of bibliographic research. I have seen as my responsibility not only the correcting of many of the errors that have crept into the history of anesthesia but also on the basis of historiography to try to present with an unbiased judgment the main contributions. This building of a synthesis is not easy and there are probably important omissions. Won't my readers please advise me of them and of other ways to improve this book?

My appreciation is extended to my library colleagues for their help in supplying source materials. Thanks are especially due to Catherine Kennedy and others of the Mayo Clinic Library, Jens Christian Bay of the John Crerar Library, James Francis Ballard of the Boston Medical Library, Colonel Harold Wellington Jones of the Army Medical Library, Washington, D. C., and Max Harold Fisch and Dorothy May Schullian of the Cleveland Branch of the Army Medical Library. Drs. Fisch and Schullian also translated many passages from the Latin.

My appreciation is likewise extended to Dr. Robert M. Stecher and Miss Ada Floyd of the Cleveland Medical Library Association for their many courtesies. Let every historian of medicine pay tribute to the possessors of the early *original* volumes of the *Philosophical Transactions of the Royal Society*, so full of important data. I believe I was one of the first to use these volumes recently acquired and a prize possession of the Cleveland Medical Library Association.

Finally I wish to express my warm thanks to Dr. and Mrs. Logan Clendening* of Kansas City. Dr. Clendening's library, one of the well known historical collections, includes a vast array of important materials on the history of anesthesia, especially the American contributions. I had the pleasure last October of spending a few days with the Clendenings and their splendid library and I learned many things. A short title list of Dr. Clendening's

*This paragraph was written shortly before Dr. Clendening's death on January 31, 1945.

library on anesthesia was published in the *Bulletin of the Medical Library Association* for January, 1945.

During the preparation of the manuscript, it was necessary to correspond with many persons. To them I express my indebtedness for their splendid co-operation.

For the advice and encouragement I received from the Division of Publications of the Mayo Clinic, for the preliminary editing by James Eckman, now Captain Eckman, and to Dr. John R. Miner, who was responsible for the editing of the revised version, I express my gratitude.

And to Henry Schuman for his painstaking advice about all the publisher's details, for his encouraging confidence that the materials now brought together and revised will meet a genuine need; and to A. Colish for producing a book of such tasteful design and quality in these difficult times.

THOMAS E. KEYS

Introductory Essay

In the midst of the closing anguish of our tentative (and may it be our last!) experiment with total war, it is fitting to reflect a bit upon the practical and specific achievement of the past hundred years on the relief of physical pain. For these fateful forties of the twentieth century are the centennial of the first successful efforts in the solution of the problem of surgical anesthesia in the fabled forties of the nineteenth. May the next hundred years be as successful in affording a capacity for relief of mental suffering!

Control of pain incident to surgical operation was a pressing problem for centuries. While alcoholic concoctions must early have been used, following recognition of their stupefying effects, they were not successful because of the delirium they produced.

Pressure was used on nerves or blood vessels, as by the early Egyptian surgeons, in order to cause insensibility in the part to be operated upon. Attempts seem even to have been made by Græco-Roman surgeons to produce what we now call carbon dioxide, to bring sleep by inhalation. Amazingly, the early Inca shamans seem to have observed and utilized in trephining the pain-relieving properties of extracts of coca leaves, made by chewing the leaves and allowing the saliva to drop upon the bashed-in area on the skull to be excised. When one thinks that many of these primitive surgeons used flint knives, one appreciates what effort must have been made to get relief from the accompanying pain!

With more knowledge, concoctions of mandragora and opium had to suffice European surgeons until the development of modern chemistry made possible the study of the effects of pure chemical agents. Of course, shock in the patient may have helped also to relieve pain. Perhaps the most important factor in the success of the pre-anesthesia surgeon was his sleight-of-hand dexterity. It is astonishing that surgery continued to be practiced at all in the face of the patient's painful struggle without anesthesia, and the almost certain fatal termination without asepsis.

The History of Surgical Anesthesia

Remarkable is the fact that so many chemical agents with anesthetic properties were known and their pain relieving actions recognized long before they were practically applied in surgical anesthesia. Ether was described about 1540 by that remarkable genius, Valerius Cordus (1515-1544). It was not effectively used for anesthesia until centuries later, although there is indication that its "sleep producing" properties were known about the time of its discovery. Ether was even included in early nineteenth century pharmacopeias, but not for anesthesia. Nitrous oxide was recognized by the young Humphry Davy (1778-1829) in 1800 as being suitable for pain relief in surgical operation, but was not utilized until forty-four years later. How many of the hundreds of thousands of compounds in *Beilstein* may have important medicinal uses, if only pharmacologists can be given the opportunity systematically to explore them!

It is not merely a matter of chance that the problem of surgical anesthesia should have been solved in a practical way by the eminently hard-headed Americans, as soon as an inkling of available means became known to them. A century ago, this country was still a rapidly expanding pioneer state. People were too busy to be bothered with the finer medical skills. The chief problem in medical practice was surgical. In spite of the rough and ready individualism of the frontier nation, there was an underlying current of rich sympathy and sentiment for suffering humanity. Surgeons were on the watch for something that would relieve the pain that made their operative procedures so difficult.

Both the physician, Crawford W. Long (1815-1878) in Georgia, and the dentist, Horace Wells (1815-1848) in Connecticut, appreciated the practical applications in surgery of casual observations of the effects of ether and nitrous oxide respectively, Long at a backwoods "ether frolic," and Wells watching the effects of "laughing gas" in an itinerant chemist show. The matter was so pressing that in spite of Wells' tragic failure with nitrous oxide before the surgeons of the Massachusetts General Hospital, his former dental partner, W. T. G. Morton (1819-1868), was sufficiently stimulated to start systematic study and

Introductory Essay

experimentation. It was Morton's persistence in working out a practical technic for the administration of ether that made satisfactory anesthesia possible. A similar practical persistence has been displayed in this country in the development of sulfa drugs, antibiotics, vitamins, barbital derivatives, and local anesthetics.

Almost exactly paralleling the development of modern chemistry and pharmacology in the last century, anesthesia has become a highly complex special field of scientific investigation in the practical application of medicine. Thousands of chemical agents are now available for the relief of pain. Many complicated technical procedures of administration of anesthetics have been proposed and utilized. The successful application of the vast knowledge which has accumulated in the field requires broad appreciation of physiological principles, biochemical reactions, modifications induced by pathology, anatomical considerations, appreciation of the objectives of the surgeon, and even profound skill and insight with regard to psychological and neuropsychiatric factors. The modern professional anesthesiologist is indeed a highly trained medical specialist.

WHAT ARE PAIN AND ANESTHESIA?

Yet anesthesia remains primarily an empirical development. Our ignorance of pain is still appalling. Yet pain is the basic factor with which anesthesia is concerned. We recognize the molecular disturbances in nerves and brain, interpreted by our conditioning as "pain," to be adaptations conducive toward survival. But even in this fundamental concept we are baffled by the perversities of some individuals who seemingly enjoy and welcome pain! We know that the sensation of pain is greatly altered by mental states. Anatomists and physiologists have been able to trace the pathways for pain and have succeeded in demonstrating many of the factors which alter conduction and perception of pain. But we still do not know what pain is!

The extent of a generation's progress in approaching the concept of pain may be judged by comparing two interesting volumes having this same title. The earlier is R. J. Behan's *Pain:*

[xv]

The History of Surgical Anesthesia

Its Origin, Conduction, Perception and Diagnostic Significance (D. Appleton, New York and London, 1914, containing sixty-two pages of references), and the more recent is The Association for Research in Nervous and Mental Disease's *Pain* (*Res. Publ. Ass. Nerv. Ment. Dis.*, 23, Baltimore, 1943, containing thirty-two separate articles by different authors). Between these two volumes there appeared another interesting publication of The Association for Research in Nervous and Mental Disease which also relates importantly to pain and anesthesia, *Sensation: Its Mechanisms and Disturbances* (*Res. Publ. Ass. Nerv. Ment. Dis.*, 15, Baltimore, 1935, containing twenty contributions on the sensory nerve endings, visceral sensations, and sensory tracts and mechanisms in the spinal cord and brain).

It is interesting that in the generation between Behan's *Pain* and the 1943 collaborative effort on the same subject, the ancient metaphysical concepts regarding pain should finally have been sloughed by medical scientists. Behan in 1914 still considers these concepts in discussing pain. In 1943 they have vanished into the thin air from which they apparently came. It is amazing, however, how semantic difficulties persist. Pain is still frequently thought to be the antithesis of pleasure, whatever that is. While anesthesia relieves pain, it can hardly be thought of as a pleasure!

Recent investigations, particularly by Nobelates Joseph Erlanger and Herbert Gasser, have demonstrated that painful sensations are carried by slow conduction in fibers of what are called the "C" group, and rapidly by "A" fibers. It has been shown that summation of painful stimuli does not occur, since as an area exposed to a painful stimulus is increased, the pain threshold is not lowered (J. D. Hardy, H. G. Wolff, and H. Goodell, Studies on Pain: A New Method for Measuring Pain Threshold: Observations on Spatial Summation of Pain, *Journ. Clin. Investig.*, 19:649, 1940). Thus it may be inferred that the intensity of pain is determined by the frequency of conduction. While it is this intensity which determines the amount of an anesthetic or analgesic necessary to use, it is agreed that the emotional state of the individual profoundly alters the threshold to pain.

Introductory Essay

Morphine, alcohol, and the barbiturates may act as analgesics by blocking synapses, thus producing disorientation with dissociation of pain perception from the usual pattern of reaction to pain. Aspirin and chemically related antipyretics may act in a similar manner in part, but they also have a significant effect in altering permeability patterns of cells so that pain resulting from swelling of tissues within a rigidly enclosed case may be relieved by their effect in withdrawing fluids from the congested area. The general inhalation anesthetics such as ether and chloroform apparently break association pathways in the cerebral cortex so as to produce complete lack of sensory perception and of motor discharge. The local anesthetic agents apparently act by disturbing cellular permeability locally at the point of application by blocking acetylcholine metabolism in such a manner that energy transfer and conduction of impulses are no longer possible.

While the generally acting anesthetic and analgesic agents may alter synaptic connections between nerve fibers, as well as produce disturbances of enzymatic energy metabolism within the cells, local anesthetics seem to act chiefly at the point of application by virtue of preventing the passage of the nerve impulse, through inhibition of enzyme chain reactions.

In a patient under the influence of a general anesthetic agent it is probable that painful stimuli continue to bombard the cerebral cortex, from the area where trauma in tissues is going forward. On the basis that this continual bombardment during operations might cause energy changes harmful to the individual and initiate the reflexes called "shock," the late Cleveland surgeon, Dr. G. W. Crile, proposed what he called "anoci-association." This is simply a combination of local and general anesthesia. The idea is to use local anesthetic agents to block painful stimuli from the operative area from reaching the brain, and to use a general anesthetic to obtain relaxation and general insensibility on the part of the patient.

In spite of voluminous discussion and vast experimentation on pain, however, we still possess little knowledge which enables us to approach the problem of its control by rational means without recourse to simple trial-and-miss experimentation. Many brilliant hypotheses on the mechanism of anesthesia have been proposed by such experimentalists as Claude Bernard (reversible protein coagulation), H. H. Meyer and C. E. Overton (lipoid solubility), R. DuBois (dehydration), H. Winterstein (asphyxia), J. Traube (capillary activity), O. Warburg (adsorption), and R. Hober and R. Lillie (surface tension and membrane permeability). As V. E. Henderson concludes (*Physiol. Rev.*, 10:171, 1930), we do not know how to explain anesthesia.

On the other hand, from such experimentation with specific chemical agents, we have learned the types of chemicals which block either the conduction or the perception and sensation of pain. Frequently we are able to modify such chemical agents to produce greater or less degrees of central nervous system depression, or to alter side effects incident to their use in blocking a nerve pathway. We strive continually to find new chemicals which will produce the desired anesthetic effect with least disturbance of other physiological activities of the organism, and of course with least possibility of any conceivable harmful effects.

Indeed, our knowledge of the relationships between chemical constitution and biological action with respect to anesthetics is now so well advanced that we can almost devise chemicals to specification for specific anesthetic purposes. This probability was what so intrigued me in developing divinyl oxide ("vinethene"). Dr. Clarence Muehlberger, with whom I first discussed the matter, agreed that we had biochemorphic knowledge enough to predict what the general biological properties of the then unknown chemical compound, divinyl oxide, would be.

However, we are still a long way from understanding how these anesthetic chemicals accomplish the purposes for which we use them. We comprehend dimly how certain physical factors such as cold may reduce metabolism of nerves and interfere with conduction of pain, but we still don't know why cold itself is painful. We remain wholly in the dark as to how altered mental states can modify the sensation or perception of pain. Of the

Introductory Essay

energy transformations concerned we can but vaguely surmise, but we can believe that they are fundamental.

Before the deep barrier of these great mysteries we can only stand humbly thankful that we are able to accomplish as much as we can in the relief of pain. The success of the past hundred years in the acquisition of knowledge with which to improve our ability to control pain, may serve as a continued stimulus to us to keep the snowball rolling during the next hundred years. If our proportionate success is as great, then we are on the brink of awe-inspiring discoveries.

ANESTHESIA COLLECTIONS

The exciting human story of the development of surgical anesthesia is sympathetically related by Thomas E. Keys. As reference librarian for the Mayo Clinic, Mr. Keys first prepared the material comprising this volume in a series of papers appearing in *Anesthesiology*. The interest and enthusiasm with which these sketches were received suggested that it would be well worth while as a contribution to the centennial of anesthesia to revise them and publish them in book form. This has been undertaken with the characteristic enthusiasm of Henry Schuman for all things historical in medicine. Meanwhile, Mr. Keys has become a Major attached to the medical work of the Army. He is assigned to the Cleveland Branch of the Army Medical Library. Here Major Keys has a rare opportunity to indulge his passion for the history of medicine.

Major Keys' keen historical sense is reflected in the affectionate care he is bestowing upon the great medical treasures entrusted to his safekeeping. Although medical men generally have intense pride in the Army Medical Library, and although they think that it is the finest repository of medical books in the world, they have been content more or less to let it go at that. The result has been that there have occurred considerable deterioration and neglect, through failure to provide sufficient funds for proper maintenance and expansion. In the present quarters of the Cleveland Medical Library Association, the rare historical

[xix]

collections of the Army Medical Library are now splendidly housed and are receiving the finest kind of attention. These collections of course include a vast amount of original material relating to the development of anesthesia. Major Keys has made ample use of these in the preparation of his monograph.

There are many admirable collections relating to anesthesia in this country. The most significant is that preserved with the "Ether Room," the old operating amphitheater at the Massachusetts General Hospital, where Horace Wells' fiasco with nitrous oxide occurred a century ago, and where W. T. G. Morton, who witnessed the tragedy as a medical student, later demonstrated real anesthesia with ether.

Among the more extensive collections is that brought together by the late Dr. Logan Clendening in Kansas City, Kansas. Sir William Osler had given great stimulus to the collecting of original anesthesia items (*Ann. Med. Hist.*, 1:329, 1917). His library at McGill, under the direction of Dr. W. W. Francis, has many fine items. A large collection of American anesthesia literature has recently been acquired by Dr. Josiah C. Trent of Durham, North Carolina. Dr. Lawrence Reynolds of Detroit has built up a splendid anesthesia collection. It is especially rich in European literature. Dr. Emmet Field Horine of Louisville, Kentucky, has also collected in this field. Dr. Harry Archer of the University of Pittsburgh School of Dentistry has developed the best collection relating to the work of Horace Wells. As might be expected, Dr. Arno B. Luckhardt in Chicago possesses a noteworthy group of anesthesia items. The best Priestley material was assembled by the late Edgar Fahs Smith at the University of Pennsylvania. The Historical Library of Yale Medical School under the direction of Dr. John F. Fulton has assembled one of the country's outstanding collections.

The Crummer Room of the University of California Medical Center in San Francisco shelters particularly fine original manuscript and association items relating to all phases of anesthesia. Dr. Ralph Waters of the University of Wisconsin has also developed an admirable historical anesthesia collection under the inspiration of the late Dr. William Snow Miller. The Frank McMechans labored heroically to afford appreciation of the romantic interest and history of anesthesia, and their efforts are being worthily maintained by Dr. Howard Dittrick in Cleveland. One of the best collections abroad on the history of anesthesia was brought together at the Radcliffe Infirmary in Oxford by Dr. R. R. MacIntosh.

It would be helpful to keep careful records of current advances in anesthesia. The original documents should be preserved and added to these special collections. At the Mayo Clinic, the brilliant work of Dr. John S. Lundy and his associates in developing effective intravenous anesthesia is properly appreciated with respect to its historical significance, and the important documents relating to this development are being preserved carefully. Under the stimulus of Dr. Paul M. Wood, the American Society of Anesthetists is promoting an important repository for historical material relating to anesthesia, at its New York office.

Personal reminiscences and correspondence relating to current developments in anesthesia deserve to be preserved. What precious anesthesia lore, for example, is to be found in the vigorous correspondence maintained for so many years between Dr. Arthur Guedel in Los Angeles and Dr. Ralph Waters in Madison! The volumes of letters of the "Water Babies" must hold many valuable suggestions and ideas in anesthesia.

PERSONAL NOTES ABOUT ANESTHESIOLOGY

These reflections suggest that indulgence might be extended toward me in such personal reminiscences as might seem to be related to recent developments in anesthesia. It has been my privilege to participate in many of these, with respect both to local and to general anesthesia, during the past quarter century.

My earliest contact with great contributors to the history of anesthesia was one which I did not appreciate at the time. I grew up in Elizabeth, New Jersey, and when I was about ten years old, I seemed to be having some difficulty in reading and seeing. Ophthalmology was then a new specialty in this country, and a number of smart young men were claiming to be specialists in this field. My mother took me to the local eye specialist and he told her that I was going blind. For $5 a week he would take care of me. This was a little too much for the family budget, so our family physician, Dr. Paul Mravlag, a Viennese who was mayor of the city, was consulted. He told my mother to take me to a real ophthalmologist whose office was on Madison Avenue in New York.

It was quite an experience for me. There was first the exciting trip to New York, then the wait in the crowded reception room, and then the short but very impressive examination in the dark room. The verdict was simply that I had astigmatism and near-sightedness. A prescription was given to me which was signed by Carl Koller.

Some twenty years later, after I had learned who Carl Koller was, I had the pleasure of returning to his office on East 59th Street to have my twenty-year-old prescription renewed. At that time, he told me much of his early associations with Sigmund Freud in Vienna, and how he had been induced to study cocaine as a possible antagonist to morphine, with the idea in mind of treating morphine addiction. Dr. Koller confided to me that he really wasn't interested in this problem at all, since he wanted to be an ophthalmologist. He said he was searching for something which he could put in the eye to anesthetize it for operations for cataract. As soon as he tasted cocaine, he said he realized the numbing effect was due to a blocking of sensation and that it might be what he was looking for.

On my persuasion, Dr. Koller wrote a full account of his part in the development of cocaine as the first efficient local anes-thetic, and this I abstracted for publication in 1925 with his pic-ture. A few years later some of us were instrumental in having him elected an Honorary Member of the American Society for Pharmacology and Experimental Therapeutics.

Introductory Essay

In 1934, the Semi-Centennial of the first use of cocaine as a local anesthetic, the Federated Societies for Experimental Medicine met at the Hotel Pennsylvania in New York. I tried hard to persuade Dr. Koller to come to the annual banquet. However, he refused because of ill health. I tried to get several popular magazines, and also the newspapers, to write some account of Dr. Koller on this occasion. It struck me as being very remarkable that the man who had contributed more than any other man then alive to the relief of human pain and suffering, should be right there in New York. It struck me also as being very remarkable that no one seemed to think that this was a very interesting or significant matter. Such are the rewards for service to humanity!

In the pharmacology laboratory of Professor A. S. Loevenhart at the University of Wisconsin, where I later worked, there was much interest in local anesthesia. In a survey of alkyl analogues of procaine, it was shown that the isopropyl derivative was probably more efficient, since it will anesthetize the intact mucous membrane, and without any increase in possible toxicity. However, since there were no patent rights involved, no commercial manufacturer seemed to be interested in developing the agent. On the other hand, one of the series which could be patented, but which was shown to be quite toxic, was widely exploited. It was in this famous laboratory that Dr. Arthur Tatum, Dr. P. K. Knoefel, and Dr. Loevenhart showed that the barbitals antagonized the toxicity of local anesthetics and that they are highly advantageous to use as a pre-anesthetic medication before the administration of a local anesthetic.

When I was a student at Princeton, I was preparing to go to medical school. However, I got sidetracked into philosophy and psychology, and then thought that I might study psychiatry. However, Andrew Fleming West, Dean of the Graduate School, threw a lot of cold water on this idea. This is probably one of the reasons why I subsequently took much interest in Woodrow Wilson! I left Princeton in March, 1917, when I was a senior, to go off with the National Guard unit to which I belonged. We were in the Twenty-Ninth Division and trained in Anniston, Alabama. However, I was transferred before the Division went overseas, to the Chemical Warfare Service, and was presently assigned to the Medical Defense Division under Dr. Walter J. Meek and Dr. J. A. E. Eyster at the University of Wisconsin. Our work on war gases necessitated the use of morphine to prevent pain in the animals we were employing. Accordingly, it was necessary to study the effects of morphine as a control on the observations we were making. When I was mustered out at the end of the war, I was generously offered the opportunity to continue with these studies.

The action of morphine has always had a peculiar fascination for pharmacologists. An immense amount of empirical information is available, but we still have little idea regarding its mode of action. From my studies it seemed to me that many of its actions are analogous to the effects of interference with oxidative processes in the body.

The effects of reduced oxygen fixation in the cells of the body had been a major project in Dr. Loevenhart's pharmacology laboratory at Wisconsin for many years. An outstanding contribution had been made by Dr. Herbert Gasser and Dr. Loevenhart on "The Mechanism of Stimulation of the Medullary Centers by Increased Oxidation" (J. Pharmacol. Exp. Therap., 5: 239-273, 1914). And Dr. Loevenhart had summarized many of his ideas on the matter in a Harvey Society lecture ("Certain Aspects of Biological Oxidation," Arch. Intern. Med., 15:1059-1071, 1915). It seemed to me that the actions of morphine could be explained on the basis of an interference with intracellular oxidative processes. While there was not much knowledge available at the time regarding the complex enzyme systems involved in intracellular oxidation, I nevertheless expressed the view that morphine exerts its effects by blocking oxidative enzyme systems. Detailed discussions with my superiors on the dangers of reasoning by analogy in scientific work inhibited me sufficiently so that these ideas were not published!

Meanwhile, I became interested in some of the effects of general anesthesia. Dr. A. E. Koehler, my wife and myself studied the effects of inhalation anesthetic agents on blood reaction. It seemed to us that the net effect was the development of a transitory diabetes. It looked again as though the general anesthetic agents interfere with intracellular enzyme systems associated with oxidation, so that the intermediate toxic products of cellular oxidation accumulate. We showed that there is a significant ketosis with ether anesthesia. Our observations on morphine and ether were interpreted quite differently from the explanation given by Dr. Yandell Henderson at Yale. However, we avoided a direct controversy, although some snappy letters passed between us.

The dramatic introduction of ethylene anesthesia by Dr. Arno Luckhardt in Chicago and its careful study by Dr. V. E. Henderson in Toronto stimulated us to study its effects on the blood reaction in comparison with nitrous oxide and other inhalation anesthetics. We obtained further evidence that blood reaction effects may be correlated with the extent of interference with oxidation.

Meanwhile, my interest had been aroused by Dr. Loevenhart and his associates on the possible relationship between chemical constitution and biological action. This had been rather extensively studied in the laboratory in relation to arsenical compounds in the chemotherapy of syphilis. It had also been involved in the study of local anesthetics. Our studies on ether and ethylene suggested that it might be of interest to determine whether or not the characteristic unsaturated carbon atom of ethylene would improve the anesthetic properties of ether if it were a part of the ether molecule. In discussing this matter with Dr. Clarence Muehlberger, we came to the conclusion that it would be worth while to obtain divinyl ether for study.

Accordingly, after failing to arouse interest among our organic chemist colleagues, I wrote to Dr. Lauder Jones, Professor of Organic Chemistry at Princeton, suggesting the problem. He asked his graduate student, Dr. Randolph Major, to undertake the synthesis of the new agent. While it had been tentatively described as having been isolated from a species of Allium, by Semmler, in 1885, it had never been synthesized nor was it certain that it had actually been isolated.

The problem of the synthesis was difficult, but eventually impure samples were obtained. Meanwhile, I had gone to San Francisco to organize the Pharmacology Laboratory of the University of California Medical School. While there, I met Dr. Sigmund Fraenkel, who was working in Dr. Herbert Evans' laboratory in Berkeley. Dr. Fraenkel was unable to synthesize divinyl ether, but he did obtain samples of other unsaturated ethers which he sent to us for study.

When the new Laboratory was organized, Dr. P. K. Knoefel came as a National Research Council Fellow, having completed his medical studies at Harvard. While at the International Physiology Congress in Boston, I met a brilliant young Chinese girl who had been born in San Francisco and wanted to come back there to work before returning to China. She was the daughter of the Minister of Education in Sun Yat Sen's Cabinet, and had studied in London. Miss Mei-yu Chen, Dr. Knoefel and myself undertook the survey of the unsaturated ethers.

By applying principles discovered by Benjamin Ward Richardson, we could predict that divinyl ether would be the most satisfactory of the unsaturated ethers for inhalation anesthesia. Experimental studies verified this prediction. Randolph Major and his associate, R. L. Ruigh, had now left Princeton to organize a research effort for Merck & Company at Rahway, New Jersey. They improved upon the method of preparing divinyl ether and worked out a procedure for stabilizing it. The product was called "Vinethene" and a patent was obtained for it. This annoyed me quite a bit, but there wasn't much I could do about it!

Meanwhile, our first reports had excited a number of scientists. Dr. Samuel Gelfan in Canada asked for the privilege of studying the effect of divinyl ether on human beings. I arranged for samples to be sent to him and for his publication to appear with the extended pharmacological report which we made. In this we attempted to cover as carefully as we could all factors of significance in the pharmacological appraisal of the new anesthetic agent. We had previously established ideal standards for the introduction of new drugs, and we were trying to live up to our own pronouncements!

My colleagues at the University of California Medical Center in San Francisco were not particularly impressed with our studies. We had demonstrations in the laboratory and there was courteous interest, but this was tempered by proper professional caution. Although the first surgical anesthesia with divinyl ether was carried out in the University of California Hospital under the direction of Dr. Dorothy Wood, the agent was not further used. Its clinical use was thoroughly studied at the instigation of the Merck Laboratories by Dr. I. S. Ravdin, Professor of Surgery at the University of Pennsylvania, and his associates. My mentors at the University of Wisconsin simply couldn't do anything with divinyl ether. It amused us to realize that they couldn't even anesthetize animals with it! Nevertheless, they appreciated its anesthetic power as demonstrated in a dramatic incident at a meeting in Milwaukee.

Meanwhile, Merck & Company established a fellowship in our laboratory for a systematic study of the various types of hydrocarbons as possible anesthetic agents. We had many long and interesting debates over details of technics. Dr. S. Anderson Peoples became interested in attempting mathematical treatment of concentration time relations. Certainly the problem became complicated. Dr. David Marsh reported in a systematic way on an extensive series of hydrocarbons, many of which he synthesized for the first time. The results showed that it was not likely that more practical inhalation anesthetic agents could be obtained than those already well known. We extended the series to include halogenated hydrocarbons in order to attempt to get an agent which would be practically useful but not inflammable or explosive. The study deserves careful consideration, but unfortunately is not yet published. It is doubtful, however, if anything practically significant will come from it.

Meanwhile, much to our chagrin, clinicians were discovering that divinyl ether is potent and, in fact, dangerous if its administration is pushed too hard or too long. Evidence of liver injury occurred, and we were all much concerned. Finally, however, its general place in short anesthesias had become established, and our interest turned to other matters.

We held many vigorous discussions on anesthesia with Dr. Arthur E. Guedel of Los Angeles and some of his associates, who would join our summer vacationing group in cool San Francisco. Often these arguments would be conducted at "Pharmaglen," a sheltered little redwood grove in the Santa Cruz Mountains along the San Lorenzo River, about sixty miles south of San Francisco. Some half-dozen cars would take twenty or thirty of us down the winding Skyline Boulevard through forest and meadow overlooking ocean and bay. We usually went for a Sunday picnic, and we would spend the day discussing factors concerned in stimulation and depression of the central nervous system, with blackboard nailed to redwood trunk.

From these discussions developed a study of the chemical adjuncts to anesthesia. We investigated the metabolic depressant action of morphine in comparison with barbitals. Dr. Hamilton Anderson took charge of most of this work. We were much inspired in our discussions by the brilliance of Dr. Gordon Alles of Los Angeles in developing benzedrine, the central stimulating action of which was so well demonstrated clinically by Dr. Anderson Peoples while in London.

These considerations led us to revise the terminology of anesthesia. We believe that much confusion in thought is caused by the traditional habit of terming the second stage of anesthesia the stage of "excitement." It is much more appropriate to refer to it as "delirium," and to reserve the term "excitement" for the effects of emotions or stimulating drugs.

Dr. George Emerson became interested in various aspects of the relations of anesthesia to oxidation, when he went to West Virginia University School of Medicine. In searching for a non-addictive pain relieving agent, he developed dinitrophenylmorphine. In spite of the careful studies we made on this compound, we could not convince the well-entrenched committee of the National Research Council that we had anything worth while in regard to morphine addiction.

Our opinion is that drug addiction is largely a psychiatric reaction to an unbearable environment. Addiction is a form of "escapism." Jack Shuman and Art Guedel argued this very effectively with us, and later Walter Treadway supported us. In spite of the fact that we were greatly interested in the relationship between chemical constitution and biological action, we could not get ourselves to believe that the addictive properties of morphine could be divorced from its pain relieving properties.

As I look back over the past twenty years, I yield to the temptation of jotting down some kaleidoscopic memories:

Anesthesia discussions at lunch time in the corner laboratory of Science Hall at the University of Wisconsin—Loevenhart's idea of stimulating brain activity by blocking oxidation by carbon dioxide administration—Wesley Bourne's confirmation of our ideas on ether acidosis—Ralph Waters' arrival at Wisconsin to develop the first Department of Anesthesiology in the uncompleted new laboratory building—Discovering that carbon dioxide will actually anesthetize as Hickman had claimed a century earlier—Meeting of the Anesthesia Research Society with the enthusiasm of the Frank McMechans—Art Guedel's endotracheal anesthesia, with the animal completely submerged in water—The startling demonstration by Hans Killian of rectal anesthesia with tribromethanol ("Avertin"), with the patient almost passing out with circulatory depression—Inauguration of resident training in anesthesia—Studying blood cell fragility under anesthesia with enthused students.

The royal gastronomic welcome of the anesthetists of San Francisco—Dr. Mary Botsford's enthusiasm for nitrous oxide, on which she was a master—Demonstrations of carbon dioxide anesthesia in the new pharmacology laboratory facing the eucalyptus forest on Parnassus Heights—Carbon dioxide inhalations in cases of catatonic dementia praecox, with the thrill of seeing some sense again in a "zombie"—Pete Knoefel's arrival in a Rolls Royce, with trips to Middletown discussing anesthesia and Blake—Art Guedel's demonstrations of carbon dioxide absorption—Enthusiasms and chagrins over divinyl ether—Ralph Waters' visits with the Travel Club—Arguments with the young Blakians on dose effect and time concentration relations—Norm David and George Emerson on morphine derivatives—Andy Peoples' still unpublished flowmeter apparatus for quantitative study of anesthetic concentrations—Nil Phatak working on local anesthetics—Pete Knoefel's explosions with paraldehyde substitutes—Ben Abreu and Milt Silverman on halogenated hydrocarbons—Early studies on barbital substitutes—Joe Swim's struggles with alcohol estimations—Zakheim's water color in 1936 of our demonstration of pentothal intravenous anesthesia—Dave Marsh's fractionating column and explosiometer.

*   *   *

The current centennial years in anesthesia are reviving widespread interest in scientific and clinical studies in this important field. Most importantly, these celebrations may focus our attention on the plain fact that we still know relatively little about pain or anesthesia. Perhaps as in every other phase of medicine, we shall learn that it is wiser to prevent the appearance of pain than to seek to relieve it after it occurs. To that noble achievement, Major Keys' book may well be a fitting prelude, and to that ideal also it may most appropriately be dedicated.

CHAUNCEY D. LEAKE

The History of Surgical Anesthesia

When, for the sake of a little more reputation, men can keep brooding over a new fact, in the discovery of which they might, possibly, have very little real merit, till they think they can astonish the world with a system as complete as it is new, and give mankind a prodigious idea of their judgment and penetration; they are justly punished for their ingratitude to the fountain of all knowledge, and for their want of a genuine love of science and of mankind, in finding their boasted discoveries anticipated, and the field of honest fame pre-occupied, by men, who, from a natural ardour of mind engage in philosophical pursuits, and with an ingenuous simplicity immediately communicate to others whatever occurs to them in their inquiries.

JOSEPH PRIESTLEY, *Experiments and observations on different kinds of air.* London, 1774. Preface.

I

The Development of Anesthesia

*"I esteem it the office of the physician not only to
restore health, but to mitigate pain and dolors."*
—SIR FRANCIS BACON

A—THE BEGINNINGS

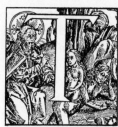HE HISTORY of the development of anesthesia
is, like the history of many other useful con-
tributions to civilization, filled with hopes and
disappointments, comedies and tragedies,
successes and failures. The bitterness of the
controversy concerning the introduction of
anesthesia with ether as well as nitrous oxide
still raging after a century is disappointing in that it has about
it the suggestion of a lack of historical perspective, as quarrels
concerning priority usually have.

It has been suggested by Archer[1] that ancient man sensed
relief from pain caused by bruises and sprains when the injured
part was exposed to cold water in a lake or stream. Other wounds
were said to have been favorably influenced by the sun's heat,
and later, by heat from fires or hot stoves.

Perhaps, as Fülöp-Miller[2] has recently observed, the first
method used to eradicate pain by primitive peoples was to treat
pain as a demon and to try to frighten the demon away. To do
this there were many methods. The skin was tattooed to keep the
demon of pain outside the body; rings were worn in the ears and
noses; talismans, amulets, tigers' claws and similar charms were
worn to ward off evil spirits.

The first anesthetist probably was a woman, for the head of
the primitive family was the Great Mother under the matriarchal
system, which has been said by some anthropologists to have

[3]

been the status of society in primitive times.* The Great Mother was priestess and sorceress, and consequently was the founder of the healing art. When a primitive sick man could not relieve his own suffering he called on the priestess. Conjurations and spells were resorted to, magic was applied, and pain was thought to be banished thereby.

Even under the patriarchal state, which some anthropologists have said subsequently developed, woman remained as a healer. Indeed, the classic example was the blonde Agamede of the Greeks, who was considered to wield exclusive power over the demons of illness and thus was able to banish pain. Gradually, however, the medicine man, conjurer or *shaman* took her place. Using different technics, he achieved the same results in the banishment of pain. He muttered magic incantations. He wrestled and fought the invisible demon. If the soul had been drawn from the body, thus causing pain, he searched for the hiding place of the soul and triumphantly returned the soul to the sufferer's body, thus relieving the patient of his pain.

Later in the development of society the medicine man was replaced by the priest, the servant of the gods. Priests have ever ministered to the sick and they relied on prayer for the alleviation of pain. Thus, the fate of the patient was entrusted to a higher power.

With the birth of Christianity came a concept for the relief of pain, based on divine healing through touch and prayer. One of the tasks of the Son of God and his followers was the banishment of suffering of all mankind. This was accomplished through the power of touch as well as prayer, which was willed down through the ages from Christ through the disciples to the Church fathers and ultimately to all those who had ministerial duties. In this manner the church of the early Middle Ages became a healing institution. Priests, monks and nuns, who to a great extent represented the church, practiced the healing art and were thought to be able to relieve pain. As some historians have shown, the early monks and their helpers not only used empirical methods for the

* For instance see Briffault, Robert: *The Mothers*, New York, Macmillan, c1931; Goldenweiser, A. A.: *Early Civilization*, New York, Knopf, 1922.

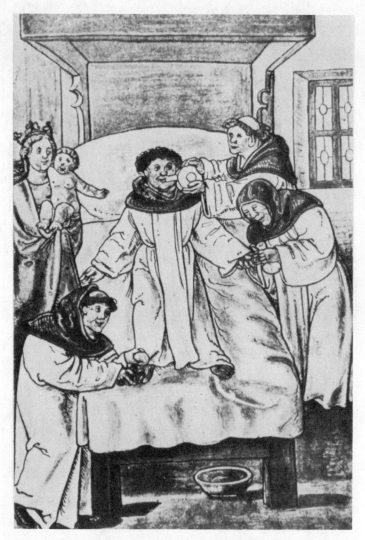

[FIG. 1] Early use of alcohol for anesthetic purposes in a monastic hospital. From Diebold Schilling's *Swiss Chronicle*, 1513.

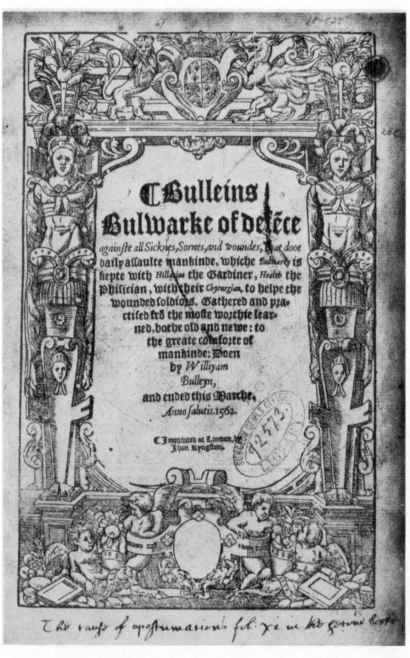

[FIG. 2] Title page to the first edition of Bullein's *Bulwarke of Defence*.
Courtesy of the Army Medical Library.

relief of pain but also developed practical aids. Indeed, as early as 1513 monks used alcohol to alleviate pain prior to and during surgical intervention (fig. 1).

The early Christian kings tried to cure the sufferings of their subjects from many diseases by the laying on of hands. This, as has been suggested, formerly was the province of the ministers of the church. But the kings usurped this privilege for their own protection. They formulated the theory of the "divine right of kings," which was convenient for many other purposes in addition to cure of the sick. Later, "touching" by monarchs was reserved for special diseases such as scrofula or the "King's evil."*

Long known to man has been the use of drugs to bring about artificial sleep. Drugs which brought about loss of consciousness were compounded from many roots, barks, herbs, berries, seeds and blossoms of flowers. Those most mentioned in the literature which were taken to relieve the pain of surgical operations were henbane, poppy, mandragora and hemp.

A Babylonian clay tablet of about 2250 B.C. reveals a remedy for the pain of dental caries, according to Prinz.[3] Cement consisting of henbane seeds in powdered form was mixed with gum mastic and applied to the cavity.

In the *Odyssey*[4] of Homer it is recorded that Helen, the daughter of Zeus, prepared a drug, possibly opium, dissolved in wine to sleep off grief and anger and to forget pain: "Now elsewhere Helen turned her thoughts, the child of Zeus. Straightway she cast into the wine of which they drank a drug which quenches pain and strife and brings forgetfulness of every ill." The Greeks also used anodyne poultices to deaden pain. Thus in the *Iliad*, Patroclus worked on Eurypylus:[4A]

> Cut out the biting shaft; and from the wound
> With tepid water cleansed the clotted blood;
> Then pounded in his hands, the root applied
> Astringent, anodyne, which all his pain
> Allay'd; the wound was dried, and stanched the blood.

* The practice of touching for the scrofula was confined in Europe to the two Royal Houses of England and France. It cannot be traced back to an earlier date than the reign of Edward III in England (1327-1377) and that of Louis IX in France (1226-1270). See *Encyclopaedia Britannica*. Ed. 14, v. 13, p. 398.

The History of Surgical Anesthesia

According to Archer,[1] Aesculapius, the god of medicine, was supposed to have used a potion, nepenthe, to produce insensibility in his patients, who were then operated upon.

The Greeks and later the Romans also resorted to a sort of local anesthesia. They placed on the region they desired to anesthetize the "stone of Memphis" treated with vinegar. According to Kleiman[5] it is possible that the anesthetic effect was obtained by dulling, for the Memphis stone was composed of carbonates which, in coming into contact with the vinegar, were said to have liberated carbon dioxide which numbed the affected part.

It is well known that the Semites compressed the veins before circumcision. Egyptian, as well as Assyrian, physicians obtained an artificial sleep for their patients by quickly compressing the carotid vessels of the neck, possibly by producing a temporary anemia.

Dioscorides,* the famous Greek physician of the first century A.D., administered the root of the mandragora plant boiled in wine to his patients before submitting them to the knife.[5] Galen used this plant experimentally to paralyze sensation and movement. Curiously enough, mandragora was employed for centuries in Asia by the Chinese and the Hebrews in cases of criminologic investigation. Criminals were compelled to drink a concoction in a form of infusion with other drugs. This produced a confused mental state which often led to a confession of crime. Mandragora also was administered, paradoxically, to aid in the relief of the sufferings and tortures endured by accused persons. In such an event it was known as the "potion of the condemned." Kleiman[5] said that Pliny observed that the "potion of the condemned" was often given to diminish the agonies of crucifixion. The potion which Jesus refused at his crucifixion is variously described by the evangelists Matthew, Mark, and John as wine or vinegar mingled with gall, myrrh, or hyssop.

The ancient Scythians, as mentioned by Herodotus, breathed

---

* For the first description in English of the properties of the mandragora of Dioscorides see p. 10. Chauncey Leake has suggested in a personal communication that mandragora contains atropine-like alkaloids which might produce dissociation of nerve pathways with resulting diminution of the sense of pain.

fumes produced by a certain form of hemp (*Cannabis indica*).
From this they obtained a state of mental excitation followed by
sleep.[6] The Egyptians, as well as the Arabians, similarly, inhaled
the fumes of this plant which they called *hashish* (that is, hemp),
from which they also obtained an exalted mental state. In the
third century, Hua T'o, the Chinese physician, utilized Indian
hemp to render his patients unconscious. This practice was also
used in many other countries.

As suggested by Garrison[30] (p. 153), Henry Sigerist found in
the Bamberg *Antidotarium* of the ninth century, a recipe for the
"soporific sponge." Karl Sudhoff found a like recipe in a Monte
Cassino *Codex* of the same period.

In the *Antidotarium* of Nicolas of Salerno who possibly lived in
the twelfth century* there is a reference to the soporific sponge
as follows:†

Spongia Somnifera

Take . . . of opium thebaicum, juice of hyoscyamine, unripened berry of
the blackberry, lettuce seed, juice of hemlock, poppy, mandragora, ivy . . .
Put these all together in a vessel and plunge therein a new sea-sponge just as
it comes from the sea, taking care that fresh water does not touch it. And put
this in the sun during the dog-days until all the liquid is consumed. And when
there is need, dip it a little in water not too warm, and apply it to the nostrils
of the patient, and he will quickly go to sleep. When, moreover, you want to
awaken him, apply juice from the root of the fennel and he will soon bestir
himself.

In the thirteenth century, Hugh of Lucca, as reported by
his son, Theodoric,[7] prepared a soporific agent with opium as the
base. It also included hemlock, henbane, leaves of mandragora,
wild ivy, and the seed of some salad plant. This mixture also was
administered on a sponge to patients and apparently was successful in producing anesthesia for some surgical procedures.
Having previously steeped the sponge in a soporific mélange, he
allowed it to dry. When this sponge was ready for use after soak-
ing in hot water, he applied it under the nose of the patient, who

---

* See Riesman, David: *The Story of Medicine in the Middle Ages.* New York, Hoeber, 1936,
p. 347.

† *Nicolaus Salernitanus*, Antidotarium. Venice, Nicolaus Jenson, 1471, f. 33b.

was instructed to breathe deeply.* To revive the patients sponges filled with vinegar were held under their noses.

That soporific draughts were sometimes an accepted prelude to surgical operations can be inferred from the fact that writers and poets talked about their use. Thus in Boccaccio's *Decameron*† in the fourth day and tenth story as told by Dioneo, there is an illustration of anesthesia produced by this method:

. . . It happened that there came to the attention of the physician [Maestro Mazzeo della Montagna] a patient with a gangrenous leg, and when the master had made an examination he told the relatives that unless a decayed bone in the leg were removed either the entire leg would have to be amputated or the patient would die; moreover, if the bone were removed, the patient might recover, but he refused to undertake the case except as if the man were already dead. To this the relatives agreed and surrendered the patient to him.

The doctor was of the opinion that without an opiate the man could not endure the pain and would not permit the operation, and since the affair was set for the evening, he distilled that morning a type of water after his own composition which had the faculty of bringing to the person who drank it sleep for as long a time as was deemed necessary to complete the operation.

The action of the medicated sponge was uncertain because there could be no standardization of the drugs used, and it therefore fell into disuse. Probably one of the reasons why anesthesia in general was so slow in developing was the fact that no drugs were standardized. No attempt was made to purify them or to regulate dosage. Often a drugged sleep resulted in death. This in itself discouraged the more staid physicians from the conquest of pain. Then, too, pain was considered in a holy light; which is to say, something that God deemed good for mankind. This was especially true in obstetrics. Babcock[8] has reported the case of

---

* The following is a literal translation from Theodoric's *Surgery* dealing with the medicated sponge (see reference 7):

Recipe for an inhalant to use in surgery as prescribed by Master Hugo. Rx. One ounce each of poppy juice, juice of unripe mulberries, henbane, juice of (coconidii?), juice of mandrake leaves, juice of tree ivy, juice of wild mulberry, half?, lettuce, seed of a sorrel which has hard round fruit, and hemlock. Mix all these together in a copper kettle, then put a new sponge into it, and let it stand in the sun in the dog days until it has completely evaporated. Then as often as needed put the sponge in warm water for an hour and apply it to the nostrils of the person to be operated upon until he falls asleep; then proceed with the surgery; and when this has been performed, to wake him up again apply another sponge soaked in vinegar repeatedly to his nostrils.

† Boccaccio, *Il Decamerone* (Firenze, Adriano Salani, 1928), v. I, Giornata Quarta, Novella Decima (pp. 436-437).

The Beginnings

Eufame MacAlyane of Edinburgh,who in 1591 was burned alive on Castle Hill for seeking the assistance of Agnes Sampson for the relief of pain at the birth of her two sons. The time was not ripe for the acceptance of anesthesia.

In the thirteenth century, Raymundus Lullius,[9] the prominent Spanish Alchemist, may have noticed a white fluid and may have called it "sweet vitriol."* Two centuries later Paracelsus, the great physician, searching for an agent that would relieve pain, mixed sulfuric acid with alcohol. He distilled this mixture and rediscovered "sweet vitriol" which was not called "ether," however, until 1730, when Frobenius[10] of Germany so named it; but as early as 1540 Valerius Cordus[11] described the synthesis of what later was to be called ether. The first written account of this appears in his *De Artificiosis Extractionibus*, Strassburg, 1561, seventeen years after his death.†

A digression to Paracelsus[12] reveals some very important evidence which supports a claim for him as the founder of anesthesia. In writing of his experiments with fowl he said:

> However, the following should be noted here with regard to this sulphur, that of all things extracted from vitriol it is most remarkable because it is stable. And besides, it has associated with it such a sweetness that it is taken even by chickens, and they fall asleep from it for a while but awaken later without harm. On this sulphur no other judgment should be passed than that in diseases which need to be treated with anodynes it quiets all suffering without any harm, and relieves all pain, and quenches all fevers, and prevents complications in all illnesses.

Perhaps the first mention of an anesthetic agent in English in a printed medical book is found in William Bullein's interesting work entitled *Bulwarke of Defence Against all Sickness* (fig. 2). This was first published in 1562. In the first several pages of this book

---

* A search through the works of Lullius does not reveal this. The best source found so far for this statement is in the ninth edition of the *Encyclopaedia Britannica* (ref. 9).

† Valerius Cordus died in Rome on Sept. 25, 1544, at the early age of 29 years. He was born in Siemershausen, Hessia, on Feb. 18, 1515, and studied medicine at the University at Wittemberg. He remained there for some time and lectured on Dioscorides. In 1542 he removed to Italy and continued his work in botany. Valerius correctly noted that ether promotes the flow of mucous secretion from the respiratory tract and that it affords relief from whooping cough. He also commented on its high volatility. For an appreciation of his contribution to anesthesia consult Chauncey Leake's article, *Valerius Cordus and the Discovery of Ether*, and G. K. Tallmadge's translation, *The Third Part of the De Extractione of Valerius Cordus* (see ref. 11).

occurs "The Booke of Simples." It is in the form of an imaginary conversation between a certain Marcellus, a surgeon, and Hillarius, a gardener. Marcellus asks Hillarius, "What is the nature of Mandragora?" Hillarius after talking at great length concerning the history and properties of the mandrake has this to say (folio 44, recto):

> The seedes of the aple, saieth *Dioscorides*, beyng drunke, will purge the bellie. The juce of this herbe pressed forthe, and kepte in a close yearthen vessel, accordyng to arte: this bryngeth slepe, it casteth men into a trauns on a depe tirrible dreame, untill he be cutte of the stone.

That same year (1562), Arthur Brooke's poem, *The Tragicall Historye of Romeus and Juliet*, was published. The earliest known version, which is an undoubted direct ancestor of Shakespeare's plot, is the history, *Giulia e Romeo*, narrated by Luigi da Porto and published in Venice about 1530. But Brooke's English poem probably supplied Shakespeare with much of the material for his own *Romeo and Juliet*.

In Brooke's poem* there is reference made to a sleeping potion as follows:

> [Friar Laurence thus speaks to Juliet (lines 2125-2142)]:
> Knowe therfore, (daughter) that / with other gyftes which I
> Haue well attained to, by grace / and fauour of the skye,
> Long since I did finde out, / and yet the way I knowe,
> Of certain rootes, and sauory herbes / to make a kinde of dowe,
> Which baked hard, and bet / into a powder fine,
> And dronke with conduite water, or / with any kynd of wine,
> It doth in halfe an howre / astonne the taker so,
> And mastreth all his sences, that / he feeleth weale nor woe:
> And so it burieth vp / the sprite and liuing breath,
> That euen the skilfull leche would say, / that he is slayne by death.
> One vertue more it hath / as meruelous as this;
> The taker, by receiuing it, / at all not greeued is;
> But painlesse as a man / that thinketh nought at all,
> Into a swete and quiet slepe / immediately doth fall;
> From which, (according to / the quantitie he taketh)
> Longer or shorter is the time / before the sleper waketh;
> And thence (theffect once wrought) / agayne it doth restore
> Him that receaued vnto the state / wherin he was before.

* Brooke, Arthur: *Romeus and Juliet* (London, Richard Tottill, 1562). Reprinted from the original work by the New Shakspere Society as *Originals and Analogues*, Series III, pt. 1. London, N. Trübner & Co., 1875, 90 pp.

The Beginnings

In Shakespeare's *Romeo and Juliet*,* the Friar does not discuss the potion in the same manner but rather his speech is a remarkable description of the signs of profound anesthesia! In speaking to Juliet the Friar continues:

> Take thou this vial, being then in bed,
> And this distilling liquor drink thou off;
> When presently through all thy veins shall run
> A cold and drowsy humour; for no pulse
> Shall keep his native progress, but surcease;
> No warmth, no breath, shall testify thou livest;
> The roses in thy lips and cheeks shall fade
> To paly ashes, thy eyes' windows fall,
> Like death, when he shuts up the day of life;
> Each part, depriv'd of supple government,
> Shall, stiff and stark and cold, appear like death:
> And in this borrowed likeness of shrunk death
> Thou shalt continue two and forty hours,
> And then awake as from a pleasant sleep.

In the works of Shakespeare there are a few references to poppy, mandragora, and "drowsy" syrups. A good example is found in *Othello* in Act 3, scene 3, lines 330-333, where the villain, Iago, speaks of Othello:

> Look, where he comes! Not poppy, nor mandragora,
> Nor all the drowsy syrups of the world
> Shall ever medicine thee to that sweet sleep
> Which thou ow'dst yesterday.

Again in *Antony and Cleopatra* (Act 1, scene 5, lines 3-6) Cleopatra addresses her attendant, Charmian:

> *Cleo.:* Ha, ha! Give me to drink mandragora.
> *Char.:* Why, madam?
> *Cleo.:* That I might sleep out this great gap of time
> My Antony is away.

At the beginning of the seventeenth century, Valverdi made use of a sort of regional anesthesia.[5] He compressed nerves and blood vessels near the region to be operated on, a procedure similar to that of the ancient Semites and Assyrians, as mentioned previously. Ambroise Paré also knew the anesthetic value of compression. Indeed, as late as 1784, James Moore[13] produced local anesthesia of a limb by compressing the nerves of the trunk.

* Act 4, scene 1, lines 93-106.

The History of Surgical Anesthesia

It is known that John Hunter used this method in a case of amputation below the knee, with some degree of success.

The Renaissance fostered a great scientific spirit which made for many remarkable advancements. Emphasis was placed on the development of chemistry and physics. Search was made in these two fields for agents to relieve pain. As will be shown later, the role of chemistry is of great importance in the history of anesthesia. In addition to genuine workers who produced valid contributions, there were many "pseudo"-scientific thinkers who speculated, often chiefly to their own benefit, regarding the cause and cure of disease. One of these, as Fülöp-Miller has so vividly described, was Franz A. Mesmer, who introduced the doctrine of vitalism. Mesmer received his degree in medicine from the University of Vienna in 1766. Vitalism was based on the assumption that some men possess the authority of transmitting what are called "the harnessed powers of the cosmic energies." These "cosmic energies" were remarkable in that they banished pain and suffering. Mesmer first used a magnet as an instrument to transmit the cosmic energy to the body of an afflicted person. He had remarkable success with the magnet, and soon thousands of patients came to him to receive the vital energies. Mesmer soon found it impossible to treat all his patients individually, so he took a wooden rod and by making passes over it invested the rod with magnetic energy. By pointing the stick at several patients he claimed that he could cure many simultaneously.

Later, Mesmer announced that the healing force emanated from his own body, and that subsequently the same beneficial results were obtained. This old healing power of the touch was rechristened "animal magnetism" (fig. 3). Absurd as Mesmer's ideas were, his confidence was shared by many leading dignitaries of the day, including Marie Antoinette, the Duke of Bourbon, and Lafayette, who recommended Mesmer's ideas to America.

Interestingly enough Benjamin Franklin,* who was at that

* See: Franklin, Benjamin: *Animal Magnetism. Report of Benjamin Franklin and other commissioners charged by the King of France with the examination of the animal magnetism as practised at Paris.* Tr. from the French . . . Philadelphia, H. Perkins, 1837, 58 pp.

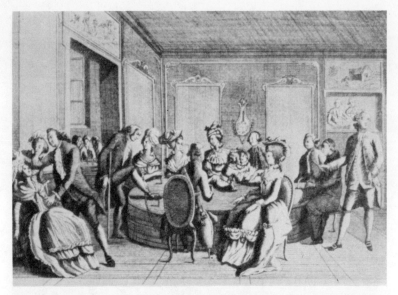

[FIG. 3] Mesmer practicing animal magnetism. From Holländer, Eugen: *Die Karikatur und Satire in der Medizin*. Ed. 2. Stuttgart, Ferdinand Enke, 1921.

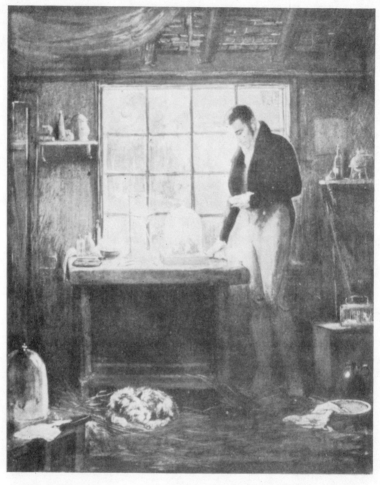

[FIG. 4] Hickman experimenting with anesthesia on animals. From an oil painting in the Wellcome Historical Medical Museum. Courtesy of the Wellcome Foundation, Ltd.

time in Paris, was skeptical about "animal magnetism" and served on a committee which exposed it as a fraud.

Mesmer was opposed by the physicians and scientists who thought of him as a quack, and he could not obtain a license to practice medicine in France. To get around this difficulty, Mesmer took in a partner, a licensed doctor, Charles Deslon. The two of them gave group treatments and after the war was ended, early in 1784, raised 340,000 livres to set up a new scientific academy. To expose the charlatanism of this partnership, the King of France appointed a commission to investigate animal magnetism as practiced by the licensed physician, Deslon. Four members of the commission were physicians of the Faculty of Paris, including Joseph-Ignace Guillotin, after whom the guillotine was named, and five members were drawn from the Academy of Sciences. These included Franklin, LeRoy, Bailly, Lavoisier and DeBory. Franklin's name headed the report which came to the conclusion that there was no such thing as "animal magnetism" and therefore no cures could be expected.

Somnambulism in Europe, a development of mesmerism, had a curious beginning. One of Mesmer's pupils, Count Maxime de Puységur of Busancy, in treating a patient who had been tied to a tree, made passes over his body to increase the magnetic influence. At the moment the treatment should have taken effect, the patient fell into a profound sleep. The count ordered him to awake and to untie himself. The patient complied and walked across a park with his eyes closed. He also obeyed all commands of the master.

After Puységur had experimented in other cases and had achieved similar results, the success of somnambulism spread over Europe. In the British Isles, James Esdaile[14] and John Elliotson[15] of Edinburgh adopted it, being convinced that it would prove an infallible agency for the relief of pain during surgical operations. James Braid[16] of Manchester also felt that hypnotism was capable either of throwing a patient into a state in which he would be unconscious of the pain of a surgical operation or of greatly moderating it.

Because the leading surgeons were skeptical of this "remedy," Esdaile journeyed to India to continue his experiments. According to Fülöp-Miller,[2] members of certain Indian castes had known for centuries of a process akin to somnambulism, calling it *Yar-Phoonk*. Esdaile said that he had removed scrotal tumors successfully from patients in this state of artificial sleep. In Europe somnambulism failed to relieve operative pain, and in America, John Collins Warren of the Massachusetts General Hospital had no success with this method.

B—FROM PRIESTLEY TO MORTON

Thus far, as has been intimated herein, no dependable means of relieving pain during surgical intervention that was generally acceptable had been discovered. To be sure, in isolated cases, it is apparent that many remedies had met with partial success. By far the most acceptable method was to offer the patient a strong drink of an alcoholic beverage and to operate swiftly. This did not abolish the sense of pain. It remained for chemistry, plus American ingenuity and resourcefulness, to provide an answer to this problem.

The pioneer who discovered carbonic acid gas (date, unknown), oxygen* (1771) and nitrous oxide (1772) was Joseph Priestley. His fundamental research on gases was the foundation of the discovery of modern surgical anesthesia, although he was unaware of it. Priestley was a dissenting Unitarian minister. In 1791 his services as a minister were abruptly terminated by riots in which his house was pillaged and burned because of his known sympathies for the French Revolution. Priestley† moved to America in 1794 to seek political and religious freedom and died in Northumberland County, Pennsylvania, in 1804. Because Priestley suggested that the inhalation of oxygen might be of

---

* Karl Wilhelm Scheele of Sweden is said to have discovered oxygen independently the same year (1771) and to have described it in 1777 in his *Chemical Essay on Air and Fire*.

† See Fulton, J. F., and Peters, Charlotte H.: *An Introduction to a Bibliography of the Educational and Scientific Works of Joseph Priestley*. Papers of the Bibliographical Society of America, 30:150-164, 1936.

benefit for certain diseases of the lungs, some members of the medical profession as well as quacks developed "pneumatic medicine." This soon became a treatment fad, and inhalations of not only oxygen but also of hydrogen and nitrogen were employed as therapy chiefly for asthma, catarrh and consumption. Later, some physicians employed inhalations of various gases for the treatment of paralysis, scurvy, hysteria and cancer.

It is of interest to note that an American chemist and physician, S. Latham Mitchill, administered nitrous oxide to animals with such dire results that he came to the conclusion that this gas was very poisonous. He also believed that nitrous oxide might possibly be the contagium for the spread of epidemics. His opinions were accepted without reservation and for many years no physician dared to make use of nitrous oxide. However, in 1795, Humphry Davy, then a young man of seventeen years, was bold enough to inhale this gas. Instead of dying, he experienced many pleasurable sensations; he felt an agreeable sense of giddiness, a relaxation of the muscles, noticed his hearing to be more acute, and in general felt so cheerful that he was compelled to laugh.

In 1800, Davy, who in early life had been a surgeon's assistant, published the results of his studies on nitrous oxide in that now much sought-after volume[17] entitled: *Researches, Chemical and Philosophical; Chiefly concerning Nitrous Oxide* . . . (fig. 5). This important book not only outlined his basic researches but also suggested the possible anesthetic qualities of nitrous oxide. In one section of the book (p. 465), Davy described his use of the gas in the temporary alleviation of the pain of inflammation of the gums induced by eruption of a wisdom tooth:

In cutting one of the unlucky teeth called dentes sapientiae, I experienced an extensive inflammation of the gum, accompanied with great pain, which equally destroyed the power of repose and of consistent action.

On the day when the inflammation was most troublesome, I breathed three large doses of nitrous oxide. The pain always diminished after the first four or five respirations; the thrilling came on as usual, and uneasiness was for a few minutes swallowed up in pleasure. As the former state of mind returned, the state of organ returned with it; and I once imagined that the pain was more severe after the experiment than before.

Later in his book (p. 556), Davy again mentioned the possibility of the use of nitrous oxide as an anesthetic agent.

As nitrous oxide in its extensive operation appears capable of destroying physical pain, it may probably be used with advantage during surgical operations in which no great effusion of blood takes place.

RESEARCHES,

CHEMICAL and PHILOSOPHICAL;

CHIEFLY CONCERNING

NITROUS OXIDE,

OR

DEPHLOGISTICATED NITROUS AIR,

AND ITS

RESPIRATION.

By HUMPHRY DAVY,

SUPERINTENDENT OF THE MEDICAL PNEUMATIC
INSTITUTION.

LONDON:

PRINTED FOR J. JOHNSON, ST. PAUL'S CHURCH-YARD.

BY BIGGS AND COTTLE, BRISTOL.

1800.

[FIG. 5] Title page to Humphry Davy's book wherein he discussed the possible use of nitrous oxide as an anesthetic agent.

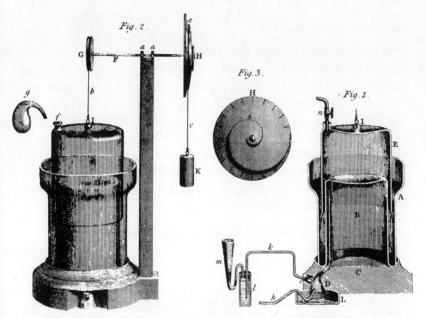

[FIG. 6] Humphry Davy's "gas machine." From the frontispiece to his book. (See Fig. 5).

Humphry Davy constructed what was perhaps one of the first modern gas machines, for in 1799 he is known to have used a gas tank for the storage of pure nitrous oxide (fig. 6). To this he attached an almost impermeable silken bag from which he inhaled the gas.*

There were others, of course, besides Davy who soon developed an interest in nitrous oxide. According to Wilks and Bettany,[18] William Allen, lecturer on chemistry at Guy's Hospital, wrote in his diary in March, 1800:

Present, Astley Cooper, Bradley, Fox, and others. We all breathed the gaseous oxide of azote. It took a surprising effect upon me, abolishing completely at first all sensation; then I had the idea of being carried violently upward in a dark cavern with only a few glimmering lights. The company

* In 1795 James Watts constructed a gas inhaler for Thomas Beddoes. See Beddoes, Thomas and Watts, James: *Considerations on the Medicinal Use, and on the Production of Factitious Aires.* Bristol, J. Johnson, 1795.

[17]

said that my eyes were fixed, face purple, veins in the head very large, apoplectic stertor. They were all much alarmed, but I suffered no pain and in a short time came to myself.

Interestingly enough, Dr. John C. Warren, who often enters into a story of anesthesia, used the inhalation of ether in 1805 as a means of relieving the last stages of pulmonary inflammation.[19]

Michael Faraday, a student of Humphry Davy, was the next investigator to make a contribution to the modern application of anesthesia. He did much original work on the isomerism of butylene with ethylene, and on the chlorides of carbon. He also liquefied many gases. While thus experimenting he noticed the soporific nature of ether vapor. In 1818 he wrote in the *Quarterly Journal of Science and the Arts*:[20]

V. *Effects of Inhaling the Vapour of Sulphuric Ether*

When the vapour of ether mixed with common air is inhaled, it produces effects very similar to those occasioned by nitrous oxide. A convenient mode of ascertaining the effect is obtained by introducing a tube into the upper part of a bottle containing ether, and breathing through it, a stimulating effect is at first perceived at the epiglottis, but soon becomes very much diminished, a sensation of fulness is then generally felt in the head, and a succession of effects similar to those produced by nitrous oxide. By lowering the tube into the bottle, more of the ether is inhaled at each inspiration, the effect takes place more rapidly, and the sensations are more perfect in their resemblance to those of the gas.

In trying the effects of the ethereal vapour on persons who are peculiarly affected by nitrous oxide, the similarity of sensation produced was very unexpectedly found to have taken place. One person who always feels a depression of spirits on inhaling the gas, had sensation of a similar kind produced by inhaling the vapour.

It is necessary to use caution in making experiments of this kind. *By the imprudent inspiration of ether, a gentleman was thrown into a very lethargic state, which continued with occasional periods of intermission for more than 30 hours,* and a great depression of spirits; for many days the pulse was so much lowered that considerable fears were entertained for his life.

Davy had suggested the anesthetic possibilities of nitrous oxide and Faraday had noticed the similar effects of ether. But the evaluation of any process is necessarily slow, and it was some time before physicians were to apply these and similar gases to the relief of pain during surgical operation.

Undoubtedly, one of the heroic figures in the development of surgical anesthesia was Henry Hill Hickman.[21] This scholarly Englishman was admitted in 1820 as a member of the Royal College of Surgeons of London, at the early age of 20 years. He was also a member of the Royal College of Surgeons of Edinburgh. In 1824 he carried out a series of experiments by operating, without causing pain, on animals after the administration of carbon dioxide gas (fig. 4). Because of the many prejudices of the era, he did not persuade surgeons either at home or abroad to allow him to try this gas as an anesthetic on their patients.* Nevertheless, he deserves the credit of having been the first of the modern investigators to prove by experimentation on animals that the pain of surgical operation could be abolished by the inhalation of a gas.

Hickman recognized that certain vapors introduced into the lungs and thence into the circulation of the blood should provide a means of bringing on an artificial sleep prior to surgical intervention. He had mice, puppies, and a mature dog inhale carbonic acid gas, and he thus obtained anesthesia for them during surgical procedures. According to Buxton, Hickman[22] further recognized the importance of maintenance of the constant flow of the blood and of the surgeon's being prepared to meet and deal with circulatory collapse.

On February 21, 1824, Hickman wrote a letter to Mr. T. A. Knight of Downton Castle, near Ludlow, giving full account of his investigations. Knight was a fellow of the Royal Society and Hickman, a personal friend, hoped to obtain recognition from this much respected body so that his work might be checked by others. In the same year Hickman published his famous pamphlet, "A letter on suspended animation" (fig. 7). In this pamphlet he suggested the possibilities of the production of anesthesia

* Interestingly enough Paul Bert over fifty years later, while studying the toxic action of carbonic acid gas and proving that it was not a heart poison, noticed its anesthetic action. This suggested to him the idea of a possible surgical application. He proved experimentally that carbonic acid gas mixed with oxygen in proportions of 40% and 60% respectively gave good results. He cautioned his readers however as follows: "I am far from believing that the preceding researches are precise and detailed enough to authorize immediate application: an experimental table upon which a dog is fastened is one thing, and the bed of a patient is another." See Bert, Paul: *Barometric Pressure; Researches in Experimental Physiology.* Tr. by Mary A. Hitchcock and Fred A. Hitchcock. Columbus, Ohio, College Book Company, 1943, pp. 921-924.

prior to surgical operations on human patients. Failing to impress his own countrymen with the importance of his investigations, he turned to the French capital. In April, 1828, he presented a memorial to King Charles X of France, in which he explained the importance of his discovery. In August of 1828 he asked the French Academy of Medicine to investigate his claims. The academy named a committee to do this, but nothing came of it.

It is hard to believe that the leading scientists of both England and France failed to recognize the contribution of Hickman or to

A

LETTER

ON

SUSPENDED ANIMATION,

CONTAINING

EXPERIMENTS

Showing that it may be safely employed during

OPERATIONS ON ANIMALS,

With the View of ascertaining

ITS PROBABLE UTILITY IN SURGICAL OPERATIONS ON THE

𝕳𝕦𝕞𝕒𝕟 𝕊𝕦𝕓𝕛𝕖𝕔𝕥,

Addressed to

T. A. KNIGHT, ESQ. OF DOWNTON CASTLE,
Herefordshire,

ONE OF THE PRESIDENTS OF THE ROYAL SOCIETY,

████ ████ ██████ ██ ██ ██ ████████ ████

———

BY DR. H. HICKMAN,
OF SHIFFNAL;

Member of the Royal Medical Societies of Edinburgh, and of
the Royal College of Surgeons, London.

———

IRONBRIDGE: Printed at the Office of W. Smith.
1824.

[FIG. 7] Title page to Hickman's pamphlet.
Courtesy of the Wellcome Foundation, Ltd.

[20]

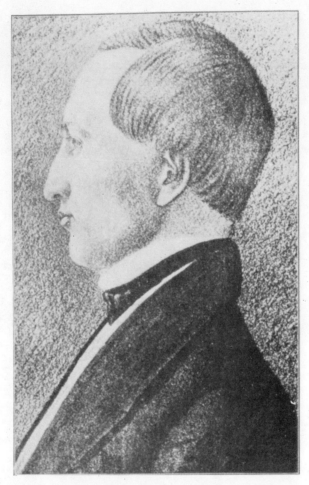

[FIG. 8]   CRAWFORD W. LONG, aged twenty-six. From a
crayon portrait made a few months after his first use of
ether as an anesthetic.

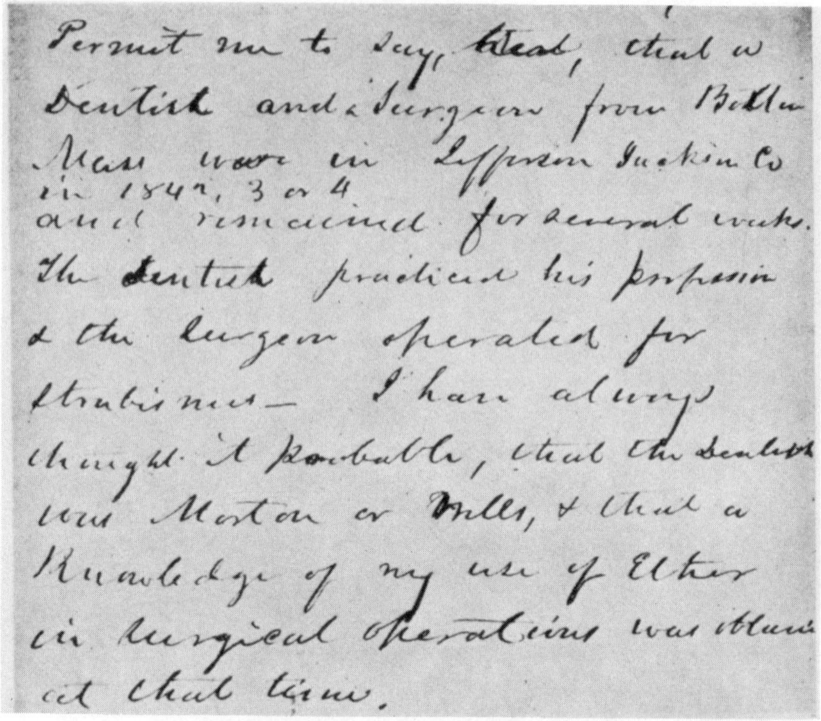

Permit me to say, that a
Dentist and a Surgeon from Boston
Mass were in Jefferson Jackson Co
in 184², 3 or 4
and remained for several weeks.
The dentist practiced his profession
& the surgeon operated for
strabismus — I have always
thought it probable, that the dentist
was Morton or Wells, & that a
knowledge of my use of Ether
in surgical operations was obtained
at that time.

[FIG. 9] Holograph letter by Crawford W. Long.
(Clendening Library.)

investigate his claims scientifically.* Even Sir Humphry Davy, who had been president of the Royal Society, failed to be impressed. In France, the brilliant Baron Larrey alone supported Hickman. He had been army surgeon under Napoleon and knew the horrors of pain caused by surgical operations. He had found that wounded soldiers suffered little pain when they were operated on in a half-frozen condition. But his colleagues outvoted him and declined to push the matter. Hickman, of course, was most disappointed. He returned to England and died prematurely on April 5, 1830.

Meanwhile, in the United States, the use of ether and nitrous oxide was developing. Stockman of New York (according to Kleiman[5]) demonstrated the exhilarating effects of nitrous oxide as early as 1819. Following the advice of men like Beddoes, American physicians employed ether in the treatment of pulmonary tuberculosis and suggested it for other conditions. But it was the employment of nitrous oxide and ether for pleasurable purposes that largely contributed to the use of these gases in anesthesia. There were many itinerant "professors"† of chemistry who traveled through the towns and villages of the country, lecturing on gases and demonstrating the exhilarating effects of nitrous oxide, especially. Many times part of the demonstration consisted of having young members of the audience inhale ether vapor or nitrous oxide. These young participants became pleasantly drunk. They lost their sense of equilibrium, talked foolishly and sometimes laughed with complete abandon.

Soon some of these young persons were amusing themselves without lectures. "Laughing-gas parties" and "ether frolics" became the vogue. Sometime during the year 1839, according to Lyman,[23] William E. Clarke, a young student of chemistry in Rochester, New York, was in the habit of entertaining his companions with inhalations of ether. While a student at Berkshire Medical College in 1841 and 1842, Clarke continued his "ether

---

* In 1928 Chauncey Leake and Ralph Waters repeated Hickman's work and confirmed it. See: Leake, C. D., and Waters, R. M.: "The Anesthetic Value of Carbon Dioxide." J. Pharmacol. and Exp. Therap. 33:280-281 (July) 1928. See also (same title) Anesth. and Analg. for Jan. 1929.
† Samuel Colt, inventor of the revolver, in his early years was one of these.

entertainments." Presumably because of these experiences, in January, 1842, having returned to Rochester, he administered ether from a towel to a young woman named Miss Hobbie, and one of her teeth was then extracted without pain by a dentist, Dr. Elijah Pope. This would appear to be the first use of ether anesthesia on record; it antedates what is at present known of the work of Long by at least two months.*

It was after a public demonstration, which he had not attended, of the effects of nitrous oxide that the young physician, Crawford W. Long (fig. 8) of Jefferson, Georgia, was moved to consider the possibility of administering ether to a patient so that he could operate without causing pain. He knew little about nitrous oxide, but had witnessed "ether frolics" while he was a medical student in the University of Pennsylvania. One of his friends, James M. Venable, who had participated in "ether frolics," had for some time been discomforted by two small tumors on his neck. Here was an opportunity to demonstrate the effectiveness of ether. After some persuasion, Venable agreed to be operated on while he was under the influence of ether, and on the afternoon of March 30, 1842, Long removed one of the small tumors from Venable's neck. The operation was performed successfully and the patient did not feel the surgeon's knife nor did he suffer any pain. Crawford Long was the first man to use ether for the purpose of producing surgical anesthesia for other than dental operations. Dr. Long continued for some time to use ether for anesthesia in his operations. He hoped to encounter patients who needed to undergo major surgical procedures so that he might make a more convincing report, but in such a small community none came his way. Dr. Long published in the issue for December, 1849, of the *Southern Medical and Surgical Journal* an account of his discovery, but Morton's work had been reported by Bigelow[24] and Warren[25] in the *Boston Medical and Surgical Journal* in 1846, as will be shown herein.

In the late Logan Clendening's collection of materials relat-

* Apparently Clarke did not consider his contribution of importance, for it is not mentioned in an account of his life in Stone, R. F.: *Biography of Eminent American Physicians and Surgeons*, Indianapolis, Carlon and Hollenbeck, 1894, p. 89.

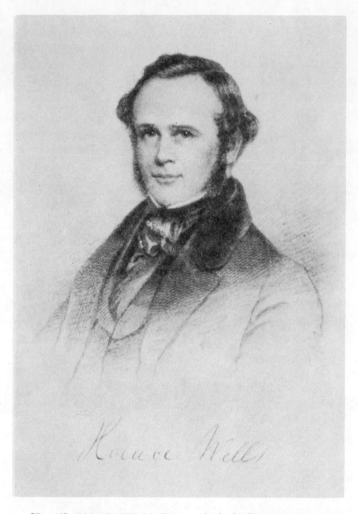

[Fɪɢ. 10] HORACE WELLS. From a print in the Clendening Library.

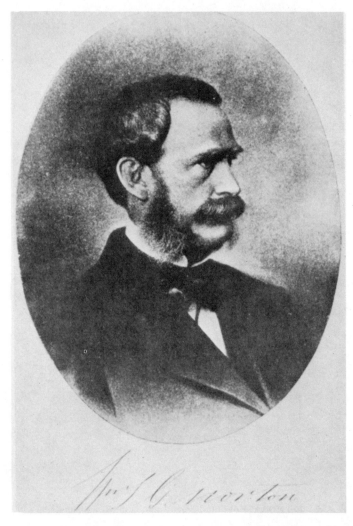

[FIG. 11] WILLIAM T. G. MORTON. From a print in the Clendening Library.

ing to the history of anesthesia is a holograph letter of Crawford W. Long, undated and unsigned (fig. 9). Its authenticity is attested by a letter written by Dr. Long's daughter, Mrs. Frances Long Taylor. Mrs. Taylor's letter presents evidence to show that this was the first draft of a letter written to Dr. G. L. McCleskey, "who was living near Jefferson, Ga., at the time of the visit of the two men from Boston and who recalls the name of one who operated upon a Miss Adeline McClendon for strabismus, Dr. [Y.] Bentley. The name of the dentist he had forgotten. They remained in town a week. I think 1844 was the time he gives as the time of their visit."

In Dr. Long's letter is the following revealing statement:

> Permit me to say then, that a Dentist and a surgeon from Boston, Mass. were in Jefferson Jackson County in 1842, 3 or 4 and remained for several weeks. The dentist practiced his profession & the surgeon operated for strabismus—I have always thought it probable, that the Dentist was Morton or Wells, & that a knowledge of my use of ether in surgical operations was obtained at that time.
>
> I have not been able to ascertain the name of the dentist, if you know the history of Dr. Wells, you can possibly asertain (*sic*) whether he travelled South at the time mentioned.

It is of interest to note in passing that Dr. Long at about the same time as Sir James Simpson (1847) began the administration of ether in obstetrical work.[26]

It was at an exhibition of the exhilarating effects of nitrous oxide gas that the next important development in the history of anesthesia took place. On the evening of December 10, 1844, Dr. Gardner Q. Colton was demonstrating the effects of "laughing gas" before an enthusiastic audience at Union Hall in Hartford, Connecticut. According to Colton's own story,[27] one of the young men who volunteered to try the gas was Samuel A. Cooley, a drug clerk. He immediately came under the influence of the gas and while jumping about, struck his leg on a wooden settee. He bruised it badly. After taking his seat he was astonished to find his leg bloody. He felt no pain until the effects of the gas had worn off. Dr. Horace Wells (fig. 10), one of the town's leading dentists, who had sat next to Cooley and had himself sniffed the gas at Colton's urging, noticed this circumstance. When the audience was retiring, Dr. Wells asked Dr. Colton why a man could not have a tooth extracted without pain while he was under the influence of this gas. Dr. Colton replied that he did not know, because the idea had never occurred to him. Dr. Wells believed that it could be done and persuaded Colton to bring a bag of the gas to his office the next morning, December 11, 1844. Dr. John M. Riggs, a colleague (for whom Riggs' disease, or alveolar pyorrhea, is named), was called in to extract one of Wells' own teeth. Dr. Colton administered the nitrous oxide and Riggs extracted a molar. Dr. Wells on recovery was said to have exclaimed: "It is the greatest discovery ever made! I didn't feel it so much as the prick of a pin!"

At Dr. Wells' request, Dr. Colton taught him how to prepare the gas and then left Wells and continued his lectures on the exhilarating powers of nitrous oxide. Dr. Wells made and tested the effects of the gas and then journeyed to Boston to make known the discovery. He called on Dr. William Thomas Green Morton (fig. 11), a former student and partner, as well as other dentists and physicians, stating his discovery. According to Colton, they treated him as a visionary enthusiast.

Wells obtained permission from Dr. John C. Warren (fig. 12) to address the class in surgery at Harvard Medical School. At the close of his remarks, Wells administered the gas to a boy and extracted a tooth. Most unfortunately, the boy screamed out, for anesthesia had not been complete. Later, the patient admitted that he had suffered no pain and did not know when the tooth had been drawn. At the time, however, the students hissed and pronounced the so-called discovery a hoax. Had Dr. Wells' demonstration proved successful to all parties concerned, nitrous oxide probably would have been adopted for surgical anesthesia. But even though Wells returned to Hartford and used nitrous oxide successfully in his dental practice in 1845, as the deposition of some forty respectable citizens of Hartford indicates, the use of this gas was abandoned until June, 1863, when Dr. Colton revived it in New Haven, Connecticut, administering it for Dr.

J. H. Smith, a distinguished dentist of that city. Although Wells had failed to convince the world of the value of nitrous oxide as an anesthetic agent, he is credited with conceiving the idea of anesthesia and publicizing the possibility of its use. William Morton had witnessed the unsatisfactory demonstration of his former partner and teacher, Horace Wells, under whom he studied dentistry. At that time Morton* had been a student at the Harvard Medical School, where he had for his preceptor Dr. Charles A. Jackson. Dr. Jackson was not only a qualified physician but also a chemist of note and among other accomplishments was well known for his researches in geology.

In the practice of dentistry, Morton, according to Miller,[28] had invented an improved process for making artificial teeth. This required that his patients submit to the painful process of having the roots of their teeth extracted before Morton's artificial teeth could be fitted. The pain of extraction of such roots was tremendous, and the procedure was unsatisfactory. Morton was constantly thinking of a means of alleviating this pain.

One day in July, 1844, a patient, Miss Parrot, asked to have a tooth filled, a process which ordinarily caused excessive pain. Many times Jackson had mentioned that ether sprinkled on the skin could relieve pain. Morton's patient could not endure the pain caused by the necessary preparation for filling. To deaden the pain locally, Dr. Morton applied sulfuric ether to the adjacent tissue as recommended by Jackson. He was able to continue his work without hurting the patient. Because the action of ether as he administered it was slow, it was necessary for the patient to return on several subsequent days. One day, in using the ether a bit freely, Morton noticed its numbing effects on the surrounding parts of the face. The idea occurred to Morton that if the whole system could be brought under the influence of this drug, a valuable means of relief might be afforded for more difficult dental surgery.

---

* Morton never received a medical degree in course. In 1852 Washington University in Baltimore granted him an honorary M.D. degree. See Morton, Elizabeth W.: "The Discovery of Anesthesia." *McClure's Magazine*, 7:311-318 (Sept.) 1896.

Morton thought of the inhalation of ether. But he thought it would endanger life. He had learned on reading Pereira's *Materia Medica* that a small amount of ether inhaled was not dangerous, but that inhalation of large amounts was dangerous. He began to experiment. First he submitted a puppy to the inhalation of ether. This was successful. Next he tried to anesthetize goldfish. He also experimented on insects, caterpillars and worms. One day the puppy sprang against a glass jar containing ether and broke it. The contents fell to the floor and Morton soaked his handkerchief in the portion that remained and applied it to his own mouth and nostrils. He felt the effects of the vapor and thought he might have had a tooth pulled without feeling pain.

Morton next tried to experiment on his two dental assistants, Thomas Spear and William Leavitt. But when they inhaled ether both students became greatly excited, not subdued. Something was wrong. He consulted Dr. Jackson. Jackson recommended that he try pure sulfuric ether. Morton professed ignorance of the use of sulfuric ether and Jackson* later based his claim to the discovery on his suggestion to Morton that ether would anesthetize the patient. Morton did find out from Jackson, however, that pure sulfuric ether would serve his purpose better than the commercial product. After experimenting on himself, he was ready for the proper patient.

On September 30, 1846, an opportunity presented itself for Morton to test his theoretic discovery. On the evening of that day a patient, Eben H. Frost, came to Dr. Morton's office. An ulcerated tooth was causing him considerable pain and he wished

---

* Dr. Jackson felt that he was the discoverer not only of anesthesia (until he heard about Long's claim) but also of the telegraph. Jackson was a passenger with Prof. Samuel F. Morse on board the ship "Sully," sailing from Le Havre to New York in October, 1832. One day after dinner there was a discussion among the company on the recent electro-magnetic discoveries. Jackson told about his experiences in Paris in witnessing the electric demonstrations of Ampère. The question was asked of Jackson if the length of wire in the coil of a magnet did not retard the passage of electricity. In proof that it did not, Jackson told how Franklin had caused electricity to travel twenty miles by means of a wire stretched up the Schuylkill River. Jackson claimed that Morse conceived the telegraph then and there, basing his claim to the discovery on this chance conversation. See Hodges, R. M.: *A Narrative of Events Connected with the Introduction of Sulphuric Ether into Surgical Use.* Boston, Little, Brown, and Co., 1891, pp. 64-65. Also Jaffe, Bernard: *Men of Science in America.* New York, Simon and Schuster, 1944, pp. 193-194.

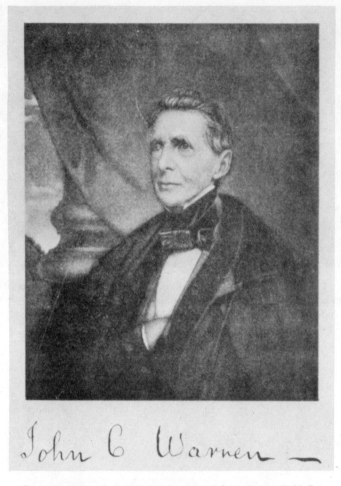

[FIG. 12] JOHN C. WARREN. Reproduced from Camac, C. N. B.
(Compiler): *Epoch-making contributions to medicine, surgery and the
allied sciences.* Courtesy of W. B. Saunders Co., 1909.

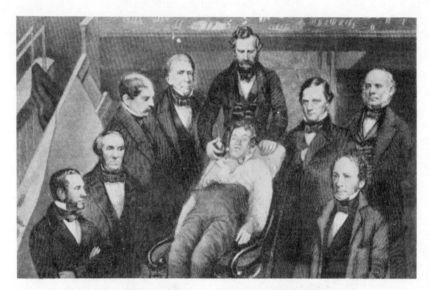

[Fig. 13] The first public demonstration of anesthesia with ether. From left to right surrounding the patient, Gilbert Abbot, are H. J. Bigelow, J. Mason Warren, A. A. Gould, J. C. Warren, W. T. G. Morton, Samuel Parkman, S. D. Townsend, and George Hayward. Engraving by H. B. Hall. Reproduced from Rice, N. P.: *Trials of a public benefactor*. New York, Pudney & Russell, 1858.

to have it extracted. Dreading the operation, Frost asked to be mesmerized. Morton said that he had something better and induced his patient to inhale sulfuric ether. The success of his first dental operation under anesthesia produced by ether is best told by the *Boston Journal* which Miller[28] said printed an account of the operation the following day:

> Last evening, as we were informed by a gentleman who witnessed the operation, an ulcerated tooth was extracted from the mouth of an individual, without giving him the slightest pain. He was put into a kind of sleep, by inhaling a preparation, the effects of which lasted about three-quarters of a minute, just long enough to extract the tooth.

Shortly after the painless extraction of Eben Frost's tooth, Morton called on Dr. John C. Warren, explained his discovery and asked permission to try it at some operation. In reply to his visit he received the following historic note from Dr. C. F. Heywood, house surgeon to the Massachusetts General Hospital:[28]

> *Dear Sir:* I write at the request of Dr. J. C. Warren, to invite you to be present on Friday morning at 10 o'clock, at the hospital, to administer to a patient who is then to be operated upon the preparation which you have invented to diminish the sensibility to pain.

> Yours respectfully, C. F. Heywood,
> *House Surgeon to the General Hospital.*

Dr. Morton, Tremont Row, October 14, 1846.

On that famous Friday morning, October 16, 1846, members of the staff of the hospital filled the operating room. Because Morton had to wait for the completion of his inhaling apparatus, which was being constructed for him by an instrument maker, he arrived a few minutes late at the hospital. Meanwhile, Dr. Warren, believing that Morton had not intended to fulfill his mission, prepared to proceed with the operation in the usual manner. Then Morton appeared on the scene and after apologizing for his slowness, induced the patient, a young man named Gilbert Abbot, to inhale the vapor from his new apparatus, the principle of which, according to Miller,[28] has been but slightly improved in all the succeeding years (fig. 13).

As to the actual operation, the removal of a tumor of the jaw, the report[25] of the surgeon, John C. Warren, may be consulted:

On October 17th [i.e., 16th], the patient being prepared for the operation, the apparatus was applied to his mouth by Dr. Morton for about three minutes, at the end of which time he sank into a state of insensibility. I immediately made an incision about 3 inches long through the skin of the neck, and began a dissection among important nerves and blood vessels without any expression of pain on the part of the patient. Soon after he began to speak incoherently, and appeared to be in an agitated state during the remainder of the operation. Being asked immediately afterwards whether he had suffered much, he said that he had felt as if his neck had been scratched; but subsequently, when inquired of by me, his statement was, that he did not experience pain at the time, although aware that the operation was proceeding.

On the next day, Dr. George Hayward performed an operation on a patient anesthetized with ether. He removed a large fatty tumor from the arm of a female. Morton was the anesthetist. The operation was a success and there was no evidence of pain, excepting some occasional groans during the last stage. The patient subsequently stated that these were the result of a disagreeable dream.

According to Garrison,[30] it was largely due to the high character of such men as Warren and Bigelow that anesthesia produced by ether was instituted all over the world. Warren conceived it to be his duty to introduce the use of anesthesia into the practice of hospitals, but learned that Morton intended to obtain an exclusive patent for its use.* On consultation with Hayward, Warren came to the conclusion that since the ethics of medicine forbade physicians to conceal any useful discovery, further use of this new invention could not be encouraged, since it was not known of what it was made and since by patent it was prohibited

* It would appear that, in spite of Morton's jealous guarding of his secret, some physicians strongly suspected the true nature of his anesthetic agent. Dr. J. D. Mansfield of South Reading, Massachusetts (*Boston M. & S. J.* 35:424-425 [Dec. 23], 1846) in a letter dated November 10, 1846, said that he himself had had experience "in a social party" with a mixture composed of "sulph. ether, water and morphine, with a few drops of diluted sulphuric acid. This mixture was inhaled through a common retort, with a ground stopper at the apex of the globe. The effects which it had on those who inhaled it were similar, if not identical, with those produced by the *vapor* now so much in vogue." Dr. Mansfield was sharply critical of Morton's decision to patent his anesthetic agent, as were several other persons. But in the fifth edition of *Morton's Letheon* (copy in the New York Academy of Medicine Library), a letter from a noted Washington lawyer, Charles M. Keller, is reprinted. This letter is dated Jan. 5, 1847. Mr. Keller said that in his opinion it was just as legal to patent Letheon as it was to patent Watt's invention of the steam engine. Daniel Webster endorsed Mr. Keller's opinion, saying (Feb. 19, 1847): "I concur in the foregoing opinion, entirely; entertaining no doubt that Dr. Morton's discovery is a new and useful art, and as such the proper subject of a patent."

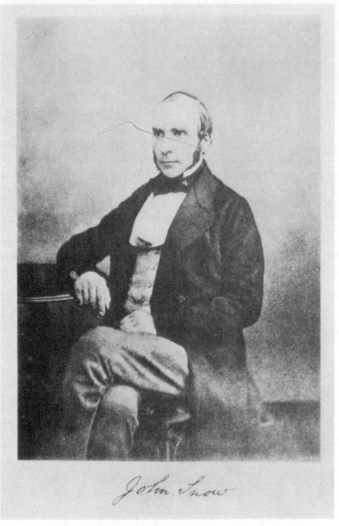

[FIG. 14] JOHN SNOW, the first physician to devote his full time to anesthesia. Reproduced from the Asclepiad, 1887, vol. 4.

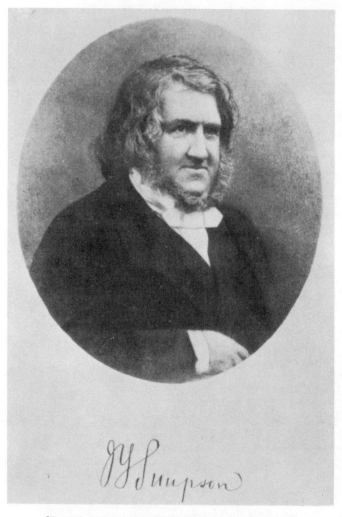

[FIG. 15] SIR JAMES YOUNG SIMPSON. Reproduced
from Gordon, H. L.: *Sir James Young Simpson and chloroform*. London, T. Fisher Unwin, 1897.

from being used freely. Morton became much alarmed at this turn of events, and declared his willingness to make known the agent employed and to supply assistance in administration of it whenever called on to do so.

On October 30, 1846, Morton requested a list from Dr. Warren of all hospitals and charitable institutions in the country, so that he might present them with the use of his new alleviator of pain. Apparently this was done, and operations conducted on patients anesthetized with ether became established at the Massachusetts General Hospital, and subsequently in other hospitals throughout the country.

The first thorough account of the use of sulfuric etherization was read by Henry Jacob Bigelow, one of the surgeons of the Massachusetts General Hospital, on November 9, 1846, before the Boston Society of Medical Improvement.[24] It was subsequently published in the *Boston Medical and Surgical Journal* for November 18, 1846, and at once provoked from the Philadelphia *Medical Examiner* the much-quoted attack on Boston physicians on the score that they were giving succor to quackery and that if such actions continued, "Physicians and quacks will soon constitute one fraternity."[31]

Stimulated by the appearance of this paper by Dr. Bigelow, Dr. F. Dana, Jr.,[32] of Boston, sent to the *Boston Medical and Surgical Journal* a spirited defense of mesmerism, in which he said that mesmerism had been tested much longer than anesthesia produced by sulfuric ether. He referred to the work of Elliotson in England (previously mentioned herein), said that the Section on Medicine of the Royal Academy of France had approved mesmerism in 1831, and claimed that Baron Cuvier, Gabriel Andral, François Broussais and Matthew Baillie all had strongly approved mesmerism. The *Boston Medical and Surgical Journal*, however, always had been contemptuous of mesmerism.

The use of anesthesia developed very rapidly in Europe. Ether was administered in Paris on December 15, and in London on December 19, 1846. On December 21 anesthesia was assured a prominent place in the world when Robert Liston[29] performed his first operation in which anesthesia was produced by ether.

Meanwhile Oliver Wendell Holmes in a letter to Morton* suggested the name "anæsthesia" for the condition and "anæsthetic" for the adjective as follows:

Boston, Nov. 21, 1846.

My Dear Sir: Every body wants to have a hand in a great discovery. All I will do is to give you a hint or two as to names—or the name—to be applied to the state produced and the agent.

The state should, I think, be called "Anæsthesia." This signifies insensibility—more particularly (as used by Linnæus and Cullen) to objects of touch. (See Good—Nosology, p. 259.)

The adjective will be "Anæsthetic." Thus we might say the state of Anæsthesia, or the anæsthetic state. The means employed would be properly called the anti-æsthetic agent. Perhaps it might be allowable to say anæsthetic agent, but this admits of question.

The words anti-neuric, aneuric, neuro-leptic, neuro-lepsia, neuro-stasis, etc., seem too anatomical; whereas the change is a physiological one. I throw them out for consideration.

I would have a name pretty soon, and consult some accomplished scholar, such as President Everett or Dr Bigelow, senior, before fixing upon the terms, which *will be repeated by the tongues of every civilized race of mankind*. You could mention these words which I suggest, for their consideration ; but there may be others more appropriate and agreeable.

Yours respectfully,

O. W. HOLMES.

Dr. Morton.

Osler[33] said that Withington told him that the word was used "first in Plato (Timaeus) and is used by Dioscorides in the modern sense." It was used, in 1718, by J. B. Quistorpius[28] in the title "De Anæsthesia." It first appeared in English in N. Bailey's dictionary of 1721 as "Anaisthesia, a loss or Defect of Sense, as in such as have the Palsy or are blasted."

The following testimony by Daniel Webster (from a photostatic reproduction in the Clendening Library) in a letter written by him to Morton is an important opinion concerning Morton's contribution:

---

* This was first printed in the 2nd edition, 2nd issue of E. Warren's *Some Account of the Letheon.* See Dr. Fulton's Appendix, p. 182.

† See Good's Nosology, p. 259.

The Acceptance of Anesthesia

Dr. W. T. G. Morton,   Washington, Dec. 20, 1851
Dear Sir,

In reply to your letter of the 17th Inst. I would say that having been called on, on a previous occasion, to examine the question of the discovery of the application of ether in surgical operations, I then formed the opinion, which I have since seen no reason to change, that the merit of that great discovery belonged to you, and I had supposed that the reports of the Trustees of the Hospital, and of the Committee of the House of Representatives of the U. S. were conclusive on this point.

The gentlemen connected with the Hospital, are well known to me, as of the highest character, and they possessed at the time of the investigation, every facility, for ascertaining all the facts in the case.

The Committee of the House were, I believe, unanimous in awarding to you the merit of having made the first practical application of ether, and a majority, by their report, awarded to you, the entire credit of the discovery.

Very respectfully
Your obd. svt.
(signed) DANL WEBSTER

c—THE ACCEPTANCE OF ANESTHESIA

"L'éther, qui ôte la douleur, ôte aussi la vie, et l'agent nouveau que vient d'acquérir la chirurgie est à la fois merveilleux et terrible."
—FLOURENS

Morton forsook the practice of dentistry and discontinued his medical courses at Harvard in order to devote his full time to anesthesia. Without doubt he therefore can be considered to be the first professional anesthetist. The first qualified physician who devoted his full time to anesthesia was John Snow of London (fig. 14).

John Snow[34] was licensed as a member of the Royal College of Surgeons in 1838. In 1843 he received the degree of Bachelor of Medicine from the University of London, and in 1844 he was granted the degree of Doctor of Medicine by the same university. Snow had for some time been interested in gases, and when late in the year of 1846 the news arrived from America that surgical operations could be performed without pain if patients previously submitted to the inhalation of sulfuric ether, he immediately became attentive.

The History of Surgical Anesthesia

According to Richardson (p. xiv, ref. 34), the first attempts at the production of anesthesia by the inhalation of ether in England* "were not so successful as to astonish all of the surgeons, or to recommend etherization as a common practice. The distrust arose from the manner in which the agent was administered. Dr. Snow at once detected this circumstance; and, as he explains in the pages of the work now in the hands of the reader, remedied the mistake by making an improved inhaler."

Equipped with his new inhaler, Snow was soon administering ether to the outpatients of St. George's Hospital, London, for the prevention of pain in the extraction of teeth. Snow's success in the production of anesthesia for dental operations was noticed by a Dr. Fuller of Manchester Square. Fuller remarked to his colleagues on the superiority of Snow's method of the administration of ether over the method currently employed. As a consequence, Snow was invited to administer ether for major surgical operations at St. George's Hospital. He began to do so on January 28, 1847. Later he administered ether at the University College Hospital for Robert Liston, the great English surgeon. Liston appreciated the efforts of his anesthetist and soon Snow became the leading anesthetist in London.

On January 19, 1847, Sir James Young Simpson (fig. 15) first used ether in his obstetric practice. About this time, as has been mentioned earlier, Long of Georgia was also using ether in obstetrics. According to Thoms,[35] the first production of *anesthésie à la reine*† (that is, the administration of ether between each pain in natural labor) occurred in the United States. Dr. Nathan Colley Keep of Boston reported his use of this procedure in a letter which was published in the *Boston Medical and Surgical Journal*, issue of April 14, 1847.

Because of the disagreeable qualities of ether, such as its per-

* On January 12, 1847, Joseph-François Malgaigne related to the French Academy of Medicine his favorable experiences in four of five cases where he had operated using ether as the anesthetic agent. (See Malgaigne: [Communications sur l'emploi d' éther] Bull. de l'Acad. Roy. de Méd. 12:262-264 (Jan. 12) 1847.) Six days later Alfred-Armand-Louis-Marie Velpeau reported to the French Academy of Science his observations, which were not at all favorable. (See "Remarques de M. Velpeau à l'occasion des précédentes communications." Compt. rend. Acad. d. sc. 24:76-78 (Jan. 18) 1847.)

† Anesthésie à la reine, literally "anesthesia in the manner of that used for the queen."

sistent odor and its tendency to irritate the bronchi, Simpson[36] searched for different agents with which to replace ether. Among those he tried on himself and his associates were the chloride of carbon, acetone, nitric ether, benzine, the vapor of iodoform and chloroform. Of all the agents he tried, chloroform was the one that seemed to be the most suitable. He campaigned vigorously for its use.

The discovery of this important anesthetic agent occurred in 1831. During that year it was described independently by Samuel Guthrie[37] of Sacket Harbor, New York, Eugène Soubeiran[38] of France and Justus von Liebig[39] of Germany. According to Robinson,[40] Soubeiran's first article on chloroform was written for the October 1831 issue of *Annales de chimie et de physique.* Liebig's initial communication was a note in *Poggendorf's Annalen* for November, 1831. Guthrie's announcement appeared in *Silliman's Quarterly* for October, 1831, which did not make its appearance, however, until January, 1832. The leading physical and chemical properties of chloroform were described by Jean Baptiste Dumas in 1835. Dumas[36] bestowed on the drug its formula and name. In March, 1847, the French physiologist, Flourens,[41] proved that the inhalation of chloroform caused in animals the same temporary type of anesthesia caused by the inhalation of ether.

The use of chloroform was suggested to Simpson by David Waldie, a chemist of Liverpool. On November 4, 1847, Simpson and his assistants, Drs. Keith and Duncan, inhaled it.* Satisfied with these preliminary experiments, Dr. Simpson at once began to use chloroform in his obstetric practice. On the tenth of the same month (November) the use of chloroform analgesia in obstetrics was made known by Simpson in an address before the Medico-Chirurgical Society of Edinburgh.

The Scottish Calvinist clergy and others objected to Simpson's use of chloroform to prevent the pain of childbirth. They contended that this pain should be endured with patience and fortitude. Many influential members of the medical profession ob-

---

* According to Clark,[41] Dr. Matthews Duncan tried chloroform a day before Simpson and his colleagues inhaled it.

jected to the use of analgesia in obstetrics, including Charles D. Meigs of Philadelphia, Francis H. Rainsbotham of the British Isles and Friedrich W. Scanzoni of Germany.[40]

Simpson waged a successful campaign in behalf of the use of analgesia in obstetrics. When his adversaries quoted the Bible to show that pain was a fore-ordained penalty, Simpson quoted the Scriptures (Genesis, II:21) to prove that God was the first anesthetist (see frontispiece).

THE

TRANSACTIONS

OF THE

AMERICAN

MEDICAL ASSOCIATION.

INSTITUTED 1847

VOL. I.

———

¹⁷²¹³

PHILADELPHIA:
PRINTED FOR THE ASSOCIATION,
BY T. K. AND P. G. COLLINS.
1848.

[FIG. 16] Title page of the transactions of the first meeting of the American Medical Association. These transactions gave much prominence to anesthesia.

[34]

The Acceptance of Anesthesia

Over two centuries previous, Du Bartas,* the French Huguenot poet, in his famous encyclopedic poem *La Semaine* (1579) translated into English by Joshua Sylvester had alluded to anesthesia in his interpretation of the creation of Eve as follows:

> Even as a Surgeon, minding off-to-cut
> Som curelefs limb; before in vfe he put
> His violent Engins on the vitious member,
> Bringeth his Patient in a fenfe-lefs flumber,
> And grief-lefs then (guided by vfe and Art)
> To faue the whole, fawes off th'infected part:
> So, God empal'd our Grandfires liuely look,
> Through all his bones a deadly chilnefs ftrook,
> Siel'd-vp his fparkling eyes with Iron bands,
> Led down his feet (almoft) to *Lethe* Sands:
> In briefe, fo numm'd his Soule's and Body's fenfe,
> That (without pain) opening his fide, from thence
> Hee tooke a rib, which rarely He refin'd,
> And thereof made the Mother of Mankind:

The quarrel lasted for several years, but when Queen Victoria (fig. 17) accepted the use of Simpson's chloroform on April 7, 1853,[35] during the birth of her eighth child, Prince Leopold, the continued use of chloroform in obstetrics was assured. Queen Victoria was attended during this confinement by Sir James Clark. John Snow served as analgesist. Chloroform was administered on a handkerchief. The drug was given intermittently and inhalation analgesia was induced for the patient, who was not unconscious at any time.†

In May of the same year in which Morton demonstrated the practicability of ether anesthesia (1846), a group of physicians met in New York City to hold a national medical convention.

---

* Du Bartas, Guillaume de Saluste: *His Diuine Weekes and Workes. A Compleate Collection of all the other moft delight-full workes.* "The Sixt Day of the First Week." Tranflated and written by the famous Philomufus, Iosvah Sylvester Gent: London, printed by Humphray Lownes, [1621], p. 137. The first English edition was published in 1598.

† There is a particularly splendid story about John Snow's method of sidestepping awkward questions when asked about his treatment of the Queen. One obstetrical patient to whom he was administering chloroform became very talkative during the period of excitement and declared she would inhale no more of the vapor unless she were told word for word what the Queen had said when she was taking it. "Her Majesty," replied Dr. Snow, "asked no questions until she had breathed very much longer than you have; and if you will only go on in loyal imitation, I will tell you everything." The patient followed Dr. Snow's request. In a few seconds she forgot about the Queen. By the time she had come to her clever witness had left the hospital. See Griffith, H. R.: "John Snow, Pioneer Specialist in Anesthesia." Anesth. and Analg. 13:45-51 (Mar.-Apr.) 1934.

Delegates from medical societies and colleges of many parts of the United States were present. This was a successful meeting and it was deemed expedient for the medical profession of the country to reconvene the following year. At this meeting, held in Philadelphia, it was agreed that the name of the new organization be the American Medical Association. Standing committees were appointed to make annual reports. Such were the preludes to the first annual meeting of the American Medical Association, held in Baltimore in May, 1848.

At this first organized meeting of the American Medical Association, much prominence was given to the subject of anesthesia. This is attested by the report of the Committee on Surgery.[42]

After a discussion of the value of keeping statistical records and an illuminating account of many operations, the committee considered in detail the various anesthetic agents. The report of the committee is a most important co-eval record of the reaction of the medical profession to the introduction of anesthesia, and for that reason it will be considered somewhat in detail (fig. 16).

According to the report, some surgeons were afraid to use anesthesia in their surgical operations, feeling that the advantages afforded by the relief of pain might be offset by the risks involved:

The great question, which still divides medical opinion, is: Can the annulling of pain by anesthetic agents be produced without risk to life, or is the hazard so inconsiderable as to justify their employment in all cases where it is desirable to prevent the pain of surgical operations?

Apparently, even at this early date (1848), the authors of this report felt that a large group of surgeons were wholly in favor of anesthesia:

They look upon the dangers of etherization as so inconsiderable as to justify the induction of this state, prior to all surgical operations in which the pain is an important consideration, while they consider the advantages of anesthetic agents to be especially manifest in all extensive ones, involving life, where the nervous shock (which they believe lessened by them) might increase the risks of a fatal issue.

The authors did, however, admit that some surgeons "would

[36]

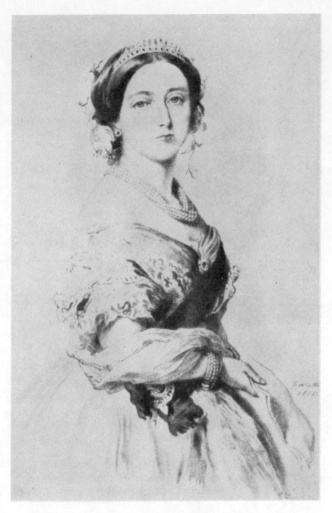

[FIG. 17] Queen Victoria in 1855. Reproduced from Lorne, V.
R. I.: *Queen Victoria—her life and empire.*
Harper & Brothers, 1902.

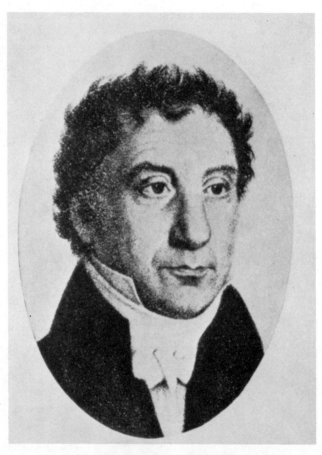

[Fɪɢ. 18] FRIEDRICH WILHELM SERTÜRNER who
discovered morphine. Reproduced from München. med.
Wchnschr. 71:77 (Jan. 18) 1924.

restrict the use of these agents to severe operations, and discourage their general employment, under a belief that their full effect cannot be attained without a degree of danger which would render their indiscriminate use unjustifiable. While a small proportion of the profession still object altogether to anæsthetics as dangerous and hurtful in their tendency . . ."

Mention is made in the report that after the introduction of ether anesthesia in Boston it was not until several months later that the method became generally popular in other communities in the United States. The favorable reports of its use in Boston and in Europe made for the more extensive use of ether anesthesia in American communities in 1847 and 1848.

The dangers of etherization were also considered. In some cases it was thought that convulsions, prolonged stupor, intense cerebral excitement, alarming depression of the vital powers and asphyxia apparently were caused by the inhalation of ether and chloroform. Secondary effects attributed to inhalation in a few cases were bronchitis, pneumonia and inflammation of the brain. Interestingly enough, according to this report (p. 190), ether was considered to be a safer drug than chloroform.

Apparently Dr. Henry W. Williams[42A] of Boston in 1850 was the first to use the anesthetic agents, ether or chloroform, prior to ophthalmic surgery.

Gradually, other anesthetic agents were developed and many improvements were made in the administration of them. These factors contributed to the welfare of the patient.

D—LOCAL, REGIONAL AND SPINAL ANESTHESIA

To discuss another type of anesthesia, in which lack of sensation is obtained by the subcutaneous injection of certain substances, it will be necessary first to refer to certain pioneer efforts made prior to the period at which this narrative has now arrived.

The unripe capsules of the white poppy when pressed and solidified form opium. This famous vegetable narcotic agent, as mentioned previously, was one of the important agents of the ancients in their production of artificial sleep. But, like the action of so many other drugs, the action of the drug was unpredictable.

On some patients large doses of this drug apparently had little effect. The action of this drug on other patients often was very dangerous, and might even result in the patient's death. Because of this danger the more conservative members of the medical profession refrained from using it.

To bring about the safe use of this drug, Friedrich Wilhelm Sertürner (fig. 18) of Paderborn, Westphalia, a chemist, devoted much of his time to research and experimentation. After experimenting with crude opium, mixing it with the better known solvents, he at one time (1806) poured liquid ammonia over the opium.[2] This produced a white crystal residue.[*] Sertürner, after experimenting on himself, found this residue, an alkaloid, to be the cause of the soporificity of opium. He named the drug "morphium" (later changed to "morphia," "morphine" and "morphin") after the Greek god of dreams, Morpheus.[43]

Lafargue, in 1836,[44] came upon a new way to deaden pain. Using a vaccination lancet, he injected morphine paste subcutaneously near the affected part, with beneficial results. In 1839, Drs. Isaac E. Taylor and James A. Washington of New York began the practice of hypodermic medication.[44] These physicians punctured the skin with a lancet and, by means of Anel's eye syringe, forced a solution of morphine under the skin for the local relief of pain. In 1845, F. Rynd[45] of Edinburgh also carried out a similar means of subcutaneous medication. In 1853, Dr. Alexander Wood of Edinburgh injected a solution of morphine under the skin in the vicinity of a painful part, affording relief from pain.

In 1853 Wood devised the modern type of the metallic hollow needle,[†] and in that same year Charles Gabriel Pravaz attached an improved hollow needle to a specially constructed syringe. On the continent this is called the "Pravaz" syringe, in honor of its inventor. In England and the United States it is commonly referred to as the "hypodermic syringe." Thus the world was

---

[*] In 1804, Seguin discovered the same substance but did not fully investigate it.

[†] The first "hollow needles" were quills. This was the type used by Sir Christopher Wren in 1656 in his intravenous injections of opium and crocus metallorum. Sigismund Elsholtz probably used a quill in 1665 also for his injections of opiates. (See p. 54.)

assured of the full benefit of the administration of morphine. According to Archer,[1] W. W. Greene of the Maine Medical School as early as 1868 advised the hypodermic use of morphine during inhalation anesthesia. He felt that his procedure prevented shock, delirium, nausea, and shortened the anesthetic influence. In 1869, according to Fülöp-Miller[2] (p. 355), the French physiologist, Claude Bernard, also advocated the same procedure.

Spessa[46] of Italy in 1871 injected a solution of morphine into a fistulous tract before surgical intervention, claiming that by doing this he was able to prevent pain during surgical operations.

The use of cocaine in anesthesia was the next important development. Its history is most interesting. According to Bumpus,[47] in ancient times the natives of Peru knew about the anesthetic qualities of the coca plant. During the severe surgical procedure of trephination they obtained local anesthesia by chewing the leaves of the coca plant and allowing the resulting saliva to run into the fresh incision.* The plant was also important in the religious and political lives of these people. Braun[48] quoted Novinny as saying that the coca plant was regarded as a gift from God which "satiated the hungry, gave renewed energy to the tired and weary, and caused the unfortunate to forget sorrows."

While on a trip to South America, Scherzer, according to Braun,[48] noticed that the leaves numbed the tongue when they were chewed. He brought back with him a large quantity of these leaves and was the first to make a report in the literature concerning their anesthetic qualities.

In 1855, Gaedicke[2]† of Germany isolated an alkaloid of the leaves of this plant, naming it erythroxylin. A few years later (1860) Albert Niemann of Germany obtained the alkaloid of coca leaves in crystalline form and named it "cocaine." He also reported the numbing effect of this drug on the tongue.

Not much attention was paid to these important discoveries

---

* Roy L. Moodie was probably the first to point this out. See his *Paleopathology, an Introduction to the Study of Ancient Evidences of Disease* (Urbana, University of Illinois Press, 1923). This book has an imaginative frontispiece by Tom Jones illustrating the practice.

† The *U. S. Dispensatory* gives the year 1844 and the investigator's name as Gaedken.

until 1873.* In that year Alexander Bennett[49] demonstrated the anesthetic properties of cocaine. Five years later (1878) Vasili Konstantinovich von Anrep[50] made a thorough study of the pharmacologic properties of cocaine. Von Anrep injected a weak solution of cocaine under the skin of his own arm. He experienced a sense of warmness which was followed by anesthesia that lasted for about thirty-five minutes. This led him to suggest the possibility of the employment of cocaine as a local anesthetic agent. He also experimented on animals. He injected a solution of cocaine into the conjunctival sac of animals, but he noticed its dilatory effect on the pupil only. However, Coupart and Borderan, in 1880, were able to demonstrate the loss of the corneal reflex in animals after the use of solutions of cocaine. According to Braun,[48] Fauvel, Saglia, and others had already learned to use coca leaves and their extracts in the treatment of painful diseases of the larynx and pharynx.

The development and use of cocaine as a local anesthetic agent was chiefly the work of Carl Koller (fig. 19). When Koller was house surgeon at the Vienna General Hospital, his friend Sigmund Freud was studying the possibility of curing patients addicted to morphine by treating them with cocaine. Both Koller and Freud studied the physiologic aspects of cocaine. Freud turned his attention away from these investigations. Koller, however, continued his studies. He injected a weak solution of cocaine into the eye of a frog and noticed that the eye became insensitive to pain. On September 15, 1884, Koller reported his observations to the Ophthalmological Congress held in Heidelberg. Soon afterward cocainization of the eye for the production of local anesthesia was generally adopted.

Not long after the acceptance of cocaine for the production of local anesthesia for surgery of the eye, cocaine was extensively used in laryngology and rhinology. Otis and Knapp used cocaine anesthesia for operations in the male urethra, and Fraenkel carried out experiments in which application of the agent to gyne-

* According to Carl Koller, in a letter to M. G. Seelig (J.A.M.A. 117:1284 [Oct. 11] 1941), Moreno y Mayz, the Peruvian army surgeon, in 1868, remarked that the sensory paralyzing effects of cocaine might be put to use in medicine.

cology was demonstrated. Cocaine was also injected in solution into the tissues, and became extensively used in dentistry and in general surgery. William S. Halsted* of the John Hopkins Hospital in 1884 injected cocaine into nerve trunks, thus obtaining "conduction" anesthesia in peripheral regions. The nerve he first blocked was the mandibular. In 1922 the American Dental Association honored Dr. Halsted for his original researches, which greatly improved the use of anesthesia in oral surgery.

In 1885, J. Leonard Corning (fig. 20)[51] of New York, having shown experimentally that cocaine had a prolonged anesthetic effect when it was administered subcutaneously, experimented on the possibilities of spinal anesthesia.[52] He injected hydrochlorate of cocaine into the space situated between the spinous processes of two of the inferior dorsal vertebrae in a dog. He obtained epidural† anesthesia, and although this procedure did not affect the anterior extremities, he was able to obtain anesthesia of the hind legs. To Corning this suggested the local action of the drug. He next worked with a man who had long been suffering from spinal weakness and seminal incontinence. This time he injected a solution of hydrochlorate of cocaine between the spinous processes of the eleventh and twelfth thoracic vertebrae. Anesthesia of the legs and genitalia resulted. Encouraged by his results, Corning[53] in 1888 injected hydrochlorate of cocaine in the vicinity of the spinal cord. According to Bumpus,[47] Corning was the originator of regional anesthesia. In 1887, he injected presumably a solution of cocaine around the median cutaneous antibrachii nerve, producing anesthesia of the skin supplied by it.

In 1891 Quincke[54] demonstrated the usefulness of spinal puncture as a diagnostic procedure.‡ Although he was unaware

---

* Halsted, W. S., "Practical comments on the use and abuse of cocaine; suggested by its invariably successful employment in more than a thousand minor surgical operations." New York Med. J. 43: 294-295, 1885.

† There are those who believe that Corning obtained spinal and not epidural anesthesia. His statement is as follows: "*Experiment* I. This was performed on a young dog . . . I injected twenty minims of a two-per-cent solution of the hydrochlorate of cocaine into the space situated between the spinous processes of two of the inferior dorsal vertebrae. Five minutes after the injection there were evidences of marked inco-ordination in the posterior extremities . . . A few minutes later there was marked evidence of weakness in the hind legs, but there were no signs whatever of feebleness in the anterior extremities." (See Ref. 52.)

‡ Dr. Essex Wynter of England discovered lumbar puncture, independently, at about this time.

of the possibilities of spinal anesthesia, he showed that the introduction of a needle through the dura was feasible. After the work of Corning and Quincke, August Bier[55] of Greifswald, Germany, in 1898 produced true spinal anesthesia in animals and then in himself and an assistant, Hildebrandt, by injecting the spinal canal with a solution of cocaine. He was soon using it for patients with complete success. Theodore Tuffier,[56] working independently of Bier, produced spinal anesthesia by injecting a solution of cocaine between the third and fourth lumbar spaces. Many other investigators reported their observations and spinal anesthesia became established on a firm basis.

A new method of anesthesia was contributed by Carl Ludwig Schleich. Before the German Congress of Surgeons in 1892, he demonstrated infiltration anesthesia by intracutaneous injection.* In 1890, according to De Takáts,[57] Réclus, Pernice and Kummer had earlier made use of infiltration anesthesia. But Schleich apparently achieved better results by the use of a very diluted solution of cocaine. Schleich's method was used in 1894 in the United States, as reported by Würdemann. In 1896 Bransford Lewis reported his use of infiltration anesthesia.

In 1897 Braun demonstrated that the toxicity of cocaine was in direct ratio to its rate of absorption and that its efficiency was in reverse ratio. He therefore recommended the addition of epinephrine to cocaine to decrease the rate of absorption and to increase the duration of anesthesia.

Meanwhile, many investigators had developed derivatives of cocaine that were not so toxic. In 1891 Giesel isolated tropacocaine. Fourneau introduced stovaine† in 1903. Einhorn, in 1904, discovered novocaine (procaine hydrochloride). Many other similar drugs were later developed.

Apparently the first surgeons in the United States to use spinal anesthesia were Tait and Caglieri[58] of San Francisco. On October 26, 1899, they performed osteotomy of the tibia with the patient under spinal anesthesia.

* Halsted anticipated Schleich's work by about five years. See Halsted's letter to Sir William Osler, reprinted in Fulton, John: *Harvey Cushing*. Springfield, Illinois, Charles C. Thomas, 1946. p. 142.
† So named because its discoverer's name means stove.

The first American to report on true spinal anesthesia was Dr. Rudolph Matas[59] (fig. 22) of New Orleans. On November 10, 1899, he first anesthetized a patient by what he termed "the spinal subarachnoid method." According to Souchon,[60] Matas has made several original contributions to the development of anesthesia. He devised an apparatus for massive infiltration anesthesia; in January, 1898, he operated on a patient anesthetized by intraneural and paraneural infiltration with cocaine and other drugs, obtaining anesthesia of the forearm and hand by this method. Matas developed a method of anesthesia of the region supplied by the second division (maxillary nerve) of the trigeminal nerve by blocking the nerve at the foramen rotundum. On April 29, 1899, using this type of anesthesia, he removed both maxillae of a patient for carcinoma. That same year (1899) he succeeded in obtaining regional anesthesia by blocking the second and third divisions of the trigeminal nerve for operations on the jaw. In 1938 Dr. Matas was awarded the first Distinguished Service Medal of the American Medical Association at its annual meeting. Wayne Babcock[61] of Philadelphia early in his career (1904) began to use spinal anesthesia. He has consistently advocated this type of anesthesia in selected cases. Bourne[62] and his associates have recently recommended spinal anesthesia for thoracic operations. But this use had been previously reported by Harlan F. Newton[62A] of Boston and Harry J. Shields[62B] of Toronto. Their first cases were operated on in 1931.

According to Matas,[59] Dr. George Washington Crile (fig. 23) of Cleveland at an early date practiced the direct open injection of nerve trunks with cocaine to produce anesthesia. On May 18, 1897, he amputated a patient's leg without causing pain after injecting the sciatic and anterior crural nerves. Dr. Harvey Cushing[63] and others in Dr. Halsted's clinic at the Johns Hopkins Hospital used this principle that same year (1897), anesthetizing the inguinal region for the radical treatment of hernia. As has been mentioned earlier herein, Halsted in 1884 had obtained conduction anesthesia by injecting the nerve trunks with cocaine.

The use of peridural or epidural anesthesia, first suggested by

[43]

Corning in 1885, is relatively new in the United States but it has been widely used in Europe and South America. The method as pointed out by Charles B. Odom[64] is a form of block anesthesia and derives its name from the space into which the anesthetic solution is injected. As the epidural space extends the entire length of the spinal canal, it is possible through a single puncture to achieve analgesia to carry out operations below the chin without puncturing the dura. This type of anesthesia was independently thought of by Fidel Pagés[65] of Spain in 1920. He used it to anesthetize the abdomen and chest. His untimely death (1921) cut short his work on this subject. In 1931, A. M. Dogliotti[66] reported on peridural anesthesia as his discovery, unaware of Corning's and of Pagés's work.

E—ANOCI-ASSOCIATION;
REFRIGERATION ANESTHESIA

Dr. Crile[67] and his associates at the H. K. Cushing Laboratory at Western Reserve University in Cleveland, Ohio, made another contribution to anesthesiology: the development of a method of combining local anesthesia with general anesthesia, first reported in 1908[68] and known as "anoci-association" or "anociation." Before a general anesthetic agent was administered they blocked off the nerve supply to the field of operation by the local or intraneural infiltration of procaine hydrochloride (novocaine). When this technic was combined with preliminary treatment involving special management of the patient (applied psychology) and the use of narcotic agents it was found that fear, pain, shock and postoperative manifestations were, to a large extent, controlled.

The use of cold as an anesthetic agent has been mentioned earlier herein. Sir Benjamin Ward Richardson,* a pupil of John Snow, according to Leake,[69] improved on this type of anesthesia

---

* Richardson made many important contributions to anesthesia. He brought into use no less than fourteen anesthetics. Of these methylene bichloride was the most employed. He invented the first double valved mouthpiece for use in chloroform anesthesia. (See Richardson, Sir Benjamin Ward: In *Dictionary of National Biography*, v. 22, Supplement, pp. 1169-1170.) Early in his career he made researches on gases, and his studies on anesthetic narcotism led him to anticipate what he afterwards made practicable by means of the lethal chamber—the painless extinction of lower animal life. Among the therapeutic substances he introduced into medical practice were hydrogen peroxide, sodium ethylate, the colloids and amyl nitrite. (See Martin, Mrs. George: "Life of Sir Benjamin Ward Richardson by his daughter . . ." In Richardson, B. W.: *Disciples of Aesculapius.* London, Hutchinson & Co., 1900, v. 1, pp. 1-12.)

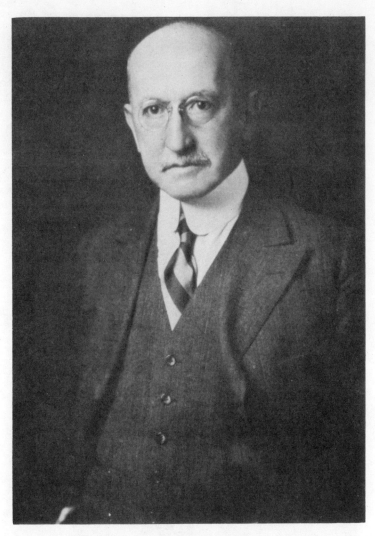

[Fig. 19] CARL KOLLER.

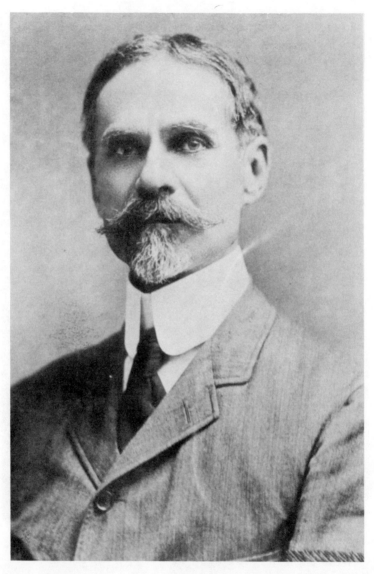

[Fig. 20] J. LEONARD CORNING. Reproduced by courtesy of the
New York Academy of Medicine.

in 1867. He introduced the ether spray for the purpose of producing local anesthesia. This was found to be satisfactory for many minor operations. It was later modified by the use of ethyl chloride which, because it evaporates more quickly, is more effective than ether in this particular technic.

Refrigeration anesthesia in amputations, employed by Severino in the seventeenth century, and known to have been used by Larrey in the nineteenth century as mentioned earlier herein, has recently proven to be a successful measure. Frederick M. Allen of New York read his first paper on this subject in August, 1941, before the meeting of the International College of Surgeons in Mexico City.[70] Dr. Allen used cracked ice, snow ice or ice-water as the sole anesthetic for forty-three amputations of lower extremities. Dr. Allen could find no evidence of shock during the period of reduced temperature before, during, and after these painless operations. Neither the pulse nor the blood pressure was disturbed. However, healing was found to be slower than with other methods. In September, 1943, Drs. Harry E. Mock and Harry Mock, Jr., published a review article[71] covering 101 cases already reported in the literature plus seventeen of their own. Their experience was similar to Allen's and left them greatly in favor of this type of anesthesia.

F—RECTAL ANESTHESIA

The modern production of anesthesia by the intestinal route was attempted shortly after sulfuric ether became more generally available as an inhalation anesthetic agent. Apparently, Nikolas Iwanowitch Pirogoff[72] (fig. 21), the famous Russian surgeon, first described this method in 1847.* Sutton[73] said that Pirogoff's original plan was to introduce liquid ether into the rectum. Magendie warned him that this might be a dangerous procedure. Pirogoff then devised a method of vaporizing the ether by heating it and administering it in its volatile form. Pirogoff was so enthusiastic about this method

* Also in 1847, Dr. Antonio Saez of Madrid administered ether as an enema before removing a huge (13¼ lb.) tumor of the breast. See García del Real, Eduardo: "Early surgical anesthesia in Spain." Brit. Med. Bull. 4 no. 2:146-147, 1946.

that he thought it would supplant the inhalation method. Roux,[74] Y'Yhedo,[75] and Dupuy[76] reported that same year on the production in animals of complete anesthesia by way of the rectum.* Liquid ether, pure or in aqueous mixture, was employed. Nevertheless, in spite of Pirogoff's enthusiasm, there does not seem to be further mention in the medical literature concerning this type of anesthesia until 1884.

In that year Daniel Mollière[77] of France reintroduced anesthesia produced by the administration of ether by way of the rectum. At first he employed a hand bellows which forced ether vapor into the intestine. Later, he warmed the ether by placing

RECHERCHES

PRATIQUES ET PHYSIOLOGIQUES

SUR

L'ÉTHÉRISATION

PAR

N. PIROGOFF

Docteur en Médecine; Académicien; Professeur à l'Académie Médico-Chirurgicale de St.-Pétersbourg; Chirurgien en chef du second Hôpital militaire; Chef des travaux anatomiques; Chirurgien consultant aux hôpitaux d'Oboukhow, de St. Marie-Madeleine et de St. Pierre et St. Paul; Conseiller d'État, Membre du Conseil Médical et Membre Correspondant de l'Académie des Sciences.

ST. PÉTERSBOURG.

IMPRIMERIE FRANÇAISE. TROÏTZKY PÉRÉOULOK. № 3.

1847.

[FIG. 21] Title page of Pirogoff's book wherein anesthesia by the intestinal route was first described. Reproduced by courtesy of the Army Medical Library.

* For an illuminating account of the contribution of Marc Dupuy, as well as some contemporary reactions to Pirogoff's work, see Proskauer, Curt: "The simultaneous discovery of rectal anesthesia by Marc Dupuy and Nikolai Ivanovich Pirogoff." J. Hist. Medicine and Allied Sciences 2:379-384 (Summer) 1947.

the container in a water bath at a temperature of 120° F. (48.8° C.). The resulting pressure forced the ether vapor into the intestine. According to Sutton,[73] in that same year (1884), Yversen, Hunter, Bull, Weir, Wancher, and Post recorded their experiences with this method. These observers reported some unfavorable results, including more or less pronounced diarrhea and melena and one death. Kleiman[5] said that this type of anesthesia produced severe injuries to the mucosa.

The discouraging results aforementioned again led to the abandonment of anesthesia produced by the colonic absorption of ether. However, in 1903, J. H. Cunningham revived the method. He introduced a new technic in which air was utilized as a means of transporting ether vapor into the intestine. With Frank Lahey[78] in 1905 he published his first article concerning the new method. Walter S. Sutton[73] improved on the work of Cunningham, and in 1910 published the results obtained with the method in a series of 140 cases. He recommended the use of oxygen instead of air as a vehicle, and developed a more satisfactory apparatus than had been available for the administration of this type of anesthesia.

On August 11, 1913, James Tayloe Gwathmey (fig. 24) read his preliminary communication on oil-ether colonic anesthesia before the seventeenth meeting of the International Medical Congress in London. He referred to his experiments with animals as well as to some clinical results. He was able to overcome irritation of the mucosa by the addition of Carron oil to the ether, by giving the mixture as an enema, slowly introduced into the rectum. This type of anesthesia was remarkably successful. The first public demonstration of oil-ether colonic anesthesia was made on September 27, 1913, at the People's Hospital in New York City, on one of Dr. I. M. Rothenberg's patients, Dr. Solomon Rothenberg operating. The work was continued at other hospitals in New York City, and spread to other sections of the United States and to other countries. On November 20, 1913, Dr. Gwathmey[79] read a paper before the New York Society of Anesthetists (now the American Society of Anesthetists), demonstrating the continued use of oil-ether anesthesia in about 100 cases. Olive oil, being found more satisfactory, was substituted for Carron oil. In 1923, by reducing the amount of ether used in oil-ether colonic anesthesia, Gwathmey developed a successful method for the relief of pain during labor. In 1930, Gwathmey[80] reported on 20,000 cases in which this method had been used successfully for the relief of the pain of childbirth. The final technic involved three intramuscular injections of magnesium sulfate, morphine sulfate being given with the first injection of magnesium sulfate, and a rectal instillation of a compound of quinine alkaloid, alcohol, ether, and petroleum liquid or olive oil. Another anesthetic agent found to be successful when administered by way of the rectum was tribromethyl alcohol in amylene hydrate (avertin). This agent was discovered by Eichholz[2] in 1917 and first clinically employed by Butzengeiger[81] in 1926.

G—TWILIGHT SLEEP

A type of analgesia once much in favor was "twilight sleep" for the relief of obstetric pain. According to Claye,[82] von Steinbüchel of Graz, stimulated by the work of Schneiderlin and Korff on scopolamine-morphine, in 1902 used for the first time this type of analgesia in his obstetric practice. Another early worker in this field was C. J. Gauss* who did much to extend the use of "twilight sleep." Von Steinbüchel found it possible, after premedication with scopolamine-morphine alone, to carry out such obstetric procedures as perineal suture, dilatation of the cervix by Bossi's method and sometimes delivery with forceps. In some cases it was necessary to repeat the hypodermic injection after not less than two hours. If the patient still felt pain, ether or chloroform was also given by inhalation. The significant contribution of von Steinbüchel, in this respect, was his discovery of how little inhalation anesthesia was required when the patient previously had had premedication with scopolamine-morphine. Because relief of pain was often inadequate, unfavorable influ-

* See, for instance: Gauss, C. J.: "Die Anwendung des Skopolamin-Morphium-Dämmerschlafes in der Geburtshilfe." Med. Klin. 2:136-138, 1906, and later articles.

ences on uterine contractions were noticed, and asphyxia frequently was encountered among babies, "twilight sleep," although it was received with tremendous enthusiasm, is today not the analgesic agent of choice in obstetrics. On the other hand, however, its importance as preliminary medication prior to general anesthesia for surgical operations, as also reported by Crile, is now becoming of marked significance.

H—ETHYLENE, DIVINYL OXIDE, CYCLOPROPANE AND CYPROME ETHER

In the field of general anesthesia other agents were being developed. Some of these were not successful enough to warrant their inclusion herein. Others have been of decided importance. Of the agents of the latter group ethylene as an anesthetic agent has an interesting history.

Apparently ethylene, or olefiant gas, as it is referred to in the earlier literature, was first prepared by Becker,[83] the exact date not being known. Another early investigator was Johannes Ingenhouss. According to Luckhardt and Lewis,[84] Ingenhouss is referred to in Joseph Priestley's book: *Experiments and Observations Relating to Various Branches of Natural Philosophy* (London and Birmingham, 1779-86, 3 v.) as the first to prepare ethylene.

Hoping to discover a more satisfactory anesthetic agent than the ones in use, Thomas Nunneley,[85] a surgeon of Leeds, reported in 1849 concerning the examination of some thirty-seven compounds. Nunneley concluded, however, that ethylene was not to be recommended as an anesthetic agent, because his results with this gas were so unsatisfactory. Coal gas, according to his experiments, was a superior agent. Nunneley did, however, report on the use of ethylene dichloride as an anesthetic agent, and apparently achieved more favorable results than those noted by Simpson, who also had used this preparation. Today, Nunneley* is chiefly remembered for his description of the anesthetic qualities

---

* Hewitt in his book, *Anæsthetics*, Ed. 3, p. 466, attributes the A. C. E. mixture to Dr. George Harley.

of a mixture of ether and an alcoholic solution of chloroform.[41] This was named the "A. C. E. mixture" (1 part alcohol, 2 parts chloroform, 3 parts ether) and was a widely used agent in the middle and later parts of the nineteenth century. In reminiscing concerning his boyhood, W. J. Mayo[86] described the use of the A. C. E. mixture in the surgical practice of his father, William Worrall Mayo. The anesthetist in this case was C. H. Mayo, at the early age of twelve years.

The next investigator to experiment with ethylene was the physiologist, Ludimar Hermann.[87] In 1864 he noted its mildly intoxicating action. Davy and Müller also studied the effects of this gas. In 1876, Eulenberg presented experimental evidence to show the anesthetic qualities of ethylene. Franz Lüssem,[88] in 1885, reported on some unsatisfactory results of experiments in which he had used a 75 per cent ethylene-oxygen mixture. These poor results were attributed to the presence, presumably, of carbon monoxide. Using a purer product, he anesthetized two dogs and a guinea-pig with an 80 per cent ethylene-oxygen mixture. He inhaled this mixture himself and after eighteen minutes noticed weakening of the arms and legs in addition to dizziness and uncertainty of gait.

About this time, according to Leake,[69] Sir Benjamin Ward Richardson, who has been referred to herein, found ethylene to be an admirable agent for general anesthesia. He felt, however, that its gaseous state was a disadvantage.

Not much more attention was paid to ethylene as an anesthetic agent until Arno B. Luckhardt[89] (fig. 25) and R. C. Thompson in 1918 gathered data which served to establish experimentally the anesthetic and analgesic qualities of a mixture of 80 per cent ethylene and 20 per cent oxygen. They began their experiments because of curiosity as to the effect of ethylene gas on animal protoplasm, stimulated by the work of William Crocker and Lee Irving Knight.[90] Crocker and Knight, in 1908, had studied the effects of ethylene on carnations. That year carnation growers had met with severe losses on their shipment of flowers to Chicago. These flowers, when placed in greenhouses, would "go to sleep" and buds showing petals would fail to open. Believing that illuminating gas was responsible for the damage to the flowers, these botanists of the Hull Botanical Laboratory studied the effect of the gas on the flowers. After much research they discovered that ethylene, which forms about 4 per cent of illuminating gas, was the chief offender.

Because of the toxic effect of ethylene on carnations, Luckhardt and Thompson studied its effects on animals. They were not able to demonstrate any toxic manifestations among laboratory animals, but did notice that ethylene had a marked anesthetic action. The first World War interrupted their studies, but in 1922, Luckhardt, working at this time with J. B. Carter, resumed the experiments. They confirmed the earlier unpublished data and extended their study. Satisfied with these investigations on various animals, Luckhardt and Carter next experimented on themselves and other volunteer workers. Later, they gave a private demonstration before an interested group of physicians and professional anesthetists at the University of Chicago. So well satisfied were the spectators as to the admirable qualities of ethylene as an anesthetic agent that in a short space of time (on March 14, 1923) ethylene, administered by Isabella Herb for the surgeon Arthur Dean Bevan, was used at the Presbyterian Hospital (Chicago) for general anesthesia. Not long thereafter, on April 27, 1923, Luckhardt and Carter[91] reported on ethylene as a general anesthetic agent in 106 surgical operations.* Meanwhile Isabella Herb[92] published her clinical study.

J. H. Cotton[93] in 1917 in the *Canadian Medical Association Journal* reported data to show that ethylenated ether had strong anesthetic and analgesic qualities, and William E. Brown,[94] also of Canada, without knowledge of the work of Luckhardt and his colleagues, in March, 1923, published his preliminary communication in which experimental evidence on the value of ethylene as an anesthetic agent was presented.

After the development of the clinical use of ethylene, many

* For a delightful story of the history of ethylene consult the following reference: Luckhardt, A. B.: "An adventure in research." Bull. Conn. State Dent. Assn., pp. 46-56 (May) 1944.

other general anesthetic agents were evolved. Chauncey D. Leake, of the University of California (fig. 27), well known for his pharmacologic studies on various anesthetic agents and his resulting discouragement of unsafe preparations, made an important hypothesis. Working with M. Y. Chen,[95] Leake suggested that it might be interesting to prepare a compound consisting of a hybrid molecule utilizing the structural characteristics of ethylene and ethyl ether. It was the feeling of these investigators that this compound would be a general anesthetic agent which might give promising results. When this prediction was made, according to Leake,[96] divinyl oxide was known only theoretically. Upon Leake's request, in 1930, Randolph Major and W. L. Ruigh, of Princeton University, sent him an impure sample of the aforementioned unsaturated ether. In 1931 they prepared pure divinyl oxide.[97] After the pharmacologic studies of Leake, P. K. Knoefel and A. E. Guedel[98] on the anesthetic action of divinyl oxide in animals, S. Gelfan and I. R. Bell[99] of the University of Alberta demonstrated its safety as an anesthetic agent for human beings. It was first employed in cholecystectomy on an obese patient at the University of California Hospital in San Francisco in 1933. Dr. Dorothy Wood served as anesthetist.

Cyclopropane, another relatively new anesthetic agent, was discovered by August Freund[100] in 1882. Freund noticed that propylene, an isomer of cyclopropane, was present as an impurity. Many years later (1928) G. H. W. Lucas and Velyien E. Henderson,[101] searching for the cause of cardiac damage in propylene anesthesia, studied cyclopropane as a possible impurity of propylene. Cyclopropane was found not to be responsible for the cardiac damage. It was found to be, experimentally, a more potent anesthetic agent than propylene. In addition, it was demonstrated in laboratory animals that cyclopropane was rapid in its action and of slight toxicity in effective concentrations and that it could be rapidly eliminated. Henderson and Lucas[102] continued their investigations. The pharmacologic action of cyclopropane was later investigated by M. H. Seevers, W. J. Meek, E. A. Rovenstine and J. A. Stiles[103] of the University of Wiscon-

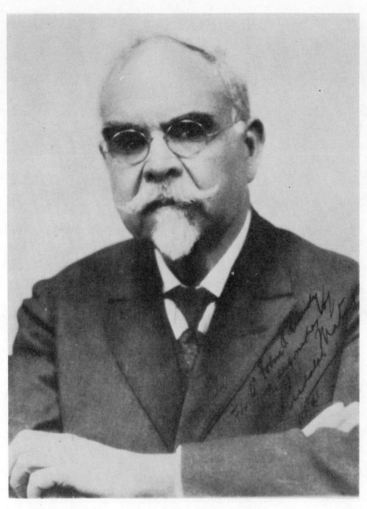

[FIG. 22] RUDOLPH MATAS.

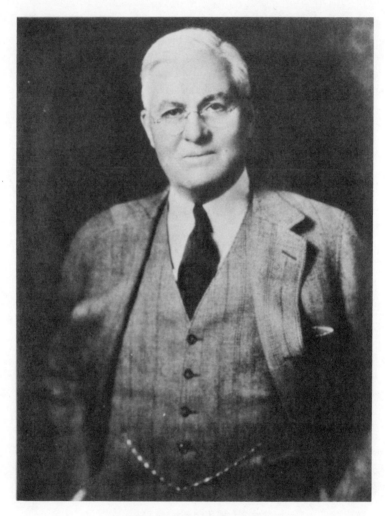

[FIG. 23] GEORGE W. CRILE.

sin. Ralph M. Waters[104] (fig. 28), head of the department of anesthesia of the same university, encouraged by the work of his associates, studied the anesthetic effects of this agent on animals. Next,Waters and his associates administered cyclopropane to each other, with satisfactory results. In 1930, they first administered it for surgical anesthesia. In October of 1933 a group of anesthetists from various parts of the country were invited to the University of Wisconsin to witness the results of this work. The demonstration met with success and the staff of the department of anesthesia of the University of Wisconsin[105] published the first clinical report of the use of cyclopropane as a general anesthetic agent.

In 1939 it occurred to John C. Krantz, Jr., C. Jelleff Carr, Sylvan E. Forman, and William E. Evans, Jr.,[106] of the department of pharmacology of the University of Maryland, that it would be of interest to prepare a hybrid molecule between ether and cyclopropane. These investigators succeeded in developing a method of synthesis for the convenient preparation of the aliphatic cyclopropyl ethers. The first member of the series that they were able to identify and consequently to prepare was cyclopropyl methyl ether. This agent they named "cyprome ether." Results of their pharmacologic studies have shown that cyprome ether is a more potent anesthetic agent than ethyl ether. After these experimental investigations, which were satisfactory enough to warrant clinical trial of the agent concerned, a volunteer hospital patient was operated on under anesthesia produced by cyprome ether. The patient's recovery was uneventful. In 1940, Constance Black, George E. Shannon and John C. Krantz, Jr.,[107] reported on the first twenty-five surgical operations performed with the patients under the influence of anesthesia produced by cyprome ether.

I—INTRAVENOUS ANESTHESIA AND RELATED PROCEDURES

The discovery of a method of conveying liquors directly into the blood stream is attributed to Sir Christopher Wren, the famous architect (fig. 29), by his contemporaries, Oldenburg[108] and Clarck.[109] The first experiments were carried out in 1656, at the home of the French ambassador, the Duc de Bordeaux. Wren was at that time professor of astronomy at the University of Oxford. Wren ligated the veins of a large, lean dog. Having made an opening on the side of the ligature toward the heart, he then introduced a syringe into this opening. The syringe, formed from an animal bladder to which a quill had been attached, was filled with a solution containing opium in this case and an infusion of crocus metallorum in another. Wren found that opium, administered intravenously, soon stupefied but did not kill the dog. A large dose of crocus metallorum, however, similarly administered to another dog, induced vomiting and death. Wren probably was unaware of the anesthetic results of his intravenous administration of opium, for his investigation was made mainly in the hope of discovering a new therapeutic procedure. According to Sturgis,[110] Wren also injected beer and wine into the blood stream, probably to determine their therapeutic effects.

Apparently, as suggested by Jarman,[111] the first genuine attempt at intravenous anesthesia was made in 1665. At that date Sigismund Elsholtz injected a solution of an opiate to obtain insensibility. At about this time (February, 1665) Richard Lower (fig. 30) transfused blood to animals for the first known time. On June 15, 1667, Jean-Baptiste Denis of Montpellier with the help of a Dr. Emmerez first transfused blood to man. The account of Dr. Lower's experiments[112] was published in the *Philosophical Transactions* of the Royal Society for December 17, 1666, and Dr. Denis' experiment[113] was published in the same *Transactions* for July 22, 1667. In all these early experiments the blood of animals, preferably lamb's blood, was used. In some of the cases of Denis, however, the blood of a calf was used. Lower and Edmund King[114] also transfused blood to a man, Arthur Coga, on November 23, 1667. In one of Denis' cases,[115] it was hoped to bring about sanity by this therapeutic measure, for the patient who underwent the procedure was demented. Because of the severe reactions which followed these early attempts at

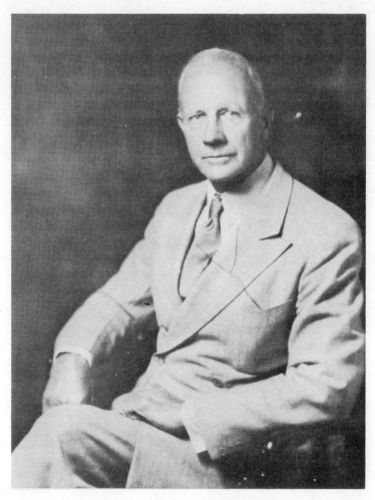

[Fig. 24] JAMES T. GWATHMEY.

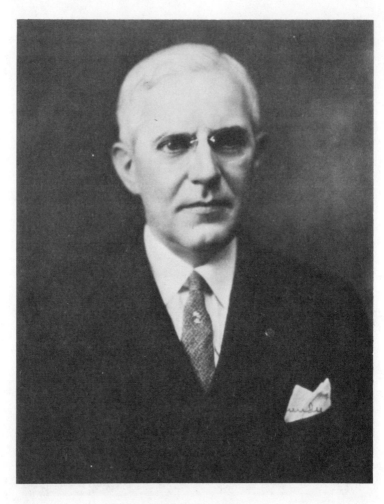

[FIG. 25] ARNO B. LUCKHARDT.

transfusion and because of the death of one of Denis' patients (probably not from the transfusion, but from poisoning) the transfusion of blood to human beings was prohibited by law in France, and in 1670 by an act of Parliament in England. The transfusion of blood was therefore abandoned for many years.

James Blundell,[116] the distinguished English obstetrician and physiologist, reopened the subject of the transfusion of blood. Many of his patients had died because of puerperal and post-partum hemorrhage. Blundell felt that transfused blood might have saved them. Postulating that when blood is to be transfused to an animal, it should be obtained only from an animal of the same species, he was the first to transfuse human blood to a patient (September 26, 1818). Unfortunately, the patient was at the point of death and could not be revived by this therapeutic measure. Blundell transfused blood on many other occasions, and, according to Sturgis,[110] of ten patients to whom blood was transfused, five died and five lived. Despite the failures, Blundell believed in the therapeutic benefits of the transfusion of blood, and predicted that the world would sometime realize its value.

Another procedure related to the transfusion of blood and to intravenous anesthesia is the intravenous administration of saline solutions to patients suffering from shock. According to Adams,[45] Latta of Leith, Scotland, introduced this practice in 1831. Many investigators in the latter part of the nineteenth century, as mentioned by Hirsh,[116] demonstrated the effectiveness of infusing a physiologic solution of sodium chloride in cases of surgical as well as traumatic shock. For a time the intravenous use of sodium chloride superseded that of whole blood, obviating the problem of coagulation as well as the problem of the procuring of blood donors.

Theodor Bischoff[117] performed some very interesting experiments in 1835. He demonstrated that when the whole blood of one animal was injected into an animal of another species, toxicity and death resulted. Bischoff found, however, that the injected animal would tolerate defibrinated blood. John Braxton-Hicks, according to Hirsh,[116] opened up the field of the use of chemical anticoagulants in 1868. He added sodium phosphate to blood used for transfusion, noting its anticoagulant properties. It was not until 1914, however, that much real progress was made in the problem of anticoagulation. At that time A. Hustin[118,119] of Belgium described a new method of transfusion in which a solution of glucose and sodium citrate was used as an anticoagulant. In the same year Professor Luis Agote[120] of Buenos Aires transfused citrated blood successfully. In 1915, Richard Lewisohn[121] of New York City reported a means of regulating the dosage of sodium citrate, so that its efficiency as an anticoagulant would be insured but its toxic characteristics would be overcome. After using the method experimentally with no ill results, he reported that he had transfused blood successfully to two patients with this new method.

Besides the problem of clotting, there remained the problem of discovering why, in the course of transfusion, some human blood was not compatible with other human blood. For even when human blood was used exclusively in transfusions, severe reactions resulted in many cases. Karl Landsteiner,[122] in 1900, and Samuel G. Shattock,[123] working independently in the same year, reported on the incompatibility of different types of human blood. In a footnote to Landsteiner's article it was pointed out that all blood could be divided into three types. The fourth type, according to Sturgis,[110] was discovered by two students, De Castello and Sturli, in 1902. Solution of the problem of the compatibility of the blood and the problem of coagulation is the basic discovery on which the successful transfusion of blood rests. Recently the blood bank, by means of which it is possible to keep blood in storage for ten days, has been developed. Blood serum and plasma are now being used to some extent to replace whole blood[124] and have been of utmost importance in war medicine.

The first monograph on intravenous anesthesia to be printed was that of Pierre-Cyprien Oré[125] (fig. 26) (1875). He had published a preliminary report on this subject in 1872.[126] Oré experimented with the intravenous injection of chloral hydrate into animals. After successful experimentation on animals he was able to produce general anesthesia in human beings by this method. On February 16, 1874, Oré reported to the French Academy of Sciences the first case in which he had employed this type of anesthesia for a human being. Oré was very enthusiastic about intravenous anesthesia with chloral hydrate, and believed it to be superior to inhalation anesthesia with ether or chloroform. But inhalation anesthesia continued to be favored and intra-

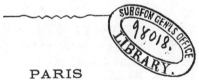

ÉTUDES CLINIQUES

SUR

L'ANESTHÉSIE CHIRURGICALE

PAR LA MÉTHODE

DES INJECTIONS DE CHLORAL DANS LES VEINES

PAR LE D' ORÉ

Lauréat de l'Institut, Chirurgien honoraire des Hôpitaux,
Docteur ès-Sciences naturelles,
Professeur de Physiologie et Lauréat de l'École de Médecine de Bordeaux,
Membre et Lauréat de l'Académie des Sciences (Médaille d'argent et Médaille d'or);
Membre honoraire de la Société de Médecine de Gand; Associé national de la Société d'Anthropologie;
Correspondant de la Société de Chirurgie, de la Société de Biologie,
de la Société des Sciences, Lettres et Arts d'Évreux,
des Sociétés de Médecine de Marseille, Caen, Metz, Poitiers; de la Société de Médecine
et de Chirurgie pratique de Montpellier, Officier de l'Instruction publique; Chevalier de la Légion d'honneur
et de l'Ordre de la Conception du Portugal.

PARIS

J.-B. BAILLIÈRE ET FILS
LIBRAIRES-ÉDITEURS DE L'ACADÉMIE DE MÉDECINE
16, rue Hautefeuille, 16

1875

[FIG. 26] Title page to the first monograph to be published on intravenous anesthesia. Reproduced by courtesy of the Army Medical Library.

[57]

venous anesthesia was not used for several years. As Greene[127] has suggested, Oré's drug (chloral hydrate) was not well suited to anesthetic purposes. Its anesthetic action was slow in disappearing and the required dosage for purposes of surgical narcosis was close to the toxic dosage.

Before and after the introduction in 1903 of the barbiturates, which were to revolutionize the use of intravenous anesthesia, other drugs were employed. In 1899, H. Dresser of Munich introduced methylpropylcarbinol urethane (hedonal),[45] and in 1905, N. P. Krawkow and his associates at St. Petersburg demonstrated the value of hedonal as an anesthetic agent for intravenous use.[45] At about this time Fedorow of St. Petersburg reported favorable results in 530 cases in which he used hedonal as an anesthetic agent in a physiologic solution of sodium chloride.[111]

In 1909 Bier[45] used the regional intravenous method to obtain anesthesia of the limbs. He injected a solution of procaine hydrochloride into the veins near the site of the proposed operation. In the same year Ludwig Burkhardt of Germany reported on the use of chloroform and ether injected intravenously for general anesthesia.[45] The difficulties in administration were so great that the intravenous use of ether and chloroform was soon discarded. In 1912 J. Goyanes of Madrid reported on the intra-arterial use of procaine hydrochloride.[45]

Paraldehyde as an anesthetic agent for intravenous use was reported on in 1913 by H. Noel and H. S. Souttar.[128] In the years after the first World War the intravenous use of paraldehyde became marked, and, according to Greene,[127] this agent has retained a small but lasting position in the field of intravenous anesthesia. It is employed chiefly to produce basal anesthesia for some major operations and to produce complete anesthesia for some minor operations.

Elisabeth Bredenfeld[129] of Switzerland in 1916 reported on the intravenous use of morphine in combination with scopolamine. In the same year C. H. Peck and S. J. Meltzer[130] suggested the clinical use of magnesium sulfate as an intravenous anesthetic agent. Another anesthetic agent that was employed intra-

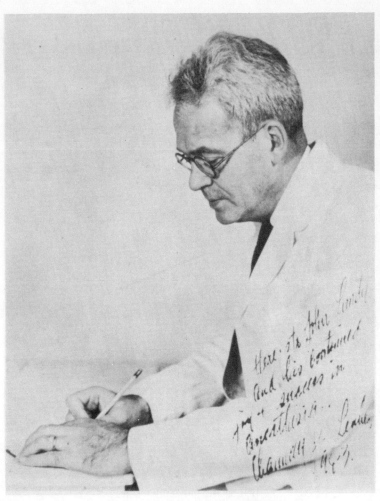

[FIG. 27] CHAUNCEY D. LEAKE.

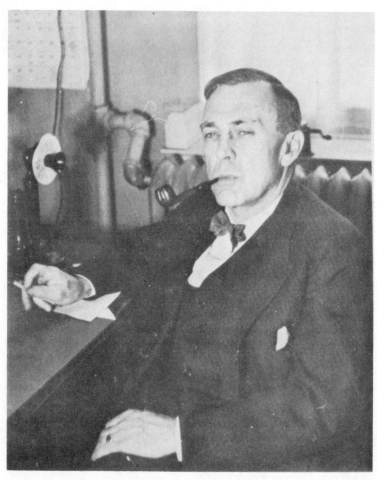

[Fig. 28] RALPH M. WATERS.

venously was ethyl alcohol. It was so used experimentally by Nakagawa[131] of Japan in 1921. M. G. Marin[47] of Mexico established the clinical use of this agent in 1929. In 1929, also, Martin Kirschner[132] reported on the intravenous use of tribromethyl alcohol in amylene hydrate (avertin).

According to Greene,[127] none of the aforementioned preparations, with the exception of paraldehyde, attained lasting favor. Anesthesia produced intravenously with these agents either could not be uniformly controlled or was not so reliable or safe as anesthesia obtained by inhalation. Furthermore, the introduction of endotracheal anesthesia in 1909 (which will be considered subsequently) made available a procedure that was safer than intravenous anesthesia,* in terms of the anesthetic agents then known.

Foundation for the relatively recent and continued success of intravenous anesthesia was the development of the barbiturates. Barbital (veronal), the first of these agents, was synthesized in 1902 by Emil Fischer[133] (fig. 32) of Berlin, one of the greatest physiologic chemists of all time. The first barbiturate was a long acting drug, very slow in producing anesthesia, and, consequently, it left patients in a deep sleep which disappeared only after twenty-four to forty-eight hours. Other long acting barbiturates included phenobarbital, soneryl, dial, and neonal. In 1920 Bardet[5] of France experimented with the anesthetic qualities of somnifene (a combination of veronal and alurate), and in 1924 Fredet[45] and Perlis introduced the intravenous technic of administration of this drug. In the same year dial (di-allyl-barbituric acid) was used as an anesthetic agent by Bogendörfer[134] of Würzburg.

The use of dial injected intraperitoneally has been recommended by John F. Fulton[135] and co-workers in their work in neurologic operations on animals. They used it first at Oxford on June 2, 1929, on the advice of John Beattie. Since coming to

---

* With the introduction of evipal sodium in 1933 and of pentothal sodium in 1934 as agents, intravenous anesthesia competed successfully with endotracheal anesthesia. For certain operations each of the above-mentioned types of anesthesia has advantages over other types in that for operations involving the face and neck, the surgeon has clear access to the operative field.

Yale in 1930, Fulton and his colleagues have used dial, sodium amytal, and pentobarbital sodium (nembutal) nearly 5,000 times as surgical anesthetics for animals with good results. Pernoston or pernocton was the first barbiturate widely used for general intravenous anesthesia. It was introduced by R. Bumm[45] of Germany in 1927. Its action was quicker and for that reason it was a more satisfactory anesthetic than the afore-mentioned barbiturates.

In 1929 somnifene, according to Geyer,[136] was injected intra-muscularly for the production of anesthesia. In the same year L. G. Zerfas, J. T. C. McCallum and their associates[137,138] reported on the intravenous use of sodium amytal for anesthesia. In 1929, also, John S. Lundy[140] (fig. 33) of the Mayo Clinic reported on the barbiturates as anesthetic, hypnotic, and anti-spasmodic agents, with special reference to sodium amytal. According to Adams,[45] this particular barbiturate was used more frequently in the United States from 1929 to 1933 than any other agent for the production of intravenous anesthesia. According to Greene, sodium amytal is still widely useful in the medical management of patients who have neurologic and psychiatric disturbances, but with the advent of even shorter acting barbiturates its use as an anesthetic agent has been displaced. Sodium amytal was used as an anesthetic agent for experimental surgery on animals, being made available in 1928. John F. Fulton[139] first used it this way on January 21, 1929. Many other laboratory workers used it about this time.

The intravenous use of pentobarbital sodium (nembutal) was reported on by R. H. Fitch, R. M. Waters, and A. J. Tatum[141] in 1930. Lundy,[142] in the same year, after an extensive study of sodium amytal and neonal, concluded that anesthesia produced intravenously with these barbiturates was not justified because of the untoward results incident to their use. In 1931,[143] however, he advocated the intravenous use of pentobarbital sodium as a hypnotic agent.

Advancement in the practical use of intravenous anesthesia was brought about by the discovery of evipan. It was first syn-

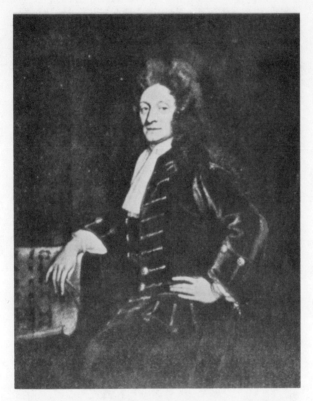

[FIG. 29] SIR CHRISTOPHER WREN, who discovered a method of administering medicine intravenously. Reproduced from the frontispiece to Ann. Med. Hist. for July, 1929. Courtesy of Paul B. Hoeber, Inc.

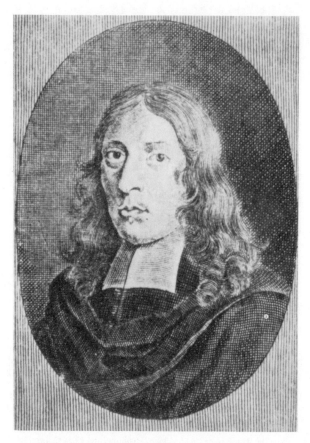

[FIG. 30] RICHARD LOWER, who was the first
man known to transfuse blood to animals. Reproduced
from Stirling, William: *Some apostles of physiology.*
London, Waterlow and Sons, 1902.

thesized by the chemists Kropp and Taub, according to Bogen-dörfer.[134] H. Weese and W. Scharpff[144] reported in 1932 on its pharmacologic and clinical effects. This new derivative of barbituric acid was very rapid in its hypnotic action. Likewise, the duration of its anesthetic effect was very short. Early in 1933 Weese[145] reported on an improved compound, evipan-natrium (evipal sodium or evipal soluble), as an anesthetic agent for intravenous use. Evipan (called evipal in the United States), because of its rapid destruction within the body, was found to produce very safe anesthesia for minor operations of short duration. According to Geyer,[136] more than 4,000,000 patients have been operated upon with the aid of this anesthetic agent, administered intravenously. One of the earliest papers on the clinical use of evipan was published by Jarman and Abel[146] in 1933.

In 1934 Lundy[147] introduced the technic of intermittent intravenous administration of pentothal sodium (sodium ethyl-methyl butyl thiobarbituric acid). He also experimented with a related barbiturate, sodium allyl secondary butyl thiobarbituric acid, but concluded that pentothal sodium was the better of these two for anesthetic purposes. Lundy also found pentothal sodium to be considerably more potent than evipal sodium. Moreover, pentothal sodium afforded better surgical relaxation than did the other barbiturates. Since its introduction in this country, pentothal sodium has been widely used. At the Mayo Clinic it had been used alone or in combination with other types of anesthetic agents in 31,931 operations[148] up to and including December 31, 1941. J. R. Fulton[149] recently recommended the intravenous use of pentothal sodium under skilled direction for wartime conditions. He also advocated the intravenous use of pentothal sodium as an anesthetic measure in the treatment of fresh burns. The Medical Research Council of Great Britain[150] has also recommended anesthesia with pentothal sodium as well as that produced with gas and oxygen, prior to the local treatment of severe burns.

Another short acting barbiturate, eunarcon, was introduced as an intravenous anesthetic agent by Otto Gandow in 1936.[151]

The use of still another barbiturate, sodium isoamyl-ethyl-thio-barbiturate, was reported in 1938 by S. C. Cullen and E. A. Rovenstine.[152] Recently new ultra-rapidly acting barbiturates are being used in England.*

Accoᵣding to Lundy and his associates,[153] the scope and safety of intravenous anesthesia have been increased by the simultane-

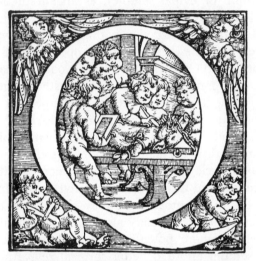

[FIG. 31] Initial Q from Vesalius's *Fabrica*, 1543, showing preliminary tracheotomy preparatory to inserting a reed tube.

ous use of oxygen or of a mixture composed of 50 per cent oxygen and 50 per cent nitrous oxide. Intravenous anesthesia also is of great value as a method of induction for other forms of general anesthesia and to supplement spinal, local, and regional anesthesia, when indicated. Recently, Mousel[154] has suggested that intravenous anesthesia be favored particularly in cases in which diathermy or cautery is to be used, for intravenous anesthesia eliminates the hazard of fire and explosion. For the same reason, intravenous anesthesia is of great value for the reduction of a

* Personal communication, Dr. Noel Gillespie, State of Wisconsin General Hospital, Madison 6, Wisconsin.

[62]

fracture under the roentgenoscope. Another advantage of intravenous anesthesia in operations on the head and neck, as suggested by Greene,[127] is elimination of anesthetic apparatus from the field of the operation. To patients undergoing short operations, the rapid and pleasant transition from consciousness to complete anesthesia constitutes the chief advantage of intravenous anesthesia.

A recent use of intravenous anesthesia is its employment in dental operations. Hubbell[155] reports 13,000 intravenous anesthesias in which a 2.5 per cent pentothal solution was the only anesthetic agent used. In 4 per cent of these cases oxygen was given during the operation. All operations were for extractions and oral surgery performed in the office. Earlier papers on this subject are those of Wycoff,[156] Bullard,[157] and Hubbell and Adams.[158]

J—ENDOTRACHEAL ANESTHESIA

It is well known that Vesalius prior to 1543 passed a tube into the trachea of an animal (fig. 31), the thorax open and the lungs exposed; by blowing air into the tube he was able to maintain artificial respiration. This important experiment appears, significantly, at the very end of the *Fabrica* as follows:

Next you will begin the section which I promised a little while ago I would describe, that on a pregnant bitch or sow, although from the point of view of the voice it is better to take a pig, since when a dog is bound for some time, no matter what you do, he neither barks nor howls after a while, and so you cannot judge the weakening or cessation of the voice . . . (Description of how to tie the animal down) . . . And then I make a long cutting in the throat with a rather sharp knife which can lay back the skin and the muscles beneath it right down to the trachea, taking care that the cutting does not slip off to the side and injure some important vein. Then with my hands I take the trachea and separating it from the superimposed muscles with my fingers only, I look for the carotid arteries on its sides and the nerves directed to it of the sixth pair of nerves of the brain, then I observe also the nerves returning on the sides of the trachea, which I sometimes intercept with a binding (ligate), sometimes cut, and this first on one side, with the result that when the nerve is tied or cut one can clearly observe how the voice perishes midway, and when both are cut, it ceases entirely, and if I release the bindings it returns again, quickly indeed . . . (Description of examination of abdomen and thorax) . . . But that life may in a manner of speaking be restored to the animal, an opening must be attempted in the trunk of the trachea, into which a tube of reed or cane should be put; you will then blow into this, so that the lung may rise again and the animal take in air. Indeed, with a slight breath in the case of this living animal the lung will swell to the full extent of the thoracic cavity, and the heart become strong and exhibit a wondrous variety of motions. So, with the lung inflated once and a second time, you examine the motion of the heart by sight and touch as much as you wish . . . (Further examination of the thoracic cavity) . . . With this observed, the lung should again be inflated, and with this device, than which I have learned nothing more pleasing to me in Anatomy, great knowledge of the differences in the beats should be acquired. For when the lung, long flaccid, has collapsed, the beat of heart and arteries appears wavy, creepy, twisting, but when the lung is inflated, it becomes strong again and swift and displays wondrous variations . . . (Description of examination of the fetus) . . . And as I do this, and take care that the lung is inflated at intervals, the motion of heart and arteries does not stop . . . (Description of examination of the auricles of the heart).*

Robert Hook[159] performed a similar experiment before the Royal Society in 1667. After these early experiments, intubation of the trachea was employed as a therapeutic procedure in asphyxia and drowning, often with dire results. John Snow,[34] whose contributions to anesthesia have been mentioned previously herein, apparently was the first to produce endotracheal anesthesia in an animal. He performed tracheotomy on a rabbit and into the resultant opening he inserted a wide-bore tube. The animal was made to breathe through this tube and into and out of a bag filled with the vapor of chloroform.

Apparently, Friedrich Trendelenburg[160] was the first to use this procedure on man. In 1869, to prevent aspiration of blood into the lungs during an operation on the upper air passages, Trendelenburg performed preliminary tracheotomy and passed a wide-bore tube into the trachea. Attached to the tube was an inflatable cuff. This provided watertight contact with the tracheal wall. The tube was connected by a length of rubber tubing to a gauze or flannel-covered funnel. Anesthesia was accomplished and continued by dropping of chloroform onto the gauze or flannel.

* This translation has been compared with that of Benjamin Farrington. (See Farrington, Benjamin: "The last chapter of the *De Fabrica* of Vesalius." Tr. Royal Society of South Africa, 20:1-14, 1932.) Farrington notes that this is the only experiment in this chapter which Vesalius claims to have originated.

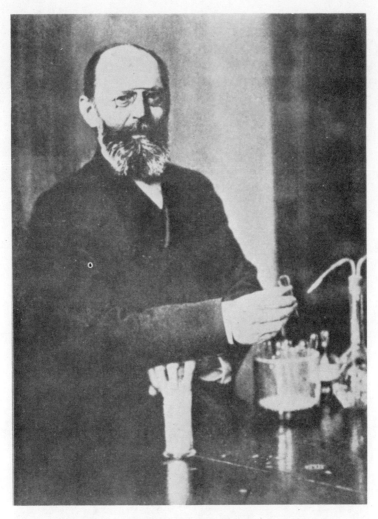

[FIG. 32] EMIL FISCHER, who synthesized the first barbiturates.
Reproduced from Moore, F. J.: *A history of chemistry*. New York,
McGraw-Hill Book Co., 1918.

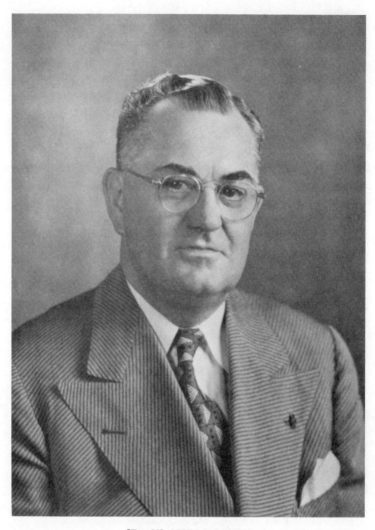

[FIG. 33] JOHN S. LUNDY.

Endotracheal Anesthesia

William Macewen[161] in 1880 found it possible to obtain endotracheal anesthesia without resorting to tracheotomy. He desired to maintain continuous anesthesia, and also to protect the respiratory tract from the possible aspiration of blood in the removal of a malignant lesion situated at the base of the tongue. To do this he inserted a metal tube into the trachea by way of the mouth. Chloroform was administered through the tube, the laryngeal opening was packed off and the operation was successfully performed.

To meet the needs of anesthesia in otorhinolaryngologic operations, Karel Maydl, professor of surgery at the University of Prague, in 1893 modified the apparatus O'Dwyer[162] had invented for intubation of the larynx for the relief of patients suffering from diphtheria. Maydl[163] connected a Trendelenburg funnel to an O'Dwyer tube, and the result apparently was satisfactory.

Using Maydl's technic, Victor Eisenmenger[164] constructed an apparatus which he described in the same year (1893) as that in which Maydl's work was done. This consisted of a wide-bore semirigid tracheal tube in which was carried an inflatable cuff modeled after that of Trendelenburg.

According to Matas,[165] Truehead of Galveston, Texas reported in 1869 on an apparatus of which the purpose was to insufflate air into the lungs by means of an intubating cannula. The mouthpiece of this apparatus was connected to a bellows which automatically injected and aspirated air in and out of the trachea. In this machine Truehead anticipated the Fell-O'Dwyer apparatus.

In 1880, O'Dwyer published his preliminary article on intubation of the larynx for the relief of asphyxia caused by acute or chronic laryngeal obstruction. Some time later, George H. Fell, of Buffalo, New York, invented an apparatus for artificial respiration. This he demonstrated at the International Medical Congress held in Washington on September 7, 1893. It consisted of a hand bellows connected to a tube which was inserted into the trachea. Fell modified his original apparatus by substituting a face mask for the tracheotomy tube. This mask fitted closely over the nose and mouth. Air was forced into the larynx through the natural passages, and expired air was allowed to escape by a side outlet in the injecting tube.

Because of the disadvantages of the oronasal apparatus of Fell, O'Dwyer made a much needed modification of it. O'Dwyer's improvement consisted of a long intubation cannula fitted with a conical tip graduated so that it would fit variations in the size of the larynx. The external end consisted of two branches; one branch received the ingoing air from the bellows; the other branch served as an exit for the air (fig. 34). Although O'Dwyer's apparatus had been anticipated by many experimenters, his machine was remarkable for its simplicity and efficiency.

Matas devoted much time and work to attempts to improve thoracic surgery. The chief difficulties encountered in surgery of the thorax previously had arisen from the making of large surgical openings in the thorax. These permitted the rapid and free entrance of air, followed by collapse of the lungs. This in turn led to cyanosis, defective oxygenation and arrested respiration. Older surgeons afforded some relief to their patients in cases of penetrating wounds of the thorax by sealing the opening. But when they were confronted by tumors of the thorax or mediastinum, most surgeons of the eighteenth and nineteenth centuries refused to operate because of the notoriously poor results of surgical intervention in such cases.

Matas, in 1897, read of the experiments of Tuffier and Hallion.[166] These investigators inserted a long copper tube attached to a bellows into the larynx of a dog. Artificial respiration being established by this means, the pleura was freely incised through an intercostal space. The edges of the wound were kept apart to allow free circulation of air. The pleural cavity was illuminated by a small incandescent lamp. It then became easy to operate on the esophagus and pneumogastric nerve without interfering with respiration.

At about this time Matas also read in the *Medical and Surgical Reports of the Presbyterian Hospital* of New York for 1896 an article

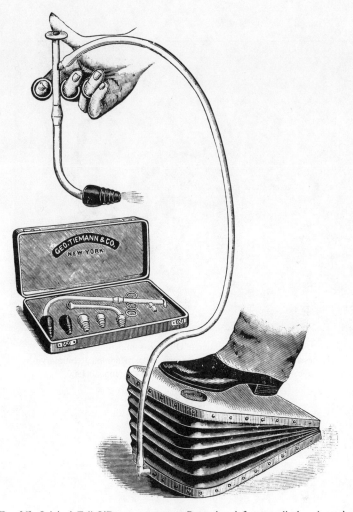

[FIG. 34] Original Fell-O'Dwyer apparatus. Reproduced from medical and surgical reports of the Presbyterian Hospital (N. Y.), 1896.

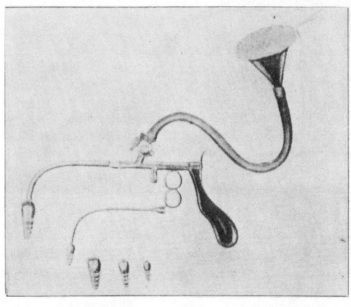

[Fig. 35] The Matas modification of O'Dwyer's intubating apparatus with anesthesia attachment. Reproduced from Matas, Rudolph: "Intralaryngeal Insufflation," J. A. M. A. 34:1468-1473 (June 9) 1900.

on the use of the Fell-O'Dwyer apparatus for the treatment of opium narcosis in nonsurgical conditions. In these cases, artificial respiration was prolonged by the use of the Fell-O'Dwyer apparatus and respiratory failure was overcome. His reading of the aforementioned two papers suggested to Matas a method for the solution of the problems of operations on the thorax. He elaborated his ideas before the Louisiana State Medical Society in 1898,[167] recommending use of the Fell-O'Dwyer apparatus to prevent the disastrous results of acute pneumothorax in thoracic operations. Dr. F. W. Parham,[168] a colleague, profited by these remarks; using the suggestions of Matas, he successfully resected the wall of the thorax for a sarcoma.

Matas not only was the first to advocate intralaryngeal insufflation for intrathoracic operations, but he also modified the Fell-O'Dwyer apparatus for the maintenance of anesthesia while artificial respiration was being applied (fig. 35). He altered the laryngeal cannula by furnishing a branch and stopcock to which a rubber tube and funnel were connected. The funnel was covered with flannel and was used as an inhaler.

Franz Kuhn of Kassel, Germany, published his first communication[169] of a series on endotracheal anesthesia in 1900, and in 1902 he published a paper on nasal intubation.[170] A few years earlier, in 1895, to abolish the idiosyncrasy of a patient to chloroform, Rosenberg[171] recommended the local application of cocaine to the nose. Kuhn also advocated the use of cocainization as a very helpful adjunct to intubation. Dr. Kuhn[172] published a book on intubation in 1911. He deserves a good deal of credit, for by 1912 his advances in endotracheal anesthesia anticipated the methods employed today.

In 1907, Barthélemy and Dufour[173] of Nancy advocated use of the insufflation principle of endotracheal anesthesia.* This study anticipated, to a large extent, the work of S. J. Meltzer and John Auer.[174] The last-mentioned investigators published the re-

* I am greatly indebted to Dr. Gillespie for many of the facts reported in this and in the two succeeding paragraphs. See: Gillespie, N. A.: *Endotracheal Anesthesia* (Madison, University of Wisconsin Press, 1941). Gillespie was the first to point out, as far as I am aware, that Barthélemy and Dufour, two years previous to Meltzer and Auer, had discovered the use of the insufflation principle of endotracheal anesthesia.—T.E.K.

sults of their researches in 1909: they demonstrated that if air were blown into the trachea of an animal whose respiratory mechanisms had been paralyzed, full oxygenation of the blood could be maintained. Not long afterward (1910) Charles A. Elsberg[175] succeeded in clinical application of the work of Meltzer and Auer. In 1912 Charles H. Peck[176] and later many others also demonstrated the application of this principle to clinical anesthesia. Meanwhile, in 1911, F. J. Cotton and Walter Boothby[177] had advocated the endotracheal insufflation of mixtures of oxygen and nitrous oxide. Chevalier Jackson's perfection of the direct-vision laryngoscope introduced by Alfred Kirstein[176A] in 1895 also contributed to the success of endotracheal anesthesia. By its use intubation was made more nearly certain and more nearly accurate.

Further improvement in insufflation endotracheal anesthesia was achieved during the first World War. At this time, I. W. Magill and E. S. Rowbotham were serving with the British Army Plastic Unit as anesthetists. For their type of patient, insufflation endotracheal anesthesia was well-suited. They also found it possible to improve upon the technic. It was found desirable to pass a second tube into the trachea to act as a return airway for the escaping vapor. For operations involving the mouth, they learned to pass the tube through the nose into the pharynx and thence, by the help of a guiding rod or forceps, into the trachea. After more experience, Magill and Rowbotham found it possible to intubate the trachea "blindly" without the use of other instruments.

It then occurred to these anesthetists that anesthesia could be more economically produced if only one wide-bore tube were inserted into the trachea and the patient were allowed to breathe in both directions through it. The early machines of Gwathmey and McKesson in the United States and that of Boyle in England, which worked on the "semi-closed" principle, were admirably suited to this form of inhalation endotracheal anesthesia. A further development in technic was that instituted by Joseph W. Gale and Ralph M. Waters.[179A] These innovators reported a method for intubating one bronchus with a tube fitted with an inflatable cuff, so that one lung could be isolated for operations such as lobectomy and pneumonectomy. The advantages of endotracheal anesthesia and the fact that this method so closely approximates physiological respiration won for it a favor which endures to the present day.

K—CARBON DIOXIDE ABSORPTION

In 1915, Dennis E. Jackson[180] (fig. 36) published an article in which he described a method for the production and maintenance of prolonged anesthesia or analgesia by means of nitrous oxide, ethyl chloride, ether, chloroform, ethyl bromide, somnoform, and others, with oxygen. Jackson's method involved the continuous process of rebreathing by the experimental animal of gaseous or volatilized anesthetic agents from which the exhaled carbon dioxide had been removed. Sodium hydrate and calcium hydrate were used to absorb the exhaled carbon dioxide. Oxygen was constantly added in proportions suitable to maintain the animal in good physical condition. Jackson did not have an opportunity to try his experiments on human beings, but suggested that human patients could be anesthetized by his method. He demonstrated his equipment at the sixty-seventh annual meeting of the American Medical Association in Detroit in 1916. There Jackson stated that the cost of this nitrous oxide-oxygen anesthesia should be approximately thirty-two cents per hour. This was considerably less expensive for patients than other technics had been, since at that time the usual cost of nitrous oxide-oxygen anesthesia was about $2.50 per hour. Very few members of his audience thought his method was practicable. At the Washington University School of Medicine in St. Louis, however, Dr. Otto Henry Schwarz and his son Dr. Otto Henry Schwarz, Junior, and Dr. Willard Bartlett gave Jackson some encouragement. The Drs. Schwarz performed a number of examinations in the obstetrics department of that university, using nitrous oxide-oxygen anesthesia produced with Jackson's machine (fig. 37). Dr. Pessel successfully produced anesthesia a number of times by the employment of Jackson's machine. Once he anesthetized a patient for Dr. Bartlett, who removed a thyroid gland. In the summer of 1918, Dr. Jackson offered his machine to the Medical Corps of the United States Army, but nothing came of this. Dr. Ralph M. Waters, then of Sioux City, Iowa, became very much interested, however. In 1920, he wrote to Jackson, asking for reprints and suggestions. Jackson coöperated and Dr. Waters[181] demonstrated clinically the work Jackson had done so well experimentally. Waters' apparatus was somewhat simpler than Jackson's. It consisted of a face mask, a container for granulated soda lime which opened into a large rubber bag, and a rubber tube leading from the bag to the nitrous oxide and oxygen tanks. The great advantage of this type of anesthesia was of course the remarked reduction in expense to the patient, as had been predicted by Jackson.

In 1924, as has been mentioned, Waters perfected Jackson's carbon dioxide absorption technic. Guedel[182] and Waters wrote concerning the importance of the inflatable cuff in 1928. The absorption technic, with the use of the inflatable cuff, made possible the development of true inhalation endotracheal anesthesia.

Brian C. Sword started to investigate the possibilities of a circle filter about 1926. According to Sword,[183] the apparatus generally employed for the carbon dioxide absorption method of anesthesia, consisting of a canister and bag at the face, was awkward in that it was too close to the field of operation. In an effort to surmount this difficulty, Sword consulted Professor Yandell Henderson, of the Yale University School of Medicine. Richard v. Foregger aided in the construction and, in 1928, the first apparatus was built. The apparatus was so made that the inspiratory and expiratory phase ran in the same direction. This required a separation by means of valves and two tubes: one for inspiration and one for expiration. The two tubes were connected by a "Y" so that they could be applied to a mask. The canister and rebreathing bag were attached 2 feet (61 cm.) away and, when this "circle" type of respiration was used, it made

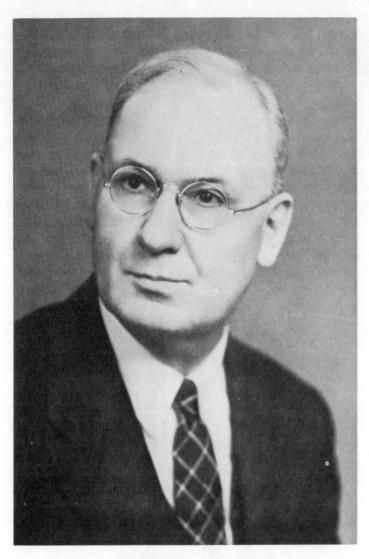

[FIG. 36] DENNIS E. JACKSON.

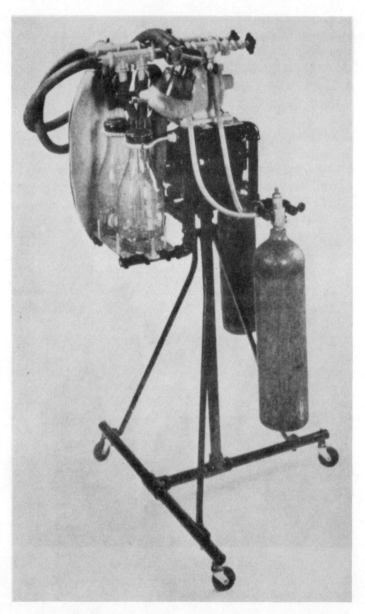

[FIG. 37] Model of Dennis Jackson's first anesthetic apparatus.

little difference where the bag was placed. It was thus removed from the field of operation.

In this connection it is interesting to note that J. A. Heidbrink's first machine, an improvement of the original Teter gas machine, provided for rebreathing. Dr. Heidbrink[184] improved on the Teter machine in 1906. The Teter machine had two bags, one for nitrous oxide and one for oxygen. Dr. Heidbrink added a third bag for rebreathing.

In 1927, Dr. Heidbrink developed a "round trip" absorber. This he displayed that year at a medical meeting in Minneapolis. He withheld it from the market for some time, believing that the absorber principle would complicate anesthetic technic. In the meantime, "round trip" absorbers were brought out by Dr. Richard v. Foregger and Dr. Ben Morgan. This required that the Heidbrink machine be supplied with an absorber; hence, their two-chamber absorber was designed and built.

L—PHYSIOLOGIC FACTORS

In 1847 Alfred-Armand-Louis-Marie Velpeau[185] and François Magendie[186] reported their general observations on the physiologic effects of ether. Ducros, according to Hahn,[186A] early in the year claimed priority in the discovery of these physiologic effects based on his work done in 1842 and in March, 1846. And Morton[186B] in 1850 published his short study. It was Magendie's illustrious pupil, Claude Bernard, however, to whom we are indebted for basic work in this field. Bernard, realizing that the successful practice of medicine must be based on sound physiological principles, carried his research into all possible lines. It was his good fortune to be working at the time that anesthesia had become accepted as a necessary and a desirable part of the practice of surgery. To be sure, the practice of anesthesia on the Continent was for the most part entrusted to mediocre assistants, a condition that is still said to exist.[187] Bernard tried hard to place anesthesiology on a scientific basis and his monograph[188] can be considered a landmark.* Bernard clear-

* Bernard in this important work which includes an excellent survey of the history of anesthesia may have been the first to suggest pre-anesthetic medication with morphine and other central depressants. Bernard also was one of the early advocates of the need for adequate oxygen supply during anesthesia.

ly recognized the dangers of anesthesia and made a careful study from the theoretical viewpoint.

As pointed out so well by Olmsted,[189] the theory of the action of anesthetic agents prevalent about 1870 was that anesthesia was merely asphyxia. Bernard did not believe this to be true and proposed a different one based on his observations of the action of chloroform on muscle and nerve tissues.[190] (He found that under chloroform anesthesia muscle first loses its excitability and then becomes rigid and opaque.) He found that nerves also became opaque under chloroform and if the action had not been pushed too far, the nerve would return to its original state when the anesthetic agent was eliminated and would again be able to conduct nerve impulses. Accordingly, Bernard[191] developed the theory that anesthesia is caused by a reversible coagulation of the constituents of the nerve cell. Interestingly enough, Bernard's theory was supported by a study published in 1930 by Bancroft[192] and Richter of Cornell University. It was severely attacked, however, two years later by Henderson and Lucas[193] of Toronto.

Edmund W. Andrews,[194] a Chicago surgeon, found some difficulty in using pure nitrous oxide as an anesthetic agent. He reasoned that the oxygen contained in nitrous oxide was not available for the proper oxidation of the blood. If any attempt was made to continue its anesthetic action, the patient began to show the signs of asphyxia. Nitrous oxide, alone, therefore, was not a satisfactory anesthetic for operations of long duration. To overcome this difficulty, Andrews experimented to see if the addition of oxygen to nitrous oxide would make for a safe anesthetic. He found that in rats a mixture of one-fourth oxygen and three-fourths nitrous oxide was satisfactory. Andrews used a mixture of one-third oxygen and two-thirds nitrous oxide (the mixture having been already compressed into cylinders) successfully for operations of short duration upon a few of his own patients. He felt, however, that the best proportion of oxygen would be one-fifth by volume, which he had computed would equal the proportion in atmospheric air.

Paul Bert (fig. 38) was one of the outstanding pupils of

Claude Bernard. Like his teacher he was keenly aware of the shortcomings of anesthesia, and searched for an anesthetic agent that would be without any danger to the patient and still have the desirable qualities. The use of nitrous oxide for operations of short duration had by his time become popular, especially for the extraction of teeth. Bert without previous knowledge of the work of Andrews found that the administration of pure nitrous oxide could not be prolonged for more than two minutes without bringing on symptoms of asphyxia of dangerous appearance.[195]

Bert, profiting by his profound knowledge of the pressures of gases, was able to remove this difficulty. He used a mixture of three-quarters nitrous oxide* and one-quarter of oxygen, having this mixture breathed under a slightly increased barometric pressure. He thus introduced into the blood of the experimental animal the quantity of oxygen necessary to maintain respiration and the quantity of nitrous oxide sufficient to maintain anesthesia. He was able, in this manner, to overcome the dangers of asphyxia.

Because of his success with animals, Bert recommended the use of nitrous oxide-oxygen anesthesia under increased atmospheric pressure for operations upon human beings. Its use proved successful, but unfortunately Bert's method while brilliantly conceived lacked practicability necessitating as it did cumbersome and expensive apparatus (fig.39).

Bert carried out his researches on other anesthetic agents, especially chloroform, but felt that nitrous oxide was the superior agent for the following reasons: (1) The absence in the use of nitrous oxide of the usual period of excitation. (2) The tranquillity it gives to the surgeon who has the assurance that the dosage of the anesthetic agent cannot change during the operation and that consequently the patient has nothing to fear. (3) The almost instantaneous return to complete sensibility even after 25 minutes of anesthesia. (4) The almost general absence of discomfort, nausea, and vomiting. (5) Its remarkable harmlessness.

* Bert later changed these proportions using a mixture of one-sixth oxygen and five-sixths nitrous oxide under an increased pressure of a fifth of an atmosphere. See Bert, Paul: Sur la possibilité d'obtenir, à l'aide du protoxyde d'azote, une insensibilité de long durée, et sur l'innocuité de cet anesthésique. Compt. rend. Acad. d. Sc. 87:728-730, 1878.

As has been suggested earlier herein, while sulfuric ether was the first agent of choice in the United States and was regarded by many surgeons as a safer anesthetic than chloroform, in England chloroform was thought to be the safer and more reliable agent. In France, Marie-Jean-Pierre Flourens[196] early called attention to the toxicity of chloroform. The use of chloroform led to many deaths and its greatest advocate, Simpson, had his share. Simpson reasoned that fatalities were due to syncope brought about by sudden failure of the circulation and asphyxia caused by the failure of respiration.

James Syme of Edinburgh, who was one of the first surgeons in Great Britain to use ether anesthesia, attributed chloroform deaths to failure of respiration alone. His view is well defined in his aphorism: "attend to the respiration, never mind the pulse." Because of Syme's influential position (his son-in-law was Lord Lister), this view dominated the administration of chloroform throughout Scotland and part of England. In London, the watchword was "watch the pulse." But even here many physicians believed in Syme's ideas. John Snow working with very limited equipment and resources reached the correct conclusion that though respiration usually ceases before the heart, sometimes the heart is the first to stop.

In 1855, however, a chloroform commission in Paris presented a report supporting Syme's idea that respiration failed before the heart. The British were not satisfied, and in 1879 a committee on anesthetics was appointed by the British Medical Association to investigate the problem further; it reached the following conclusions in regard to chloroform: (1) that lowering of the blood pressure is due to the weakening of the heart's action, (2) that this effect is given by chloroform and not by ether, (3) and that death may occur any time during chloroform inhalation by sudden stoppage of the heart. This report had wide acceptance and threw Syme's ideas into the background.

Interest in the Syme theory was revived, however, by one of his favorite students, Lt. Col. Edward Lawrie. It was Lawrie, according to Osborne,[201] who organized the first Hyderabad[197]

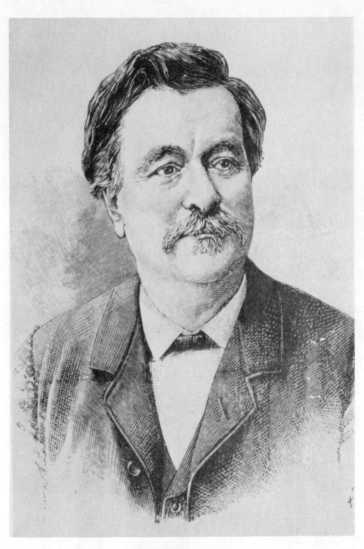

[Fig. 38] PAUL BERT.

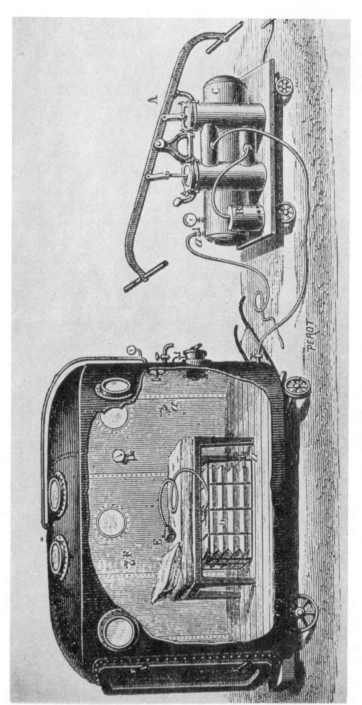

[FIG. 39] Paul Bert's anesthetic apparatus.

commission with himself as director. Lawrie did not possess the proper qualifications for research other than an unbounded enthusiasm for the project and for his preconceived idea that Syme was right. Needless to say, Lawrie's report supported Syme's contentions. The medical world did not support the findings of the first Hyderabad commission, whereupon in 1889 the second Hyderabad commission was organized.

Because of his brilliant success in other fields of investigation, Lauder Brunton was chosen to direct the second commission's research. A glance at the conclusions of this report[198] suggests that it would have been better to have had a director with more scientific training. Brunton concluded (1) Failure of respiration is the only means by which the heart's safety is jeopardized, (2) The heart never stops before respiration, (3) The vagus action of the heart is beneficial, preventing a too great distribution of the chloroform, (4) Chloroform does not directly injure the heart substance, (5) The fall of blood pressure during anesthesia is beneficial to the heart, (6) The Glasgow committee used faulty methods and ascribed to chloroform what was really due to asphyxia.

It was in the midst of this state of confusion that Edward Henry Embley of Melbourne, Australia, carried out his important experimental work. His first paper on the subject was entitled: "The question of safety in Syme's teaching in chloroform anæsthesia."[199] Here Embley announced that not only Syme but also the renowned Hyderabad commission were wrong in their conclusions. Embley continued his studies and his great contribution was published in the British Medical Journal in 1902.[200] It meant the final defeat of the work of the Hyderabad commission and consequently the renouncement of the Syme doctrine and experimental proof of Simpson's conjectures. Embley stated that (1) Heart muscle is very sensitive to chloroform poisoning, (2) The drug raises the excitability of the vagus, (3) Deaths in the induction stage of anesthesia are syncopal and unconcerned with respiration, (4) Failure of respiration is mainly due to fall of blood pressure, (5) In the post induction stages of anesthesia there is a general depression of all activities and no longer syncope through excited vagus action. According to Osborne,[201] the only important point that Embley missed was the fibrillation of the heart caused by deep chloroform poisoning. Later on, after further experimentation, he was able to prove that under chloroform anesthesia there was not only an arrest of the muscular activity of the heart, but also an arrest of the muscular activity of the arterioles.

As pointed out so well by Hoff[202] of New Haven, the final solution of the chloroform problem was brought about by A. G. Levy. In his preliminary report, Levy[203] outlined the solution as follows: (1) In properly organized laboratory experiments, syncope and sudden death were produced during light chloroform anesthesia. (2) The cause of syncope was the sudden onset of ventricular fibrillation. (3) Intravenous injection of adrenalin was almost always fatal in light chloroform anesthesia, and that such sudden death was produced by ventricular fibrillation. Later, Levy[204] elaborated on these points and demonstrated their relation to the clinical problem.

Arthur E. Guedel (fig. 40) in the fall of 1941 was the recipient of the third award of the Henry Hill Hickman Medal. So that the reader may gain some idea of the importance of this award, it can be said that on November 17, 1931, the Royal Society of Medicine accepted from the Henry Hill Hickman Memorial Committee the sum of 200 pounds for the creation of a bronze medal in commemoration of Hickman. The medal was and is awarded by the Council of the Royal Society of Medicine on the recommendation of the Council of the Section of Anæsthetics. It is granted not oftener than triennially for original work of outstanding merit in anesthesia or in subjects relating thereto. This medal was first awarded in 1935 to Wesley Bourne of Montreal (figs. 41 and 42a and 42b). The second award was made in 1938, to Ivan Whiteside Magill, of London, whose contributions already have been discussed. The fourth award was made in 1944 to Ralph M. Waters, Professor of Anesthesia in the University of Wisconsin.

Physiologic Factors

The interest of Guedel in anesthesia can be traced back for many years. In 1909 he devised the technic of the self-administration of nitrous oxide and air for obstetrics and for minor surgical operations that could be performed in the physician's office. His first report[205] on this subject appeared in 1911. This type of anesthesia was especially valuable in obstetric cases. As the patient received warning of an approaching pain, she placed the inhaler to her nose and breathed deeply a few times; then began to breathe normally. Intermittent anesthesia was thereby induced with each pain. In his pamphlet,[206] "The Self-Administration of Nitrous Oxide," Guedel said that about 75 per cent of the mixture is rebreathed. His apparatus contained a respiratory valve which regulated the percentage of air to be mixed with the gas and the amount of the gas mixture to be rebreathed.

Although Dr. Guedel has made important contributions in the development of new anesthetic agents, such as in demonstrating the anesthetic action of divinyl oxide, earlier referred to herein, and his work on cyclopropane, as well as his work on carbon dioxide absorption, his outstanding contribution has been his emphasis on the importance of the physiologic factors in inhalation anesthesia. In May, 1920, his first paper on this subject appeared in print.[207] This paper was a reflection of his experiences with the American Expeditionary Forces during World War I. In France he found it convenient to teach his colleagues the significance of certain reflexes under various stages of anesthesia. Guedel's conceptions of the "signs of anesthesia"* have been brought up to date in his recent monograph.[208] Dr. Guedel also has classified the various physical

---

* Dr. Noel Gillespie has suggested in his article, "The Signs of Anæsthesia" (Anes. & Analg. 22:275-282 [Sept.-Oct.] 1943), that the reflex signs of anesthesia are as important as the respiratory.

In the above-mentioned article, Gillespie points out that Plomley in the *Lancet* for January 30, 1847, first attempted to define the "stages" of anesthesia. A few months later, John Snow defined the "five degrees of narcotism." (See Snow, John: *On the Inhalation of the Vapour of Ether in Surgical Operations*. London, Churchill, 1847, pp. 1-4.) From the time of Snow to that of Hewitt (and continuing in England until 1928) anesthesia was divided into four stages as follows: I. *Induction;* II. *The stage of struggling, or breath-holding, or delirium, or dreams;* III. *Surgical anæsthesia;* IV. *Overdose, or stage of bulbar paralysis.*

[77]

reactions which occur at various stages of anesthesia. These include respiration, activity of the eyeballs and the pupils, the eyelid reflex, the "area of swallowing" and the "area of vomiting." Guedel's contribution was his excellent description of the planes into which the third stage is subdivided.

Albert H. Miller,[209] of Providence, Rhode Island, in 1925 published the results of his study of ascending respiratory paralysis as it occurs when the patient is under the influence of general anesthesia.* Dr. Miller was able to demonstrate that at the commencement of anesthesia, respiration is of the usual or mixed type. As anesthesia deepens, after a period of delayed thoracic respiration, the abdominal type of respiration appears. After a few inspirations, thoracic inspiration begins; it commences midway in the period of abdominal inspiration. A little later, thoracic inspiration occurs, but still is further delayed. Finally, abdominal inspiration begins. If the anesthetic dosage is further increased, paralysis of the costal muscles becomes more complete, and the condition of exaggerated abdominal respiration occurs. This is an indication of the presence of profound anesthesia.

There. are other terms familiar to many anesthetists that deserve an emphasis in this historical study. Such a term is "balanced anesthesia." This was suggested by Lundy[210] in 1926 to indicate the use of a combination of anesthetic agents and methods so balanced that part of the burden of relief of pain is borne by preliminary medication, part by local anesthesia and part by one or more general anesthetic agents. Lundy[211] recently has suggested that as more anesthetic agents become available, the tendency may be to use several agents and methods during a single operation. The advantage of this newer development is that it leads to greater flexibility and more (relative) safety.

"Ether percentages" and "anesthetic tension" are subjects

---

* The phenomenon of intercostal paralysis was first described by John Snow in 1858. (See Snow, John: *On Chloroform and Other Anæsthetics.* London, Churchill, 1858, p. 42.)

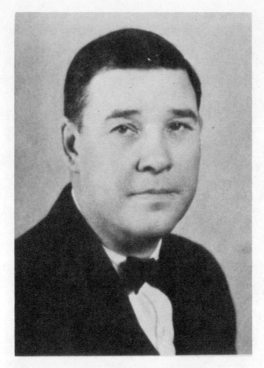

[Fig. 40] ARTHUR E. GUEDEL.

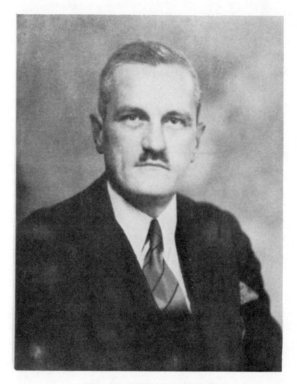

[Fig. 41] WESLEY BOURNE.

that need some clarification. Dr. Walter Boothby, who was in charge of the metabolism laboratory at the Peter Bent Brigham Hospital for several years and who served as lecturer on anesthesia in the Harvard Medical School from 1914 to 1916, did much work in and developed the aforementioned subjects. He has made important contributions to the physiology of anesthesia, in addition to his assistance of a technical nature. Boothby's interest in anesthesia machines dates back to about 1910. He was stimulated by the enthusiasm of Dr. F. J. Cotton on the basis of Cotton's observations made at the Cleveland Clinic. Accordingly, with the help of Cotton and that of Albert Ehrenfried, Boothby[212] designed the Cotton-Boothby nitrous oxideoxygen ether apparatus. As has been mentioned earlier, Cotton and Boothby[177] also developed the use of nitrous oxide-oxygen anesthesia produced by endotracheal insufflation. Karl Connell, with the use of the anesthetometer, which he devised in 1913, showed that anesthetic tension, that is, the tension of ether vapor necessary to produce narcosis in man, is about 50 mm. of mercury. Boothby[213] confirmed Connell's work and found that the optimal dosage of ether vapor for man is between 47 and 53 mm. of mercury. He further demonstrated that patients vary but slightly in their susceptibility to ether.

The anesthetometer of Connell was also found to be useful in the determination of ether percentages. Boothby[214] suggested that surgical anesthesia depends on the establishment in the blood and tissues of a definite ether tension corresponding to about 15 per cent of ether vapor in the alveolar air. He further demonstrated that in order to induce anesthesia quickly, air containing approximately 30 per cent of ether vapor should be administered for a period of from two to twelve minutes.

Frank Mann,[215,216] using the Connell apparatus, tested the vascular reflexes of dogs with various tensions of ether vapor. He found that the physiologic reactions which occur during anesthesia with ether vary with remarkable constancy. The lowest ether tension that will allow operative work on dogs is about 36 mm. of mercury. Any tension between 36 and 45 mm. of mercury is safe so far as the life of the animal is concerned, but tensions between 48 and 50 mm. are likely to prove fatal.

M—PHARMACOLOGIC FACTORS

The honor of being the recipient of the first award of the Hickman Medal belongs, as has been mentioned, to Wesley Bourne, anesthetist to the Royal Victoria Hospital, Montreal, and lecturer on pharmacology at McGill University. Bourne also has the distinction of being the first to receive the degree of Master of Science in Pharmacology, for work on Anesthetics. This was conferred upon him by McGill University. His thesis was entitled, "Heat Regulation and Water Exchange: the Influence of Ether on Dogs."[217] The first degree of Master of Science in Anesthesia to be awarded, and the first to be granted in the United States, so far as the author is aware, was conferred on Dr. Edward B. Tuohy[218] in 1936 by the University of Minnesota. Several of these degrees have been awarded since. It is of interest to note here than in 1935 the Royal College of Physicians and Surgeons (England) instituted a diploma in anesthetics.

Dr. Bourne has made many contributions of a physiologic and pharmacologic nature to the development of anesthesia. A few of his outstanding observations will be reviewed briefly. Early in his career Bourne,[219] working with Stehle, proved that pure ether possessed to the highest degree the anesthetic qualities usually attributed to it. There had been those who believed that impurities sometimes found in ether were the important factors. Bourne next studied the impurities[220] when added to ether used in anesthesia. He found that small concentrations of impurities were not harmful in ether anesthesia. Some of the commercial houses had claimed these impurities to be harmful. Later Storm Van Loewen and his co-workers and Sir Henry Dale, working separately, confirmed Bourne's findings. Bourne concluded, on the basis of work carried out in the preparation of his thesis, that dogs, under the influence of ether anesthesia, lose the factor which regulates bodily temperature. In considering the

THE ROYAL SOCIETY OF MEDICINE
(Patron: HIS MAJESTY THE KING).
1. WIMPOLE STREET,
LONDON, W.1

24th May 1935.

Dear Sir,

It is my pleasant duty to inform you that
the Council of the Royal Society of Medicine has
unanimously decided to make the first award of the
Hickman Medal to you upon the recommendation of the
Council of the Section of Anaesthetics of this Society.

The Hickman Medal was founded in 1931 and
its award is made for original work of outstanding
merit in anaesthesia or in subjects directly connected
therewith. The Deed of foundation lays down that the
first award should be made in 1935 and subsequent
awards at intervals of not less than three years.
The award is open to any person of any nationality.
I enclose a reproduction of both sides of the medal
which is struck in bronze.

I am having the Medal prepared and despatched
to you as soon as possible.

May I ask you to accept my personal
congratulations on this first Award.

Believe me,

Yours faithfully,

P. R. Edwards.

Secretary,
Royal Society of Medicine.

Wesley Bourne Esq., M.D.,
Royal Victoria Hospital,
Manchester.

enclo.

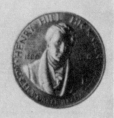

[FIG. 42a] Letter from the Royal Society of Medicine to Dr. Bourne,
announcing the first award of the Hickman Medal.

THE ROYAL SOCIETY OF MEDICINE
(Patron HIS MAJESTY THE KING)
1. WIMPOLE STREET,
LONDON W 1

24th June 1935.

Dear Sir,

Thank you for your kind letter which I will lay before my Council at its next meeting.

(herewith) I am to-day sending you under separate cover, the Hickman Medal.

This Medal is carried out in bronze, is designed by H. Paget and is struck for us at the Royal Mint.   On the one side is a portrait of Henry Hill Hickman and on the other side is an allegorical representation of Pain being banished by Anaesthesia. For this purpose we have personified Anaesthesia as a beautiful women, Pain as a kind of devil who has held the patient by his chain.   Anaesthesia has, as you will see, broken the chain binding the patient to Pain and is banishing him with an imperious gesture.   He scowls at her holding his broken chain and his now useless scourge.

Yours faithfully,

Geoffry R. Edwards

Secretary.

Wesley Bourne Esq., M.Sc.,M.D.,
      32, Holton Avenue,
         Westmount,
            Montreal, Canada.

[FIG. 42b] Letter from the Royal Society of Medicine to Dr. Bourne, explaining the Hickman Medal.

problem of the acidosis which occurs during anesthesia, Bourne,[221] working with Stehle, established on the basis of data concerning human beings the fact that phosphoric acid is the responsible factor. Bourne[222] also was able to show that the acidosis of anesthesia could be reduced by the rectal administration of copious quantities of a specially balanced solution of alkaline sodium and potassium phosphate, immediately after operation. About this time, too, Chauncey Leake[223-225] was working on the problem of acidosis, especially the blood reaction in ethylene-oxygen anesthesia and nitrous oxide-oxygen anesthesia.

Bourne[226-229] and his associates also studied the effects of anesthetic agents upon the liver. They concluded that ethylene was the anesthetic agent of choice for operations carried out in the presence of severe hepatic disease. Neither sodium amytal nor tribromethyl alcohol in amylene hydrate (avertin) influenced hepatic function, according to them. Stehle and Bourne[230] also made a study of the changes in the activity and appearance of the kidney as brought about by anesthesia.

Although they did not believe that restorative agents should be used routinely in anesthesia, Raginsky and Bourne[231] nevertheless found ephedrine to be of value clinically in overcoming profound anesthesia produced with tribromethyl alcohol in amylene hydrate (avertin). In a recent communication, Bourne[232] and his associates, in discussing the use of spinal anesthesia for thoracic surgical operations, found the use of analeptic measures justified in instances of anesthesia in which there is a marked decrease in blood pressure, accompanied by an increase in pulse rate.

Another study originating from the Department of Pharmacology at McGill University is that of Bourne[233] and his colleagues on the action of anesthetic and sedative agents upon the inhibited nervous system. These investigators concluded that amytal, pentobarbital sodium, alcohol, and tribromethyl alcohol in amylene hydrate (avertin) quickly abolish most of the signs of inhibitory neurosis in dogs. They[234] also studied the changes in conditioned reflexes in dogs brought about by anesthetic and sedative agents.

Because of its great importance, the subject of pre-anesthetic medication and post-anesthetic care must be mentioned. As pointed out earlier herein, Claude Bernard (p. 39) was one of the pioneers in this field. Other early contributors included von Steinbüchel (p. 48), Crile (p. 44), Elizabeth Bredenfeld (p. 58), Lundy (p. 60), and Bourne (p. 43).

In 1930 Chauncey Leake[234A] read a paper entitled "Chemical Adjuncts to General Anesthesia." Here Leake pointed out that chemical agents were indicated not only for pre-anesthetic hypnosis but also for the regulation of pre-operative metabolism, for aid in the induction of, maintenance of and rapid recovery from direct anesthesia, for the relief of post-anesthetic nausea, and for post-operative analgesia. Leake indicated the need for an extended critical pharmacological and clinical evaluation of the various agents proposed. Leake[234B] carried out such a study on depressant drugs used for pre-anesthetic medications and strongly condemned routine pre-anesthetic medication.

P. K. Knoefel[234C] in 1933 called attention to the fact that delayed shock produced by prolonged anesthesia with ether and chloroform is due to a concentration and reduction in the volume of the circulating blood resulting from the general stimulation of the sympathetic nervous system including the outpouring of adrenin. Knoefel suggested that possibly amytal with related substances might as pre-medication agents counteract the tendency to produce shock.

A. L. Tatum, A. S. Atkinson, and K. H. Collins[234D] of the University of Chicago studied acute cocaine poisoning which frequently follows the clinical use of cocaine as a local anesthetic. They were able to reduce greatly the risk of anesthetic toxicity by the prophylactic administration of a mixture of barbital sodium and paraldehyde in laboratory animals. P. K. Knoefel, R. P. Herwick and A. S. Loevenhart[234E] of the University of Wisconsin also worked on the problem of the prevention of local anesthetic poisoning. Working with animals they found sodium amytal of the greatest prophylactic value. They also demonstrated the effectiveness of hypnotic drugs in preventing the convulsant type of intoxication as well as the ineffectiveness of these and other drugs in preventing the paralytic type of intoxication.

N—ANESTHETIC APPARATUS*

Perhaps the first modern gas inhaler was the one that James Watts, an engineer, constructed for Thomas Beddoes.[235] Humphry Davy's "gas" machine is illustrated on page 17 (fig. 6). According to Miller,[236] this, too, was constructed for Davy by Watts.

The ether inhalers in the United States, such as the one perfected by Morton, were soon discarded and replaced by the ether sponge. The sea sponge, probably similar to the sponge of Theodoric of the thirteenth century, was hollowed to fit the face, as mentioned by Miller. It was then saturated with ether. It provided by its extensive surface sufficient ether vapor for the purpose of anesthesia.

In England, closed inhalers were the favored apparatus. The achievement of John Snow and his inhaler has been mentioned. His successor, Joseph T. Clover, published in 1862 an account of his chloroform inhaler by means of which the percentages of chloroform and air could be more accurately regulated than heretofore. Clover, according to Barbara Duncum,[236A] following the death of Snow was the acknowledged leader of the anesthetic profession in England.

Mixtures of ether and chloroform were used for anesthesia in the late 1860's. As has been mentioned earlier herein, Colton reintroduced the use of nitrous oxide for anesthetic purposes, during the extraction of teeth. In 1867 D. H. Goodwille's patented inhaler for nitrous oxide gas, ether and chloroform was advertised. This inhaler was similar to that of John Snow and covered the nose as well as the mouth. It was important in that it permitted the mixture of air with the gas.

In the S. S. White Dental Manufacturing Company's catalogue for 1867, according to Miller,[236] is pictured a complete nitrous oxide gas machine. In the same catalogue there is also a picture of an inhaler designed to cover both the mouth and nostrils.

---

* For an excellent series of illustrations showing the development of anesthetic apparatus see King, A. Charles: "The evolution of anaesthetic apparatus. A brief pictorial survey." Brit. Med. Bull. 4, no. 2:132-139, 1946.

Dr. Edmund W. Andrews, as has already been mentioned, introduced the use of a mixture of oxygen with nitrous oxide into the practice of anesthesia in 1868. The feasibility of this method, however, was not demonstrated until Sir Frederic Hewitt many years later adapted it. Hewitt was the first to develop an apparatus that was practicable. By using semi-elastic bags, he overcame the terrific pressures of nitrous oxide and oxygen. The bags were kept almost full from the high pressure tanks by means of an intermittent flow of the gases. The gases were controlled directly by hand valves and the tanks which acted against the high pressures.

Joseph Clover[178] reported in 1874 a supplemental bag which provided for rebreathing a portion of the anesthetic agent, and Clover[237] in 1876 introduced the gas-ether sequence. To do this he added to the bag of his inhaler a tap through which nitrous oxide could be admitted for the production of anesthesia.

S. J. Hayes, a Pittsburgh dentist, in 1882, patented an apparatus for generating and applying anesthetic agents. Ether and chloroform were mixed and heated by means of a water bath.

In 1885, Frederic Hewitt[179] described a face piece used for rebreathing nitrous oxide.

The S. S. White Dental Manufacturing Company in 1899 brought out a machine which measured the relative quantities of the gases. This was their nitrous oxide-oxygen apparatus. It was constructed similarly to a machine that Hewitt had perfected in England.

Charles K. Teter,[238] a Cleveland dentist, while practicing his profession in Upper Sandusky, Ohio, became interested in developing an apparatus for administering nitrous oxide and oxygen as well as other anesthetic agents. His first machine was manufactured in 1903 by the Cleveland Dental Manufacturing Company. It was very well liked, and it is due to some extent to Teter's influence that the use of nitrous oxide-oxygen anesthesia became widespread. Dr. Teter has administered nitrous oxide and oxygen anesthesia more than 100,000 times for the extraction of teeth and the removal of tonsils, without a single fatality.

In 1909, Dr. Teter was appointed chief anesthetist at St. Luke's Hospital in Cleveland. In 1912 he was appointed to the position of special anesthetist at Lakeside Hospital in the same city.

About 1909, according to Heidbrink,[239] the A. C. Clarl machine was developed. By means of this machine the maintenance of constant pressure in the bags was attempted. A central valve with a slot for each gas was supposed to proportion the gases. This did not have fine enough control to give good results in gas anesthesia.

From 1906 to 1910, E. I. McKesson, of Toledo, and J. A. Heidbrink, to whom many references have already been made herein, worked independently on an attempt to build a machine which would provide better control of the gases. McKesson invented a machine which produced pressure on the bags individually. This was similar to the Clark machine, but it had a better proportioning valve. In 1910 McKesson perfected the first "intermittent flow" nitrous oxide and oxygen anesthesia machine. It contained an accurate percentage control for the two gases. In 1910 McKesson[240] introduced the principle of fractional rebreathing. He found it possible to save the first part of each expiration for rebreathing. The expiratory valve made provision for the escape of the last part of each expiration.

Meanwhile, Heidbrink was developing his machines. He perfected a machine called the "oo." Later, after a few minor changes, this machine was called the model "T." Heidbrink made use of the reducing valve on his machine as a flowmeter. He was an early exponent of "timed anesthesia."

Willis D. Gatch,[241] in 1910, published his important article on nitrous oxide-oxygen anesthesia produced by his rebreathing method. His apparatus is described therein. Gatch also provided for a sight-feed dropper, and in some cases ether was administered after the gas. Karl Connell also invented a gas machine about this time. In 1918 a government order for gas machines was divided among McKesson, Connell, von Foregger and Heidbrink.

In 1911 J. T. Gwathmey[242] and William C. Woolsey began

experimenting with gas machines. They had a nitrous oxide-oxygen apparatus built for them by Langsdorf in 1912. That same year the Ohio[243] monovalve anesthesia machine was put on the market by the Ohio Chemical and Manufacturing Company of Cleveland. This year, too, was the date of the appearance of the Boothby-Cotton sight-feed apparatus.[244] To insure an even flow of gas, this machine provided for the use of automatic reducing valves. In 1914, Boothby furnished accurate calibration for the sight-feed valves.

Richard v. Foregger in 1914 built a nitrous oxide-oxygen machine without a reducing valve. The first Gwathmey apparatus built by von Foregger without reducing valves, but with control valves for oxygen and nitrous oxide, appeared in 1915. H. E. G. Boyle* modified the early Gwathmey machine and it proved so useful that with the addition of a few improvements it is still the standard machine in use in England.

As Miller[236] has said, many others during the period from 1910 to 1920 developed gas machines. These included Coburn, Cunningham, Flagg, Guedel, Peariro, Miller and Morgan.

In 1923, John S. Lundy specified the first Seattle model gas machine. This was a four-valve apparatus for the utilization of oxygen, nitrous oxide, carbon dioxide and ethylene. This was the first apparatus to have all four gases. Dr. Lundy in 1925 worked with Dr. Heidbrink on the first Lundy-Heidbrink Model. One of the first machines was delivered to the Mayo Clinic on August 20, 1925. This was followed in 1932 by the Lundy-Heidbrink kinetometer gas machine, which was better adapted for absorber use.

O—RECORDS AND STATISTICS

As stressed by Beecher,[245] the introduction of anesthesia into the clinic altered the practice of medicine perhaps more than any other single advance. Record keeping, that is the description and charting of the patients' course during anesthesia, is, therefore, of first importance. While the early historical accounts are in their essence records, as far as can be determined no exact chartings were made until 1894. On November 30, 1894 (pos-

* Personal communication from Dr. Noel Gillespie.

sibly earlier), E. A. Codman of the Massachusetts General Hospital at the suggestion of F. B. Harrington, his superior, began to make individual charts. These charts gave the following information: (1) Name of operation, (2) Name of surgeon, (3) Exact time the ether administration was begun, (4) Exact time the ether administration was ended, (5) Amount of ether necessary to anesthetize the patient, (6) Drugs previously administered, (7) The amount of mucus, (8) Condition of the heart, (9) A recording of the pulse rate throughout the entire operation and (10) A charting of the respiration throughout the entire operation. Harvey Cushing also was impressed early in his career by the importance of keeping individual anesthetic records, being convinced that it would aid his technic of ether administration. Beecher found an anesthesia chart dated by Cushing as of July 17, 1895. His chart was somewhat different from Codman's since he thought the most important thing to be observed was the careful recording of the pulse rate throughout the entire operation. His charts stressed temperature, pulse, and respirations. Cushing also added in his own handwriting things he thought were significant for each case, such as vomitus—time and amount, time when the patient came out of the ether, behavior, the time when pulse came down, and so forth.

On a trip to Italy in 1901, Cushing[246] met Dr. Orlandi, a colleague of Scipione Riva-Rocci. Dr. Riva-Rocci had introduced his sphygmomanometer in 1896, and at the time of Dr. Cushing's visit a "home-made" adaptation of Riva-Rocci's blood-pressure apparatus was in routine daily use at the bedside of every patient at the old Ospedale di S. Matteo in Pavia. Dr. Orlandi presented a model of the inflatable armlet which they employed to Dr. Cushing and Cushing introduced practically the same form of this apparatus at Johns Hopkins Hospital. He insisted on its routine use for all of his operations, and Cushing's efforts can be said to mark the beginnings of blood pressure determinations in this country.

G. W. Crile also was quick to sense the importance of blood pressure determinations. After Cushing brought the Riva-Rocci apparatus to Crile's attention, the latter employed it in a series of experimental and clinical cases where before he had used the Gärtner tonometer. Crile[247] in one of his studies, working with dogs, determined arterial pressure under complete anesthesia. His findings are of interest. He found the minimal pressure to be 80; the maximal pressure 170; the medium pressure 125. For this experimental study on blood pressure in surgery, Crile was awarded in 1923 the Cartwright prize of the Alumni Association of the College of Physicians and Surgeons, New York City.

Following the early reports of Codman and Cushing, as well as those of Crile, McKesson[248] in 1907 began to keep accurate records of blood pressure during anesthesia. Other anesthetists were soon to follow his lead. Gilbert Brown,[249] of Adelaide, Australia, wrote a paper for the *Lancet* in 1911 built around his anesthesia records on 300 cases. John Lundy[250] popularized the use of record keeping in the Pacific Northwest as early as 1923. Waters in 1927 kept extensive records including pre- and post-operative data. In 1934 E. A. Rovenstine[251] of Madison, Wisconsin, pointed out that statistical reports relating to anesthesia lacked convincing (that is, statistically reliable) evidence. He stressed the need for uniformity in collecting, correlating and reporting statistics of anesthesia. He recommended a system for collecting comprehensive data for surgical and anesthetic procedures and the use of tabulating cards and a sorting machine to make data immediately available for statistical studies. In 1933 he brought out the first *Annual Statistical Report* based on these methods, and this has appeared annually ever since. In 1937 Nosworthy[252] wrote on the value of anesthetic records. Since that time much progress has been made in making records uniform, but there is still much to be done. The American Society of Anesthetists in 1936 established a committee on records to study this problem. It established a uniform method for the keeping of anesthetic records and this system is now fairly widely employed.[253] Approximately thirty-five anesthetists or institutions in this country have expressed a desire to employ this method. Anesthetists in England and Australia have also shown an interest.

Concluding Comments

That the use of records and statistics has met with a great deal of enthusiasm is suggested by the following important recent contributions. Eisenhart, Simpson, and Gillespie[254] of the Departments of Mathematics and Anesthesia, the University of Wisconsin, cooperated on a mathematical analysis, a statistical comparison of circulatory complications after abdominal operations in which ether or cyclopropane was used as the anesthetic agent. Nosworthy[255] suggested a simple method of grouping records by means of cards. Saklad, Gillespie, and Rovenstine[256] have recommended a method for the collection and analysis of statistics in cases of inhalation therapy. And finally, Majors Wangeman and Martin[257] have presented an interesting study indicative of the successful use of the modified Hollerith punch card systems at two Army General Hospitals in the recording of surgical and anesthetic dangers.

P—CONCLUDING COMMENTS

A recent addition to the anesthetists' armamentarium is curare. This new agent prevents impulses from the motor nerves to the muscles without affecting the circulation. As pointed out by Dittrick,[258] curare was well known in the sixteenth century and reported on by botanists and explorers. Certain Indian tribes have used curare for centuries in South America in hunting and fighting. T. Spencer Wells[259] in 1859 reported its use in three cases of tetanus. It is now used as a complementary agent in general anesthesia. Griffith and Johnson[260] in 1942 and S. C. Cullen[261] in 1943 reported its use in the successful abolition of muscular rigidity in abdominal operations.

This account will be concluded with the evidence at hand which suggests that anesthesiology has reached a state of maturity. The untiring and ceaseless effort of the late Francis Hoeffer McMechan (1879-1939) and of Mrs. McMechan of Cleveland in developing the professional aspects of anesthesia throughout the world has had its lasting effects. McMechan helped in the organization of the American Association of Anesthetists in 1912. Feeling that a journal on anesthesia was greatly needed, he appealed to Dr. Joseph MacDonald, the publisher of the *American Journal of Surgery*. Subsequently McMechan edited a *Quarterly Supplement of Anesthesia and Analgesia*, which was added to the *American Journal of Surgery*, from 1914 until 1922. In 1922 the International Anesthesia Research Society was organized and Dr. McMechan became the editor of its official organ, *Current Researches in Anesthesia and Analgesia*, the first professional journal of the specialty. After McMechan's death in 1939, Howard Dittrick became the editor, and Dr. McMechan's wife, Laurette van Varseveld McMechan, the assistant editor. Mrs. McMechan, a direct descendant of the sister of Baron Larrey, and Dr. Dittrick have carried on McMechan's work in a way that has endeared them to the profession.

One development in technic may be mentioned. This is the method for continuous spinal anesthesia using a malleable needle, as suggested by William T. Lemmon. Lemmon[262] has observed during the past several years that sometimes spinal anesthesia has failed to take effect, and that in many cases the effect, once produced, is dissipated too soon. To remedy this, he devised an apparatus and injected procaine hydrochloride into the spinal fluid. As the effect of the first injection disappears, subsequent injections are carried out. To prevent or ameliorate a toxic condition which sometimes occurs, a 10 per cent solution of glucose is administered intravenously to the patient. The advantage of the Lemmon method is that it makes possible the administration of minimal effective doses, thereby helping to make intrathecal administration more flexible and thus endowing it with one of the main advantages of inhalation anesthesia.

Edwards and Hingson,[263] by virtue of Hingson's familiarity with continuous spinal anesthesia, developed continuous caudal analgesia for obstetrics, a recent contribution. Edward B. Tuohy[263A] added an improvement to the technic of Edwards and Hingson. He uses an ureteral catheter instead of a malleable needle. The first accounts of caudal anesthesia are those of Sicard[264] and Cathelin,[265] published in 1901.

Concluding Comments

Two important contributions have been made to increase the safety of the use of anesthetic gases. Because of a fatal explosion of an anesthetic agent in Boston in 1938, Philip Woodbridge,[266] then of the Lahey Clinic, J. Warren Horton, of the Massachusetts Institute of Technology, and the late Karl Connell, of Branch, New York, made an investigation. The fatal explosion seemed to have been caused by the ignition of anesthetic gases by static spark. These investigators concluded that the ideal method for the prevention of any spark discharge which might ignite an explosive mixture would be to interconnect all objects and persons by conductors between these bodies or from these bodies to a connecting floor. They felt that this method was impracticable, however. They developed "high resistance intercoupling" and by its use in the operating room found it possible to reduce certain specific hazards of frequent occurrence.

G. W. Jones, R. E. Kennedy and G. J. Thomas[267] have investigated the explosive properties of cyclopropane. This was a co-operative project between the United States Bureau of Mines and representatives from the School of Mines at the University of Pittsburgh, the American Society of Heating and Ventilating Engineers and various hospitals and industries in and around Pittsburgh. This committee advised that the practice of using a mixture of 20 per cent cyclopropane and 80 per cent oxygen be discouraged because such mixtures are violently explosive and have led to fatal accidents. A means of eliminating explosion hazards was found. It consisted in reducing the oxygen content of the anesthetic mixture by the addition of inert gases. With continued dilution of the mixtures with inert gases, a concentration of oxygen is finally reached at which the mixtures are no longer explosive or inflammable.*

In this country, two events of significance were the formation

---

* Some anesthetists believe that if this plan were adopted it would result in more fatalities from anoxia than there are now from explosions. They base their statements on their belief that the remedy results in a lower oxygen content than that of a normal atmosphere.

in 1937 of the American Board of Anesthesiology, Inc.,* as an affiliate of the American Board of Surgery, Inc. In 1941, the American Board of Anesthesiology, Inc., was established as a separate major board. Secondly, the first meeting of the Section on Anesthesiology of the American Medical Association was held in 1941.

Perhaps the best evidence in the literature which tends to show that anesthesia has matured is that recently offered by Ralph Waters.[268] Waters emphasized the viewpoint that clinical practice in anesthesia is handicapped by failure to correlate and utilize existing knowledge. Such an observation by a mature thinker in this field shows that anesthesiology is now concerning itself not only with new developments in technics and new drugs, important as these are, but also with such matters as the one mentioned by Waters: "Permanent improvement will develop in the future, as it has come in the past, mainly through consideration of scientific facts—laborious learning, imaginative insight and accumulative application."

---

* There are now fifteen American Boards in the various medical specialties. The purpose of these boards is to improve the standards of graduate medical education, the training and the practice of medical specialties in the United States and Canada. Each of the boards certifies as specialists those candidates whose general qualifications, professional standing, and special training and practice meet with their approval. In addition successful candidates must pass comprehensive examinations before they are made diplomates.

References for Section I

1. Archer, W. H.: The history of anesthesia. Proc. Dental Centenary Celebration. (Mar.) 1940. pp. 333-363.

2. Fülöp-Miller, René: Triumph over pain. Translated by Eden and Cedar Paul. New York, The Literary Guild of America, Inc., 1938. 438 pp.

3. Prinz, Herrmann: Dental Chronology . . . Philadelphia, Lea and Febiger, 1945. p. 15.

4. Homer: Odyssey. Translated by George Herbert Palmer. Cambridge, Massachusetts, Houghton Mifflin Company, 1929. p. 42.

4A. Homer: Iliad. Rendered into English blank verse by Edward, Earl of Derby. Philadelphia, Henry T. Coates & Co. n.d. v. I, Book XI, lines 963-967.

5. Kleiman, Marcos: Histoire de l'anesthésie. Anesth. et analg. 5:122-138 (Feb.) 1939.

6. Herodotus, Book 4, Chapter 75, for original description.

7. [Theodoric]: Cyrurgia Theodorici, Liber IV, Cap. VIII. In: Collectio chirurgica Veneta. Venice, 1498, folio 146.

8. Babcock, Myra E.: Brief outline of the history of anesthesia. Grace Hosp. Bull. 10:16-21 (Apr.) 1926.

9. Encyclopaedia Britannica, Ed. 9, 1888, v. 8, p. 568.

10. Frobenius: An account of a spiritus vini aethereus . . . Phil. Tr. Roy. Soc. 36:283-289 (Mar.-Apr.) 1730.

11. Leake, C. D.: Valerius Cordus and the discovery of ether. Isis. 7:14-24, 1925. See also Tallmadge, G. K.: The third part of the De Extractione of Valerius Cordus. Isis. 7:394-411, 1925.

11A. Turner, Matthew: An account of the extraordinary medicinal fluid, called aether . . . London, J. Wilkie, [1743?]. 16 pp.

12. Paracelsus: Opera medico-chimica sive paradoxa . . . Franckfurt, 1605. p. 125.

13. Moore, James: A method of preventing or diminishing pain in several operations of surgery. London, T. Cadell, 1784. 50 pp.

14. Esdaile, James: Mesmerism in India, and its application in surgery and medicine . . . London, Longman, Brown, Green, and Longmans, 1846. xxxi, 287 pp.

15. Elliotson, John: Numerous cases of surgical operations without pain in the mesmeric state; with remarks upon the opposition of many members of the Royal Medical and Chirurgical Society and others to the reception of the inestimable blessings of mesmerism . . . Philadelphia, Lea and Blanchard, 1843. 56 pp.

16. Braid, James: Neurypnology; or the rationale of nervous sleep, considered in relation with animal magnetism. Illustrated by numerous cases of its successful application in the relief and cure of disease. London, John Churchill, 1843. xxii, 265 pp.

17. Davy, Humphry: Researches, chemical and philosophical; chiefly concerning nitrous oxide, or dephlogisticated nitrous air, and its respiration. London, J. Johnson, 1800. 580 pp.

18. Wilks, Samuel, and Bettany, G. T.: A biographical history of Guy's Hospital. London, Ward, Lock, Bowden and Co., 1892. pp. 388-389.

19. Rice, N. P.: Trials of a public benefactor, as illustrated in the discovery of etherization. New York, Pudney and Russell, 1858. p. 82.

20. Faraday, Michael: Effects of inhaling the vapors of sulphuric ether. In: Quart. J. Sc. and the Arts. Miscellanea (art. XVI). 4:158-159, 1818.

21. Wellcome Historical Medical Museum, London: Souvenir, Henry Hill Hickman, Centenary Exhibition, 1830-1930, at the Wellcome Historical Medical Museum. London, Wellcome Foundation, Ltd., 1930. 85 pp.

22. Buxton, D. W.: Foreword. In: Wellcome Historical Medical Museum, London. Souvenir, Henry Hill Hickman, Centenary Exhibition, 1830-1930, at the Wellcome Historical Medical Museum. London, Wellcome Foundation, Ltd., 1930. pp. 13-17.

23. Lyman, H. M.: Artificial anæsthesia and anæsthetics. New York, William Wood and Co., 1881. p. 6.

24. Bigelow, H. J.: Insensibility during surgical operations produced by inhalation. Boston M. & S. J. 35:309-317 (Nov. 18) 1846.

25. Warren, J. C.: Inhalation of ethereal vapor for the prevention of pain in surgical operations. Boston M. & S. J. 35:375-379 (Dec. 9) 1846.

26. Taylor, Frances L.: Crawford W. Long

and the discovery of ether anesthesia. New York, Paul B. Hoeber, Inc., 1928. p. 81.

27. COLTON, G. Q.: Anæsthesia. Who made and developed this great discovery? New York, A. G. Sherwood and Co., 1886. 15 pp.

28. QUISTORPIUS, J. B.: G.D.S.P., Disputatio inauguralis medica de anæsthesia (von dem unempfindlich seyn) . . . Rostochii, J. Wepplingi, 1718. Collation A-F⁴, 24 ll.

29. COCK, F. W.: The first operation under ether in Europe. University College (London) Hosp. Mag. 1:127-144 (Feb.) 1911.

30. GARRISON, F. H.: An introduction to the history of medicine. Ed. 4. Philadelphia, W. B. Saunders Co., 1929. p. 506.

31. *Medical intelligence:* Insensibility during surgical operations produced by inhalation. Boston M. & S. J. 35:413-414 (Dec. 16) 1846.

32. DANA, F., JR.: Mesmerism. Boston M. & S. J. 35:425-428 (Dec. 23) 1846.

33. OSLER, WILLIAM: The first printed documents relating to modern surgical anæsthesia. Proc. Roy. Soc. Med. (Sect. Hist. Med.). 11:65-69 (May 15) 1918. Reprinted in Ann. M. Hist. 1:329-332, "1917" (1918).

34. SNOW, JOHN: On chloroform and other anæsthetics: their action and administration. Edited, with a memoir of the author, by Benjamin W. Richardson. London, John Churchill, 1858. 443 pp.

35. THOMS, HERBERT: "Anesthésie à la Reine," a chapter in the history of anesthesia. Am. J. Obstet. & Gynec. 40:340-346 (Aug.) 1940.

36. SIMPSON, J. Y.: The obstetric memoirs and contributions of James Y. Simpson. Edited by W. O. Priestley and Horatio R. Storer. Philadelphia, J. B. Lippincott and Co., 1856. Vol. 2, 733 pp.

37. GUTHRIE, SAMUEL: New mode of preparing a spirituous solution of chloric ether. Silliman J. 21:64-65; On pure chloric ether, 22:105-106, 1832.

38. SOUBEIRAN, EUGÈNE: Recherches sur quelques combinaisons du chlore. Ann. de Chim. 48:113-157, 1831. Also in J. de Pharm. 17:657-672, 1831; 18:1-24, 1832.

39. VON LIEBIG, JUSTUS: Ueber die Verbindungen, welche durch die Einwirkung des Chlors auf Alcohol, Aether, ölbildnes Gas und Essiggeist entstehen. Liebig's Annalen. 1:182-230, 1832. Also in Ann. de Chim., 49:146-204, 1832, and in Poggendorf's Annalen, 24:245-295, 1832.

40. ROBINSON, VICTOR: Pathfinders of medicine. New York, Medical Life Press, 1929. 810 pp.

41. CLARK, A. J.: Aspects of the history of anæsthetics. Brit. M. J. 2:1029-1034 (Nov. 19) 1938.

42. Anæsthetic agents. Tr. A. M. A. 1:176-224, 1848.

42A. WILLIAMS, H. W.: On the value of the operation of extraction of cataract, and on the use of anæsthetic agents in ophthalmic surgery. Boston Med. Surg. J. 44:389-391 (June 18) 1851.

43. SERTÜRNER, F. W.: Ueber das Morphium, eine neue salzfähige Grundlage, und die Mekonsäure als Hauptbestandtheil des Opiums. Gilbert's Ann. d. Physik. 55:56-89, 1817.

44. BARTHOLOW, ROBERTS: Manual of hypodermic medication. Ed. 2. Philadelphia, J. B. Lippincott & Company, 1873. 170 pp.

45. ADAMS, R. C.: Intravenous anesthesia: chemical, pharmacologic and clinical consideration of the anesthetic agents including the barbiturates. Thesis, University of Minnesota, Graduate School, 1940.

46. SPESSA, A.: Modo di rendere insensibile una parte nella quale devesi praticare qualche atto operatorio. Bull. d. sc. med., Bologna. s. 5. 11:224-226, 1871.

47. BUMPUS, H. C.: History of regional anesthesia in urology. J. A. M. A. 96:83-88 (Jan. 10) 1931.

48. BRAUN, HEINRICH: Local anesthesia, its scientific basis and practical use. Ed. 2. Philadelphia, Lea & Febiger, 1924. 411 pp.

49. BENNETT, ALEXANDER: An experimental inquiry into the physiological actions of theine, caffeine, guaranine, cocaine, and theobromine. Edinburgh M. J. Pt. 1. 19: 323-341 (Oct.) 1873.

50. VON ANREP, V.: Ueber die physiologische Wirkung des Cocaïn. Arch. f. d. ges. Physiol. 21:38-77, 1880.

51. CORNING, J. L.: On the prolongation of the anæsthetic effects of the hydrochlorate of cocaine when subcutaneously injected. An experimental study. New York M. J. 42:317-319 (Sept. 19) 1885.

52. ——: Spinal anæsthesia and local medication of the cord. New York M. J. 42:483-485 (Oct. 31) 1885.

53. ——: A further contribution on local medication of the spinal cord, with cases. M. Rec. 33:291-293 (Mar. 17) 1888.

54. QUINCKE, H.: Die Lumbalpunction des Hydrocephalus. Berl. klin. Wchnschr. 28: 929-933 (Sept. 21); 965-968 (Sept. 28) 1891.

55. BIER, AUGUST: Versuche über Cocainisirung des Rückenmarkes. Deutsche Ztschr. f. Chir. 51:361-369 (Apr.) 1899.

References

56. TUFFIER: Analgésie chirurgicale par l'injection sous-arachnoïdienne lombaire de cocaïne. Compt. rend. Soc. de biol. 51:882-884, 1899.

57. DE TAKÁTS, GÉZA: Local anesthesia: a short course for students and surgeons. Philadelphia, W. B. Saunders Company, 1928. 221 pp.

58. TAIT, DUDLEY, and CAGLIERI, GUIDO: Experimental and clinical notes on the subarachnoid space. Tr. Med. Soc. California. Abstracted J. A. M. A. 35:6-10 (July 7) 1900.

59. MATAS, RUDOLPH: Local and regional anesthesia with cocain and other analgesic drugs, including the subarachnoid method, as applied in general surgical practice. Philadelphia M. J. 6:820-843 (Nov. 3) 1900. See also Report of successful spinal anesthesia, J. A. M. A. 33:1659 (Dec. 30) 1899.

60. SOUCHON, EDMOND: Original contributions of Louisiana to medical science; a bibliographic study. New Orleans, Louisiana, privately printed, 1916. 12 pp.

61. BABCOCK, W. W.: Spinal anesthesia, an experience of twenty-four years. Am. J. Surg. 5:571-576 (Dec.) 1928.

62. BOURNE, WESLEY; LEIGH, M. D.; INGLIS, A. N., and HOWELL, G. R.: Spinal anesthesia for thoracic surgery. Anesthesiology. 3:272-281 (May) 1942.

62A. NEWTON, H. F.: Spinal anesthesia in thoracoplastic operations for pulmonary tuberculosis. J. Thorac. Surg. 4:414-428 (April) 1935.

62B. SHIELDS, H. J.: Spinal anesthesia in thoracic surgery. Anesth. and Analg. 14:193-198 (Sept.-Oct.) 1935.

63. CUSHING, H. W.: Cocaine anæsthesia in the treatment of certain cases of hernia and in operations for thyroid tumors. Johns Hopkins Hosp. Bull. 9:192-193 (Aug.) 1898.

64. ODOM, C. B.: Epidural anesthesia. Am. J. Surg. 34:547-558 (Dec.) 1936.

65. PAGÉS, FIDEL: Anestesia metamérica. Rev. san. mil., Madrid. 11:351-365 (June); 385-396 (July) 1921.

66. DOGLIOTTI, A. M.: Eine neue Methode der regionären Anästhesie: die peridurale segmentäre Anästhesie. Zentralbl. f. Chir. 58:3141-3145 (Dec. 12) 1931.

67. CRILE, G. W.: Phylogenetic association in relation to certain medical problems. Boston M. & S. J. 163:893-904 (Dec. 8) 1910.

68. ———: Surgical aspects of Graves' disease with reference to the psychic factor. Ann. Surg. 47:864-869 (June) 1908.

69. LEAKE, C. D.: The historical development of surgical anesthesia. Scient. Mthly. 20:304-328 (Mar.) 1925.

70. ALLEN, F. M.; CROSSMAN, L. W.; HURLEY, VINCENT; WARDEN, C. E., and RUGGIERO, WILFRED: Refrigeration anesthesia. J. Internat. Coll. of Surgeons. 5:125-131 (Mar.-April) 1942.

71. MOCK, H. E., and MOCK, H. E., JR.: Refrigeration anesthesia in amputations. J. A. M. A. 123:13-17 (Sept. 4) 1943.

72. PIROGOFF, N. [I.]: Recherches pratiques et physiologiques sur l'éthérisation. St. Pétersbourg, F. Bellizard & Cie., 1847. 109 pp.

73. SUTTON, W. S.: Anesthesia by colonic absorption of ether and oil-ether colonic anesthesia. Part I. Anesthesia by colonic absorption of ether. In: Gwathmey, J. T.: Anesthesia. Ed. 2. New York, Macmillan Co., 1924. pp. 433-438.

74. ROUX: Quoted by Sutton, W. S. (see 73).

75. Y'YHEDO: Quoted by Sutton, W. S. (see 73).

76. DUPUY, MARC: Note sur les effets de l'injection de l'éther dans le rectum. L'Union Médicale 1:34 (March 23) 1847.

77. MOLLIÈRE, DANIEL: Note sur l'éthérisation par la voie rectale. Lyon méd. 45:419-423 (Mar. 30) 1884.

78. CUNNINGHAM, J. H., and LAHEY, F. H.: A method of producing ether narcosis by rectum, with the report of forty-one cases. Boston M. & S. J. 152:450-457 (Apr. 20) 1905.

79. GWATHMEY, J. T.: Oil-ether anesthesia. Lancet. 2:1756-1758 (Dec. 20) 1913.

80. ———: Obstetrical analgesia; a further study, based on more than twenty thousand cases. Surg., Gynec. & Obst. 51:190-195 (Aug.) 1930.

81. BUTZENGEIGER, O.: Klinische Erfahrungen mit Avertin (E 107). Deutsche med. Wchnschr. 53:712-713 (Apr. 22) 1927.

82. CLAYE, A. M.: The evolution of obstetric analgesia. New York, Oxford University Press, 1939. 103 pp.

83. BECKER: Quoted by Luckhardt, A. B., and Lewis, Dean (see 84).

84. LUCKHARDT, A. B., and LEWIS, DEAN: Clinical experiences with ethylene-oxygen anesthesia. J. A. M. A. 81:1851-1857 (Dec. 1) 1923.

85. NUNNELEY, THOMAS: Quoted by Luck-hardt, A. B. (see 89).

86. MAYO, W. J.: Discussion of paper by T. E. Keys entitled "The medical books of William Worrall Mayo, pioneer surgeon of the American Northwest." Coll. Papers, Mayo Clin. & Mayo Foundation. 30:938-943, 1938.

87. HERMANN, LUDIMAR: Ueber die physiologischen Wirkungen des Stickstoffoxydulgases. Arch. f. Anat. u. Physiol. pp. 521-536, 1864.

88. LÜSSEM, FRANZ: Experimentelle Studien über die Vergiftung durch Kohlenoxyd, Methan und Aethylen. Ztschr. f. klin. Med. 9:397-428, 1885.

89. LUCKHARDT, A. B.: Ethylene anesthesia. In: Gwathmey, J. T.: Anesthesia. Ed. 2. New York, Macmillan Co., 1924. pp. 711-731.

90. CROCKER, WILLIAM, and KNIGHT, L. I.: Effect of illuminating gas and ethylene on flowering carnations. Botanical Gaz. 46: 259-276 (Oct.) 1908.

91. LUCKHARDT, A. B., and CARTER, J. B.: Ethylene as a gas anesthetic; preliminary communication. J. A. M. A. 80:1440-1442 (May 19) 1923.

92. HERB, ISABELLA: Ethylene: notes taken from the clinical records. Anesth. & Analg. 2:230-232 (Dec.) 1923.

93. COTTON, J. H.: Anæsthesia from commercial ether-administration and what it is due to. Canad. M. A. J. 7:769-777 (Sept.) 1917.

94. BROWN, W. E.: Preliminary report; experiments with ethylene as a general anæsthetic. Canad. M. A. J. 13:210 (Mar.) 1923.

95. LEAKE, C. D., and CHEN, M. Y.: The anesthetic properties of certain unsaturated ethers. Proc. Soc. Exper. Biol. & Med. 28:151-154 (Nov.) 1930.

96. ———: The rôle of pharmacology in the development of ideal anesthesia. J. A. M. A. 102:1-4 (Jan. 6) 1934.

97. RUIGH, W. L., and MAJOR, R. T.: The preparation and properties of pure divinyl ether. J. Am. Chem. Soc. 53:2662-2671 (July) 1931.

98. LEAKE, C. D.; KNOEFEL, P. K., and GUEDEL, A. E.: The anesthetic action of divinyl oxide in animals. J. Pharmacol. & Exper. Therap. 47:5-16 (Jan.) 1933.

99. GELFAN, SAMUEL, and BELL, I. R.: The anesthetic action of divinyl oxide on humans. J. Pharmacol. & Exper. Therap. 47:1-3 (Jan.) 1933.

100. FREUND, AUGUST: Über Trimethylen. Monatshefte f. Chemie. 3:625-635, 1882.

101. LUCAS, G. H. W., and HENDERSON, V. E.: A new anæsthetic gas: cyclopropane; a preliminary report. Canad. M. A. J. 21: 173-175 (Aug.) 1929.

102. HENDERSON, V. E., and LUCAS, G. H. W.: Cyclopropane: a new anesthetic. Anesth. & Analg. 9:1-6 (Jan.-Feb.) 1930.

103. SEEVERS, M. H.; MEEK, W. J.; ROVENSTINE, E. A., and STILES, J. A.: A study of cyclopropane anesthesia with especial reference to gas concentrations, respiratory and electrocardiographic changes. J. Pharmacol. & Exper. Therap. 51:1-17 (May) 1934.

104. WATERS, R. M., and SCHMIDT, E. R.: Cyclopropane anesthesia. J. A. M. A. 103: 975-983 (Sept. 29) 1934.

105. STILES, J. A.; NEFF, W. B.; ROVENSTINE, E. A., and WATERS, R. M.: Cyclopropane as an anesthetic agent: a preliminary clinical report. Anesth. & Analg. 13:56-60 (Mar.-Apr.) 1934.

106. KRANTZ, J. C., JR.; CARR, C. J.; FORMAN, S. E., and EVANS, W. E., JR.: Anesthesia. I. The anesthetic action of cyclopropyl methyl ether. J. Pharmacol. & Exper. Therap. 69:207-220 (July) 1940.

107. BLACK, CONSTANCE; SHANNON, G. E., and KRANTZ, J. C., JR.: Studies with cyclopropyl methyl ether (cyprome ether) in man. Anesthesiology. 1:274-279 (Nov.) 1940.

108. [OLDENBURG, HENRY]: An account of the rise and attempts, of a way to conveigh liquors immediatly into the mass of blood. Phil. Tr. Roy. Soc. 1:128-130 (Dec. 4) 1665.

109. [CLARCK, TIMOTHY]: A letter, written to the publisher by the learned and experienced Dr. Timothy Clarck, one of his majesties physicians in ordinary, concerning some anatomical inventions and observations, particularly the origin of the injection into veins, the transfusion of blood, and the parts of generation. Phil. Tr. Roy. Soc. 3:672-682 (May 18) 1668.

110. STURGIS, C. C.: The history of blood transfusion. Bull. M. Library A. 30:105-112 (Jan.) 1942.

111. JARMAN, RONALD: History of intravenous anesthesia with six years' experience in the use of pentothal sodium. Post-Grad. M. J. 17:70-80 (May) 1941.

112. [LOWER, RICHARD]: The method observed in transfusing the blood out of one animal into another. Phil. Tr. Roy. Soc. 1:353-358 (Dec. 17) 1666.

113. DENIS, J[EAN-BAPTISTE], and EMMEREZ, ——]: A letter concerning a new way of curing sundry diseases by transfusion of blood . . . Phil. Tr. Roy. Soc. 2:489-504 (July 22) 1667.

References

114. [LOWER, RICHARD, and KING, EDMUND]:
An account of the experiment of trans-
fusion, practised upon a man in London.
Phil. Tr. Roy. Soc. 2:557-559 (Dec. 9) 1667.

115. [DENIS, JEAN-BAPTISTE]: An extract of
a letter written by J. Denis, Doctor of
Physick, and Professor of Philosophy and
the Mathematicks at Paris, touching a late
cure of an inveterate phrensy by the transfusion of bloud. Phil. Tr. Roy. Soc. 2:617-
624 (Feb. 10) 1667/8 (i.e., 1668).

116. HIRSH, JOSEPH: The story of blood
transfusion: its civilian and military history. Mil. Surgeon. 88:143-158 (Feb.) 1941.

117. BISCHOFF, T. L. W.: Beiträge zur Lehre
von dem Blute und der Transfusion dessel-
ben. Arch. f. Anat. Physiol. u. wissensch.
Med. pp. 347-372, 1835.

118. HUSTIN, A.: Note sur une nouvelle
méthode de transfusion. Ann. et bull. Soc.
roy. d. sc. méd. et nat. de Bruxelles. 72:
104-111 (Apr.) 1914.

119. ———: Principe d'une nouvelle méthode
de transfusion muqueuse. J. méd. de
Bruxelles. 19:436-439 (Aug.) 1914.

120. AGOTE, LUIS: Un nuevo método de
transfusion de sangre. An. Inst. modelo de
clín. méd. 1:25-30 (Jan.) 1914-15.

121. LEWISOHN, RICHARD: A new and greatly
simplified method of blood transfusion: a
preliminary report. M. Rec. 87:141-142
(Jan. 23) 1915.

122. LANDSTEINER, KARL: Zur Kenntnis der
antifermentativen, lytischen und agglutin-
ierenden Wirkungen des Blutserums und
der Lymphe. Zentralbl. f. Bakt. 27:357-362
(Mar. 23) 1900.

123. SHATTOCK, S. G.: Chromocyte clump-
ing in acute pneumonia and certain other
diseases, and the significance of the buffy
coat in the shed blood. J. Path. & Bact.
6:303-314, 1900.

124. Editorial: Transfusion of blood and of
blood substitutes. J. A. M. A. 117:1627-
1629 (Nov. 8) 1941.

125. ORÉ, [P.-C.]: Études cliniques sur
l'anesthésie chirurgicale par la méthode
des injections de chloral dans les veines.
Paris, J.-B. Baillière et Fils, 1875. 154 pp.

126. ———: Des injections intra-veineuses de
chloral. Paris, Bull. Soc. Chir. 1:400-412,
1872.

127. GREENE, B. A.: Intravenous anesthesia
and analgesia; critical review and sum-
mary. M. Times, New York. 68:356-371
(Aug.) 1940.

128. NOEL, H., and SOUTTAR, H. S.: The
anæsthetic effects of the intravenous injection of paraldehyde. Ann. Surg. 57:64-67
(Jan.) 1913.

129. BREDENFELD, ELISABETH: Die intra-
venöse Narkose mit Arzneigemischen.
Ztschr. f. exper. Path. u. Therap. 18:80-90
(Apr. 4) 1916.

130. PECK, C. H., and MELTZER, S. J.:
Anesthesia in human beings by intravenous
injection of magnesium sulphate. J. A. M.
A. 67:1131-1133 (Oct. 14) 1916.

131. NAKAGAWA, KOSHIRO: Experimentelle
Studien über die intravenöse Infusions-
narkose mittels Alkohols. Tohoku J. Exper.
Med. 2:81-126 (May 3) 1921.

132. KIRSCHNER, M.: Eine psycheschonende
und steuerbare Form der Allgemeinbe-
täubung. Chirurg. 1:673-682 (June 15)
1929.

133. FISCHER, EMIL, and MERING, J.: Ueber
eine neue Classe von Schlafmitteln. Therap.
d. Gegenw. n.s. 5:97-101, 1903.

134. BOGENDÖRFER, L.: Ueber lösliche Schlafmittel der Barbitursäurereihe (Dial löslich)
Schweiz. med. Wchnschr. 54:437-438 (May
8) 1924.

135. FULTON, J. F.; LIDDELL, E. G. T., and
RIOCH, D. McK.: "Dial" as a surgical
anæsthetic for neurological operations; with
observations on the nature of its action.
J. Pharmacol. & Exper. Therap. 40:423-
432 (Dec.) 1930.

136. GEYER, GUIDO: Zur Geschichte der intravenösen Narkose. Med. Klin. 37:497-
499 (May 9) 1941.

137. ZERFAS, L. G., and McCALLUM, J. T.
C.: The analgesic and anesthetic properties of sodium isoamylethyl barbiturate:
preliminary report. Indiana State M. A. J.
22:47-50 (Feb.) 1929.

138. ———; McCALLUM, J. T. C.; SHONLE,
H. A.; SWANSON, E. E.; SCOTT, J. P., and
CLOWES, G. H. A.: Induction of anesthesia
in man by intravenous injection of sodium
iso-amyl-ethyl barbiturate. Proc. Soc. Exper. Biol. & Med. 26:399-403 (Feb.) 1929.

139. FULTON, J. F.: Personal communication to the author.

140. LUNDY, J. S.: The barbiturates as anesthetics, hypnotics and antispasmodics: their
use in more than 1000 surgical and non-
surgical clinical cases and in operations on
animals. Anesth. & Analg. 8:360-365 (Nov.-
Dec.) 1929.

141. FITCH, R. H.; WATERS, R. M., and
TATUM, A. L.: The intravenous use of the
barbituric acid hypnotics in surgery. Am.
J. Surg. 9:110-114 (July) 1930.

142. LUNDY, J. S.: Intravenous anesthesia:
particularly hypnotic, anesthesia and toxic
effects of certain new derivatives of barbituric acid. Anesth. & Analg. 9:210-217
(Sept.-Oct.) 1930.

143. ———: Experience with sodium ethyl (1-methylbutyl) barbiturate (nembutal) in more than 2,300 cases. S. Clin. North America. 11:909-915 (Aug.) 1931.

144. WEESE, H., and SCHARPFF, W.: Evipan, ein neuartiges Einschlafmittel. Deutsche med. Wchnschr. 2:1205-1207 (July 29) 1932.

145. ———: Pharmakologie des intravenösen Kurznarkotikums Evipan-Natrium. Deutsche med. Wchnschr. 1:47-48 (Jan. 13) 1933.

146. JARMAN, RONALD, and ABEL, A.: Evipan: an intravenous anesthetic. Lancet. 2:18-20 (July 1) 1933.

147. LUNDY, J. S.: Intravenous anesthesia: preliminary report of the use of two new thiobarbiturates. Proc. Staff Meet., Mayo Clin. 10:536-543 (Aug. 21) 1935.

148. ———: Personal communication to the author.

149. FULTON, J. R.: Anesthesia in naval practice. S. Clin. North America. 21:1545-1558 (Dec.) 1941.

150. E. M. S. MEMORANDUM: Local treatment of burns. Brit. M. J. 1:489 (Mar. 29) 1941. Lancet. 1:425-426 (Mar. 29) 1941.

151. GANDOW, OTTO: Erfahrungen mit "Eunarcon." Zentralbl. f. Gynäk. 60:1701-1719 (July 18) 1936.

152. CULLEN, S. C., and ROVENSTINE, E. A.: Sodium thio-ethylamyl anesthesia: preliminary report of observations during its clinical use. Anesth. & Analg. 17:201-205 (July-Aug.) 1938.

153. LUNDY, J. S.; TUOHY, E. B.; ADAMS, R. C., and MOUSEL, L. H.: Clinical use of local and intravenous anesthetic agents: general anesthesia from the standpoint of hepatic function. Proc. Staff Meet., Mayo Clin. 16:78-80 (Jan. 29) 1941.

154. MOUSEL, L. H.: Modern trends in anesthesia. Kansas M. Soc. J. 41:279-287 (July) 1940.

155. HUBBELL, A. O.: Intravenous anesthesia in dentistry. Ann. Dent. 3:84-93 (Dec.) 1944.

156. WYCOFF, B. S.: Intravenous anesthesia in oral surgery. Am. J. Orthodontics. 24:875-877 (Sept.) 1938.

157. BULLARD, O. K.: Intravenous anesthesia in office practice . . . Anesth. & Analg. 19:26-30 (Jan.-Feb.) 1940.

158. HUBBELL, A. O., and ADAMS, R. C.: Intravenous anesthesia for dental surgery . . . J. Am. Dent. A. 27:1186-1191 (Aug.) 1940.

159. [HOOK, ROBERT]: An account of an experiment made by M. Hook, of preserving animals alive by blowing through their lungs with bellows. Phil. Tr. Roy. Soc. 2:539-540 (Oct. 21) 1667.

160. TRENDELENBURG, FRIEDRICH: Beiträge zur den Operationen an den Luftwegen. 2. Tamponnade der Trachea. Arch. f. klin. Chir. 12:121-133, 1871.

161. MACEWEN, WILLIAM: Clinical observations on the introduction of tracheal tubes by the mouth instead of performing tracheotomy or laryngotomy. Brit. M. J. 2:122-124 (July 24); 163-165 (July 31) 1880.

162. O'DWYER, JOSEPH: Fifty cases of croup in private practice treated by intubation of the larynx, with a description of the method and of the dangers incident thereto. M. Rec. 32:557-561 (Oct. 29) 1887.

163. MAYDL, K.: Ueber die Intubation des Larynx als Mittel gegen das Einfliessen von Blut in die Respirationsorgane bei Operationen. Wien. med. Wchnschr. 43:57-59 (Jan. 7); 102-106 (Jan. 14) 1893.

164. EISENMENGER, VICTOR: Zur Tamponnade des Larynx nach Prof. Maydl. Wien. med.Wchnschr. 43:199-201 (Jan. 28) 1893.

165. MATAS, RUDOLPH: Intralaryngeal insufflation for the relief of acute surgical pneumothorax. Its history and methods with a description of the latest devices for this purpose. J. A. M. A. 34:1468-1473 (June 9) 1900.

166. TUFFIER and HALLION: Opérations intrathoraciques avec respiration artificielle par insufflation. Compt. rend. Soc. de biol. 48:951-953 (Nov.21) 1896.

167. MATAS, RUDOLPH: On the management of acute traumatic pneumothorax. Ann. Surg. 29:409-434, 1899.

168. PARHAM, F. W.: Thoracic resection for tumors growing from the bony wall of the chest. Tr. South. S. A. 11:223-363, 1898.

169. KUHN, FRANZ: Der Metallschlauch bei der Tubage und als Trachealkanüle. Wien. klin. Rundschau. No. 28, 1900.

170. ———: Die pernasale Tubage. München. med. Wchnschr. 49:1456-1457 (Sept. 2) 1902.

171. ROSENBERG, PAUL: Eine neue Methode der allgemeinen Narkose. Berl. klin. Wchnschr. 32:14-18 (Jan. 7); 34-38 (Jan. 14) 1895.

172. KÜHN, FRANZ: Die perorale Intubation; ein Leitfaden zur Erlernung und Ausführung der Methode mit reicher Kasuistik. Berlin, Karger, 1911. 162 pp.

173. BARTHÉLEMY and DUFOUR: L'anesthésie dans la chirurgie de la face. Presse méd. 15:475-476 (July 27) 1907.

174. MELTZER, S. J., and AUER, JOHN: Con-

References

tinuous respiration without respiratory movements. J. Exper. Med. 11:622-625 (July) 1909.

175. ELSBERG, C. A.: The value of continuous intratracheal insufflation of air (Meltzer) in thoracic surgery: with description of an apparatus. M. Rec. 77:493-495 (Mar. 19) 1910.

176. PECK, C. H.: Intratracheal insufflation anæsthesia (Meltzer-Auer). Observations on a series of 216 anæsthesias with the Elsberg apparatus. Ann. Surg. 56:192-200 (July) 1912.

176A. KIRSTEIN, ALFRED: Autoskopie des Larynx und der Trachea. Berlin Klin. Wchnschr. 32:476-478, 1895.

177. COTTON, F. J., and BOOTHBY, W. M.: Anæsthesia by intratracheal insufflation. Advances in technique; a practicable tube-introducer; nitrous oxide-oxygen as the anæsthetic. Surg., Gynec. & Obst. 13:572-573 (Nov.) 1911.

178. CLOVER, J. T.: Remarks on the production of sleep during surgical operations. Brit. M. J. 1:200-203 (Feb. 14) 1874.

179. HEWITT, F. W.: A new method of administering and economising nitrous oxide gas. Lancet. 1:840-841 (May 9) 1885.

179A. GALE, J. W., and WATERS, R. M.: Closed endobronchial anesthesia in thoracic surgery: preliminary report. Anesth. and Analg. 11:283-287 (Dec.) 1932.

180. JACKSON, D. E.: A new method for the production of general analgesia and anæsthesia with a description of the apparatus used. J. Lab. & Clin. Med. 1:1-12 (Oct.) 1915.

181. WATERS, R. M.: Clinical scope and utility of carbon dioxid filtration in inhalation anesthesia. Anesth. & Analg. 3:20-22; 26 (Feb.) 1924.

182. GUEDEL, A. E., and WATERS, R. M.: A new intratracheal catheter. Anesth. & Analg. 7:238-239 (July-Aug.) 1928.

183. SWORD, B. C.: The closed circle method of administration of gas anesthesia. Anesth. & Analg. 9:198-202 (Sept.-Oct.) 1930.

184. HEIDBRINK, J. A.: Personal communication to the author.

185. VELPEAU, [A-A-L-M.]: Sur les effets de l'éther. Compt. rend. Acad. d. sc. 24:129-134 (Feb. 1) 1847.

186. MAGENDIE, [FRANÇOIS]: Remarques de M. Magendie à l'occasion de cette communication. Compt. rend. Acad. d. sc. 24:134-138 (Feb. 1) 1847.

186A. HAHN, ANDRÉ: The beginnings of surgical anæsthesia in France: ether and

chloroform. Brit. Med. Bull. 4, no. 2:144-146, 1946.

186B. MORTON, W. T. G.: On the physiological effects of sulphuric ether, and its superiority to chloroform. Boston, D. Clapp, 1850. 24 pp.

187. ACKERKNECHT, ERWIN H.: Personal communication to the author.

188. BERNARD, CLAUDE: Leçons sur les anesthésiques et sur l'asphyxie . . . Paris, J. B. Baillière et Fils, 1875: VII, 536 pp.

189. OLMSTED, J. M. D.: Claude Bernard, physiologist. New York, Harper & Brothers, 1938. p. 214.

190. BERNARD, op. cit., p. 153.

191. BERNARD, CLAUDE: Phénomènes de la vie. Tome I, p. 265 (v. 16, Oeuvres).

192. BANCROFT, W. D., and RICHTER, G. H.: Claude Bernard's theory of narcosis. Proc. Nat. Acad. Sc. 16:573-577 (Sept. 15) 1930.

193. HENDERSON, V. E., and LUCAS, G. H. W.: Claude Bernard's theory of narcosis. J. Pharmacol. & Exper. Therap. 44:253-267 (Feb.) 1932.

194. ANDREWS, E. [W.]: The oxygen mixture, a new anæsthetic combination. Chicago Med. Exam. 9:656-661 (Nov.) 1868.

195. BÉRILLON, EDGAR: L'œuvre scientifique de Paul Bert . . . Paris, Picard-Bernheim; Auxerre, Georges Rouillé, 1887. 115 pp. The author is indebted to Mrs. Fred Hitchcock of Columbus, Ohio, for furnishing him with an excellent translation of this work.

196. FLOURENS, M. J. P.: Note touchant l'action de l'éther sur les centres nerveux. Compt. rend. Acad. d. sc. 24:340-344, 1847.

197. HYDERABAD CHLOROFORM COMMISSION: Report of the first Hyderabad chloroform commission. Lancet. 1:421-429 (Feb. 22) 1890.

198. ———: Report of the second Hyderabad chloroform commission. Lancet. 1:149-159 (Jan. 18); 486-510 (Mar. 1); 1369-1393 (June 21) 1890.

199. EMBLEY, E. H.: The question of safety in Syme's teaching in chloroform anæsthesia. Intercol. M. J. Australia. 1:660-664, 1896.

200. ———: The causation of death during the administration of chloroform. Brit. M. J. 1:817-821 (Apr. 5), 885-893 (Apr. 12), 951-961 (Apr. 19) 1902.

201. OSBORNE, W. A.: E. H. Embley memorial lecture. M. J. Australia. 1:755-760 (May 28) 1932.

202. HOFF, H. E.: Ether versus chloroform. New England J. Med. 217:579-592 (Oct. 7) 1937.

203. Levy, A. G.: Sudden death under light chloroform anæsthesia. Proc. Physiological Soc. In: J. Physiol. 42:III-VII (Jan. 21) 1911.

204. ———: Chloroform anæsthesia. London, John Bale Sons & Danielsson, 1922. VII, 159 pp.

205. Guedel, A. E.: Nitrous oxide air anesthesia self administered in obstetrics; a preliminary report. Indianapolis M. J. 14:476-479 (Oct.) 1911.

206. ———: The self administration of nitrous oxide. Indianapolis, Indiana, privately printed, c1913; c1915, 80 pp.

207. ———: Third stage ether anesthesia: a sub-classification regarding the significance of the position and movements of the eyeball. Nat. Anesth. Res. Soc. Bull. No. 3 (May) 1920. 4 pp.

208. ———: Inhalation anesthesia: a fundamental guide. New York, Macmillan Co., 1937. 172 pp.

209. Miller, A. H.: Ascending respiratory paralysis under general anesthesia. J. A. M. A. 84:201-202 (Jan. 17) 1925.

210. Lundy, J. S.: Balanced anesthesia. Minnesota Med. 9:399-404 (July) 1926.

211. ———: Clinical anesthesia . . . Philadelphia, W. B. Saunders Co., 1942. p. 559.

212. Boothby, W. M.: Nitrous oxide-oxygen anesthesia, with a description of a new apparatus. M. Communicat. Massachusetts M. Soc. 22:126-138, 1911. Boston M. & S. J. 146:86-90 (Jan. 18) 1912.

213. ———: Ether anesthesia. In: Keen, W. W.: Surgery, its principles and practice by various authors. Philadelphia, W. B. Saunders Co., 1921. Vol. 8, pp. 824-835.

214. ———: Ether percentages. J. A. M. A. 61:830-834 (Sept. 13) 1913.

215. Mann, F. C.: Vascular reflexes with various tensions of ether vapor. Am. J. Surg. Anesth. suppl. 31:107-112 (Oct.) 1917.

216. ———: Some bodily changes during anesthesia; an experimental study. J. A. M. A. 67:172-175 (July 15) 1916.

217. Barbour, H. G., and Bourne, Wesley: Heat regulation and water exchange. IV. The influence of ether on dogs. Am. J. Physiol. 67:399-410 (Jan.) 1924.

218. Tuohy, E. B.: A comparative study of the physiological activity of cobefrin and epinephrine. Thesis. Graduate School of University of Minnesota, 1935.

219. Stehle, R. L., and Bourne, Wesley: The anesthetic properties of pure ether. J. A. M. A. 79:375-376 (July 29) 1922.

220. Bourne, Wesley: On the effects of acetaldehyde, ether peroxide, ethyl mercaptan, ethyl sulphide, and several ketones —di-methyl, ethyl-methyl, and di-ethyl— when added to anæsthetic ether. J. Pharmacol. & Exper. Therap. 28:409-432 (Sept.) 1926.

221. ———, and Stehle, R. L.: The excretion of phosphoric acid during anesthesia. J. A. M. A. 83:117-118 (July 12) 1924.

222. ———: On an attempt to alleviate the acidosis of anesthesia. Proc. Roy. Soc. Med. Section of Anæsthetics. 19:49-51 (July) 1926.

223. Leake, C. D., and Hertzman, A. B.: Blood reaction in ethylene and nitrous oxid anesthesia. J. A. M. A. 82:1162-1165 (Apr. 12) 1924.

224. ———: Anæsthesia and blood reaction. Brit. J. Anæsth. 2:56-71 (Oct.) 1924.

225. ———: The effect of ethylene-oxygen anesthesia on the acid-base balance of blood: a comparison with other anesthetics. J. A. M. A. 83:2062-2065 (Dec. 27) 1924.

226. Bourne, Wesley; Bruger, M., and Dreyer, N. B.: The effects of sodium amytal on liver function; the rate of secretion and composition of the urine; the reaction, alkali reserve, and concentration of the blood; and the body temperature. Surg., Gynec. & Obst. 51:356-360 (Sept.) 1930.

227. Rosenthal, S. M., and Bourne, Wesley: The effect of anesthetics on hepatic function. J. A. M. A. 90:377-379 (Feb. 4) 1928.

228. Bourne, Wesley: Anesthetics and liver function. Am. J. Surg. 34:486-495 (Dec.) 1936.

229. ———, and Raginsky, B. B.: The effects of avertin upon the normal and impaired liver. Am. J. Surg. 14:653-656 (Dec.) 1931.

230. Stehle, R. L., and Bourne, Wesley: The effects of morphine and ether on the function of the kidneys. Arch. Int. Med. 42:248-255 (Aug.) 1928.

231. Raginsky, B. B., and Bourne, Wesley: The action of ephedrine in avertin anesthesia. J. Pharmacol. & Exper. Therap. 43:209-218 (Sept.) 1931.

232. Bourne, Wesley; Leigh, M. D.; Inglis, A. N., and Howell, G. R.: Spinal anesthesia for thoracic surgery. Anesthesiology. 3:272-281 (May) 1942.

233. Dworkin, Simon; Raginsky, B. B., and Bourne, Wesley: Action of anesthetics and sedatives upon the inhibited nervous system. Anesth. & Analg. 16:238-240 (July-Aug.) 1937.

References

234. ——: Bourne, Wesley, and Raginsky, B. B.: Changes in conditioned responses brought about by anesthetics and sedatives. Canad. M. A. J. 37:136-139 (Aug.) 1937.

234A. Leake, C. D.: Chemical adjuncts to general anesthesia. Cal. and West. Med. 33:714-717 (Oct.) 1930.

234B. ——: Some pharmacologic aspects of pre-anesthetic medication. Northwest Med. 29:561-565 (Dec.) 1930.

234C. Knoefel, P. K.: The nature of anesthetic shock and the value of pre-medication. Cal. and West. Med. 39:344 (Nov.) 1933.

234D. Tatum, A. L.; Atkinson, A. S., and Collins, K. H.: Acute cocaine poisoning, its prophylaxis and treatment in laboratory animals. J. Pharmacol. and Exp. Therap. 26:325-335 (Dec.) 1925.

234E. Knoefel, P. K.; Herwick, R. P., and Loevenhart, A. S.: The prevention of acute intoxication from local anesthetics. J. Pharmacol. and Exp. Therap. 39:397-411 (Aug.) 1930.

235. Beddoes, Thomas, and Watts, James: Considerations on the medicinal use and on the production of factitious airs. Bristol, 1795.

236. Miller, A. H.: Technical development of gas anesthesia. Anesthesiology. 2:398-409 (July) 1941.

236A. Duncum, B. M.: An outline of the history of anæsthesia, 1846-1900. Brit. Med. Bull. 4, no. 2:120-128, 1946.

237. Clover, J. T.: On an apparatus for administering nitrous oxide gas and ether, singly or combined. Brit. M. J. 2:74-75 (July 15) 1876.

238. Teter, C. K.: Personal communication to the author.

239. Heidbrink, J. A.: Personal communication to the author.

240. McKesson, E. I.: Fractional rebreathing in anesthesia; its physiologic basis, technic and conclusions. Am. J. Surg. Anesth. suppl. 29:51-57 (Jan.) 1915.

241. Gatch, W. D.: Nitrous oxid-oxygen anesthesia by the method of rebreathing: with especial reference to the prevention of surgical shock. J. A. M. A. 54:775-780 (Mar. 5) 1910.

242. Gwathmey, J. T.: Personal communication to the author.

243. Cook, E. H.: Personal communication to the author.

244. Cotton, F. J., and Boothby, W. M.: Nitrous oxide-oxygen-ether anæsthesia: notes on administration; a perfected apparatus. Surg., Gynec. & Obst. 15:281-289 (Sept.) 1912.

245. Beecher, H. K.: The first anesthesia records (Codman, Cushing). Surg., Gynec. & Obst. 71:689-693 (Nov.) 1940.

246. Cushing, H. W.: On routine determinations of arterial tension in operating room and clinic. Boston M. & S. J. 148:250-256 (March 5) 1903.

247. Crile, G. W.: Blood-pressure in surgery, an experimental and clinical research . . . Philadelphia, J. B. Lippincott, 1903. 422 pp.

248. McKesson, E. I.: Blood pressure in general anesthesia. Am. J. Surg. Anesth. suppl. 30:2-5 (Jan.) 1916.

249. Brown, Gilbert: Notes on 300 cases of general anæsthesia combined with narcotics. Lancet. 1:1005-1006 (April 15) 1911.

250. Lundy, J. S.: Keeping anesthetic records and what they show. Am. J. Surg. (Quart. Suppl. Anes. and Analg.) 38:16-25 (Jan.) 1924.

251. Rovenstine, E. A.: A method of combining anesthetic and surgical records for statistical purposes. Anesth. & Analg. 13:122-128 (May-June) 1934.

252. Nosworthy, M. D.: The value of anæsthetic records. St. Thomas's Hosp. Rep. 2:54-66, 1937.

253. Saklad, Meyer; Gillespie, Noel, and Rovenstine, E. A.: Inhalation therapy, a method for the collection and analysis of statistics. Anesthesiology. 5:359-369 (July) 1944.

254. Eisenhart, C.; Simpson, R. A., and Gillespie, N. A.: Ether versus cyclopropane (a statistical comparison of circulatory complications after abdominal operations). Brit. J. Anæsth. 18:141-159 (July) 1943.

255. Nosworthy, M.: Method of keeping anæsthetic records and assembling results. Brit. J. Anæsth. 18:160-179 (July) 1943.

256. Saklad, Meyer; Gillespie, Noel, and Rovenstine, E. A.: Inhalation therapy, a method for the collection and analysis of statistics. Anesthesiology. 5:359-369 (July) 1944.

257. Wangeman, C. P., and Martin, S. J.: The recording of surgical and anesthetic data in two Army general hospitals. Anesthesiology. 6:64-80 (Jan.) 1945.

258. Dittrick, Howard: From the jungle to the operating room. Anesth. & Analg. 23:132 (May-June) 1944.

259. Wells, T. S.: Three cases of tetanus in which "woorara" was used. Proc. Roy.

Med. Chir. Soc. London. 3:142-157 (Nov. 22) 1859.

260. GRIFFITH, H. R., and JOHNSON, G. E.: The use of curare in general anesthesia. Anesthesiology. 3:418-420 (July) 1942.

261. CULLEN, S. C.: The use of curare for improvement of abdominal muscle relaxation during inhalation anesthesia; report on 131 cases. Surgery. 14:261-266 (Aug.) 1943.

262. LEMMON, W. T.: A method for continuous spinal anesthesia: a preliminary report. Ann. Surg. 111:141-144 (Jan.) 1940.

263. EDWARDS, W. B., and HINGSON, R. A.: Continuous caudal anesthesia in obstetrics. Am. J. Surg. n.s. 57:459-464 (Sept.) 1942.

263A. TUOHY, E. B.: Continuous spinal anæsthesia: its usefulness and technic involved. Anesthesiology 5:142-148 (March) 1944.

264. SICARD, M. A.: Les injections médicamenteuses extra-durales par voie sacrococcygienne. Compt. rend. Soc. de biol. 53:396-398 (April 20) 1901.

265. CATHELIN, M. F.: Une nouvelle voie d'injection rachidienne. Méthodes des injections épidurales par le procédé du canal sacré. Applications à l'homme. Compt. rend. Soc. de biol. 53:452-453 (April 27) 1901.

266. WOODBRIDGE, P. D.; HORTON, J. W., and CONNELL, KARL: Prevention of ignition of anesthetic gases by static spark. J. A. M. A. 113:740-744 (Aug. 26) 1939.

267. JONES, G. W.; KENNEDY, R. E., and THOMAS, G. J.: Explosive properties of cyclopropane: prevention of explosions by dilution with inert gases. U. S. Dept. of the Interior, Bureau of Mines. Report of Investigations. R. I. 3511 (May) 1940. 17 pp.

268. WATERS, R. M.: The evolution of anesthesia I & II. Proc. Staff Meet., Mayo Clin. 17:428-432 (July 15); 440-445 (July 29) 1942.

II

A Chronology of Events

RELATING TO

Anesthesiology and Allied Subjects

1. 4004 B.C. according to the good Bishop Ussher. Old Testament
   "And the Lord God caused a deep sleep to fall upon Adam, and he slept; and He took one of his ribs, and closed up the flesh instead thereof."— *Genesis* II:21.

2. *c*2250 B.C. Nippur
   Babylonian clay tablet reveals remedy for pain of dental caries. Cement used was made by mixing henbane seed with gum mastic.

3. *c*1200 B.C. Greece   Aesculapius
   The God of Medicine was supposed to have used a potion called *nepenthe* to produce insensibility for his surgical patients.

4. 1149 B.C.(?) Greece   Helen of Troy
   The daughter of Zeus, according to the Odyssey, cast a drug (opium?) into wine "to assuage suffering, and to dispel anger, and to cause forgetfulness of all ills."

5. *c*550 B.C. India
   Susruta mentions the use of henbane and hemp to produce insensibility to pain.

6. *c*450 B.C. Greece   Herodotus
   Inhalation of the vapor of hemp by the Scythians.

7. *c*255 B.C. China   Pien Ch'iao
   A Chinese physician who, according to the *Chinese Annals of History*, performed major operations on patients drugged with wine (to which hemp probably was added).

8. 54-68 A.D. Roman Empire   Pedanius Dioscorides
   The Greek army surgeon, in the service of Nero, recommended the oral administration of mandragora wine for insomnia or the pain of surgical operations and cauterization.

9. 79   Roman Empire   Pliny
   Description of the mandragora wine. "Yet it may be used safely ynough for to procure sleepe, if there be a good regard had in the dose . . . Also it is an ordinarie thing to drinke it against the poyson of serpents: likewise before the cutting, cauterizing, pricking or launcing of any member, to take away the sence and feeling of such extreame cures."

10. 220(?)   China   Hua T'o
    Famous Chinese surgeon administered wine containing a soporific effervescent powder (seed kernel of hemp?) to patients before major operations. Intoxication and complete insensibility were produced.

11. *c*800   Bavaria
Sigerist has found that a recipe for the "sophoric sponge" was contained in the Bamberg *Antidotarium* of the 9th century.

12. *c*800   Italy
Sudhoff found a similar recipe in a Monte Cassino *Codex* of the same period. The sponge was steeped in a mixture of opium, hyoscyamus, mulberry juice, lettuce, hemlock, mandragora and ivy, and dried. When the sponge was moistened, the vapor it produced was ready to be inhaled by the patient.

13. *c*950   Spain   Abū Bekr Hāmidb, Samajūn
Composed important book on drugs, *Collection of sayings of old and new physicians and philosophers on simple drugs.*

14. *c*1100   Italy   Nicolaus Salernitanus
Recommends use of soporific sponge to induce anesthesia.

15. *c*1200   Italy   Hugh of Lucca
Preparation of a soporific agent with opium, hemlock, henbane and mandragora for anesthetization of patients by use of somniferous sponge for minor operations. To revive them, a sponge filled with vinegar was placed under the nostrils.

16. *c*1275   Spain   Raymundus Lullius
Discovery of "sweet vitriol."

17. *c*1363   France   Guy de Chauliac
Report of the use of narcotic agents, especially opium and the "sleeping sponge," to relieve pain during surgical procedures. The untoward effects that sometimes resulted from their use were asphyxia, "congestions" and death.

18. *c*1540   Switzerland   Paracelsus
Discovery of the soporific effect of sweet vitriol and recommendation of its use for painful diseases.

19. 1540   Germany   Valerius Cordus
Description of the synthesis of ether.

20. 1562   England   William Bullein
First known mention in an English printed book of an anesthetic agent.

21. *c*1564   France   Ambroise Paré
Obtained local anesthesia by compression of nerves.

22. 1589   Italy   Giambattista della Porta
Continuation of the use of inhalation anesthesia. An infusion of the various soporific drugs was made and the vapor of this infusion was inhaled by the patient. A deep sleep resulted, the operation was performed and the patient, on awakening, did not remember what had happened to him.

23. *c*1600   Italy   Valverdi
Use of a kind of regional anesthesia, by compression of the nerves and the blood vessels of the region to be operated on.

24. 1646   Italy   Marco Aurelio Severino
The use of freezing mixtures of snow and ice for surgical anesthesia.

A Chronology of Events

25. 1656   England   Sir Christopher Wren
First experiments with intravenous therapy.

26. 1665   Germany   Johann Sigismund Elsholtz
First attempt at intravenous anesthesia.

27. 1665   England   Richard Lower
Transfused blood to animals, first known time.

28. 1667   France   Jean B. Denis
First transfusion of animal blood to man.

29. 1730   Germany   W. G. Frobenius
"Sweet vitriol" was named "ether."

30. 1766- France   Franz Anton Mesmer
    1800   Development of the theory of "vitalism," a revamping of the doctrine of the "power of divine touch" for the prevention of human suffering.

31. 1771   England   Joseph Priestley
Discovery of oxygen.

32. 1771   Sweden   Carl Wilhelm Scheele
Independent discovery of oxygen.

33. 1772   England   Joseph Priestley
Discovery of nitrous oxide.

34. 1779   Holland-England Johannes Ingenhousz
Discovery of ethylene.

35. 1784   England   James Moore
Production of local anesthesia of the extremity by compression of the nerve trunks.

36. 1794   England   Richard Pearson
Use of inhalation of ether in the treatment of phthisis.

37. 1795   England   James Watts
Construction of a gas inhaler for Thomas Beddoes.

38. 1798   England   Sir Humphry Davy
Discovery of the analgesic and exhilarating effects of nitrous oxide.

39. 1799   England   Sir Humphry Davy
Introduction of nitrous oxide into medical practice at Beddoes' Pneumatic Institute.

40. 1800   England   William Allen
Lecturer on chemistry at Guy's Hospital, demonstrated in the presence of Astley Cooper and others the results of inhalation of nitrous oxide, noting especially the loss of sensation to pain.

41. 1805   United States   John C. Warren
The use of ether by inhalation to relieve the last stages of pulmonary inflammation.

42. 1806   Prussia   Friedrich A. W. Sertürner
The extraction of morphine from opium.

The History of Surgical Anesthesia

43. 1807   France   D. J. Larrey
No pain in amputations done on battlefield at very low temperatures (—19° C.).

44. c1815   Germany   Maxime de Puységur
"Discovery" of somnambulism, which was used to relieve the pain of surgical operations.

45. 1818   England   Michael Faraday
Publication of an account of the pain-allaying effects of ether in the *Journal of Science and Art.*

46. 1819   United States   Stockman
Demonstration of the exhilarating effects of nitrous oxide.

47. 1824   England   Henry Hill Hickman
Painless operations carried out on animals after the administration of carbon dioxide gas.

48. 1831   Scotland   Latta
Introduction of the practice of intravenous infusion of saline solution to patients suffering from shock.

49. 1831   United States   Samuel Guthrie
Discovery of chloroform.

50. 1831   France   Eugène Soubeiran
Discovery of chloroform.

51. 1831   Germany   Justus von Liebig
Discovery of chloroform.

52. 1835   France   Jean Baptiste Dumas
Definition of the physical and chemical properties of chloroform.

53. 1839   United States   Isaac Ebenezer Taylor and James Augustus Washington
Practice of hypodermic injection by puncture of the skin with a lancet and use of a syringe to throw the agent (solution of morphine) under the skin.

54. c1840   Scotland and India.   John Elliotson and James Esdaile
Painless operations in many cases through the use of somnambulism reported.

55. 1842   United States   W. E. Clarke
Administration of ether to Miss Hobbie for the painless extraction of one of her teeth by Dr. Elijah Pope (January, 1842). (See Lyman, H. M.: *Artificial anæsthesia.* N. Y., Wood, 1881, p. 6.)

56. 1842   United States   Crawford Williamson Long
James Venable submitted to an operation on March 30, 1842, for removal of a small tumor of the neck while he was under the influence of ether.

57. 1844   United States   Horace Wells
Inhalation of nitrous oxide, administered by G. Q. Colton, for the extraction of Wells' tooth by Dr. John Riggs. (Dec. 11, 1844.)

58. 1845   United States   Horace Wells
Lecture before Dr. John C. Warren's class at Harvard on "The use of nitrous oxide for the prevention of pain." In the evening he demonstrated the use of the agent as an anesthetic agent for the extraction of a tooth. The demonstration was not entirely successful.

A Chronology of Events

59. 1846   United States   Charles T. Jackson

Suggestion of the use of pure ether as an anesthetic agent to Morton, who successfully administered it for the painless extraction of a tooth.

60. 1846   United States   William T. G. Morton

Demonstration of the practicability of ether anesthesia in an operation performed by Dr. J. C. Warren in the Massachusetts General Hospital, October 16.

61. 1846   England   Robert Liston

Two operations performed at University College Hospital, London, under ether greatly stimulated the use of ether on the continent.

62. 1846   England   Peter Squire

Constructed the first British ether inhaler. Morton of the U.S. constructed the first ether inhaler.

63. 1847   France   M. J. P. Flourens

Description of the anesthetic action of chloroform in animals.

64. 1847   England   Jacob Bell

Description of the anesthetic action of chloroform.

65. 1847   Scotland   Sir James Simpson

Introduction of ether analgesia in childbirth.

66. 1847   Russia   N. I. Pirogoff

Description of rectal anesthesia with ether.

67. 1847   England   John Snow

The first physician anesthetist began the administration of ether at St. George's Hospital, London. Published his book on ether.

68. 1847   Scotland   Sir James Simpson

Successful use of chloroform as an anesthetic agent for major operations and midwifery.

69. 1848   England   Thomas Nunneley

Description of the anesthetic qualities of a mixture of ether and an alcoholic solution of chloroform. This was named the "A. C. E." mixture.

70. 1849   France   V. Regnault and J. Reiset

Experimentation on carbon dioxide absorption.

70A. 1851   United States   J. F. B. Flagg

Publication of the first American "textbook" on anesthesia.

71. 1853   England   John Snow

Successful administration of chloroform to Her Majesty, Queen Victoria, at the birth of Prince Leopold. The physician was Sir James Clark. This event greatly stimulated the use of analgesia in obstetrics.

72. 1853   United States   Edward R. Squibb

Manufacture of ether by the revolutionary method involving the continuous passage of steam heat through lead coils.

73. 1853   Scotland   Alexander Wood

Invention of the modern metallic hollow needle. Wood also injected a solution of morphine under the skin near the vicinity of the painful part to afford relief from pain.

74. 1853   France   Charles Gabriel Pravaz

Development of the hypodermic syringe.

75. 1855   Germany   Gaedicke
Isolation of the alkaloid of the leaves of the coca plant, which was called erythroxylin.

76. 1856   England   John Snow
Discovery of the anesthetic properties of amylene.

77. 1858   England   John Snow
Posthumous publication of his textbook, *On chloroform and other anæsthetics.*

78. 1860   Germany   Albert Niemann
The alkaloid of coca leaves obtained in pure form and called "cocaine." Report of the numbing effect of this drug on the tongue.

79. 1862   England   J. T. Clover
Published account of new chloroform inhaler for regulation of the percentile mixture of chloroform and air.

80. 1863   United States   G. Q. Colton
Popularization of the use of pure nitrous oxide in dental operations. The use of this gas had been almost abandoned since its introduction by Wells in 1844.

81. 1867   United States   S. S. White Dental Manufacturing Co.
Introduction of inhaler covering nose and mouth.

82. 1868   United States   Edmund W. Andrews
Introduction of the use of oxygen with nitrous oxide in anesthetic practice.

83. 1868   United States   W. W. Greene
Advocacy of the hypodermic use of morphine during inhalation anesthesia.

84. 1868   England
Suggestion that nitrous oxide be compressed into liquid form was made in the *British Medical Journal.*

85. 1869   Germany   F. Trendelenburg
Use of preliminary tracheotomy as a mode of administration of an endotracheal anesthetic.

86. 1871   United States   Henry Pickering Bowditch
Investigation of the biologic properties of blood plasma and serum.

87. 1871   United States   Johnston Brothers
Compression of nitrous oxide into wrought iron cylinders.

88. 1871   Italy   A. Spessa
Injection of a solution of morphine into a fistulous tract before surgical intervention.

89. 1872   France   P. C. Oré
Chloral hydrate injected intravenously to induce general anesthesia.

90. 1873   Scotland   Alexander Bennett
Demonstration of the anesthetic properties of cocaine.

90A. 1875   France   Claude Bernard
Pre-anesthetic medication with morphine suggested.

91. 1876 England   J. T. Clover
    Introduction of gas-ether sequence.

92. 1877 England   J. T. Clover
    Introduction of portable inhaler with regulation of flow of ether.

93. 1878 Germany   V. von Anrep
    Investigation of the pharmacology of cocaine.

94. 1878 Scotland   William Macewen
    Introduction of anesthesia produced by tracheal tube inserted through the mouth.

95. 1880 Russia   Klikovich
    Introduction of the use of nitrous oxide in obstetrics.

96. 1881 India   Alexander Crombil
    Advocacy of the injection of morphine prior to the administration of chloroform. This was probably the first type of preanesthetic medication.

97. 1881 France   R. Moutard-Martin and Charles Richet
    First injection of gum saline into the whole animal body.

98. 1882 United States   S. J. Hayes
    An apparatus for generating and applying anesthetic agents was patented. Ether and chloroform mixtures were heated by means of a water bath. Air which was pumped through the mixture was charged with the anesthetic vapor.

99. 1882 Germany   August von Freund
    Discovery and description of cyclopropane.

100. 1884 Bohemia & United States   Carl Koller
    The value of cocaine for local anesthesia was expounded.

101. 1884 France   Daniel Mollière
    Rectal anesthesia re-introduced, but because of the severe injuries to the mucosa which resulted, the method was discarded.

102. 1885 United States   William Stewart Halsted
    Introduction of nerve block anesthesia with cocaine.

103. 1885 United States   J. Leonard Corning
    Spinal anesthesia was attempted by injection of the anesthetic agent between the spinous processes of the lower thoracic vertebrae. Anesthesia in the legs and genitalia resulted. This is the first recorded instance of successful peridural anesthesia.

104. 1885 United States   J. Leonard Corning
    Published his book *Local Anæsthesia.*

105. 1887 United States   J. Leonard Corning
    Production of regional anesthesia by injection around the cutaneous antibrachii medialis nerve and production of anesthesia of the skin supplied by it.

106. 1887 England   Sir Frederick W. Hewitt
    Devised a machine for administration of nitrous oxide and oxygen.

107. 1888 Switzerland   Redard
    Ethyl chloride used as a local anesthetic agent.

108. 1888 England   Sir Frederick W. Hewitt
Published handbook, *Select methods in the administration of nitrous oxide and ether.*

109. 1889 United States(?) G. H. Hurd
Apparatus for mixing chloroform vapor and nitrous oxide introduced.

110. 1891 Germany   Giesel
Tropacocaine isolated.

111. 1891 Germany   Heinrich Quincke
Lumbar puncture demonstrated.

112. 1892 Germany   Carl Ludwig Schleich
Demonstration of infiltration anesthesia by intracutaneous injection of dilute solutions of various drugs.

113. 1892 England   Sir Frederick W. Hewitt
Introduced the first practical gas and oxygen apparatus.

114. 1893 England   Sir Frederick W. Hewitt
First edition of *Anæsthetics* published.

115. 1893 England
Society of Anæsthetists (London) founded.

116. 1894 Sweden   H. J. Carlson
Discovery that ethyl chlorate produced a sound sleep in some dental patients. Confirmation by Thiessing. Ethyl chlorate was subsequently used for general anesthesia.

117. 1894 United States   E. A. Codman
Introduction of records especially of pulse rate during anesthesia.

118. 1894 United States   J. Leonard Corning
Introduction of cocaine directly into the medullary canal.

119. 1895 Germany   Alfred Kirstein
Introduction of intratracheal tubes via the first direct-vision laryngoscope.

120. 1897 United States   John Abel
Discovery of epinephrine.

121. 1897 Germany   Heinrich Braun
Advocated the addition of epinephrine to cocaine solution to decrease the rate of absorption and to increase the duration of anesthesia.

122. 1897-98 United States   Rudolph Matas
Modification of the Fell-O'Dwyer apparatus for the relief of acute surgical pneumothorax. This provided for the maintenance of anesthesia during artificial respiration.

123. 1898 Germany   August Bier
First successful clinical use of spinal anesthesia.

124. 1899 United States   S. S. White
Gas machine which proportioned gases.

125. 1899 France   Théodore Tuffier
Development of spinal anesthesia.

126. 1899 Germany   H. Dresser
     Introduction of methyl-propyl-carbinol-urethane (hedonal).

127. 1899 Germany   Korff
     Basis of "twilight sleep." Recommendation of injection of combination of
     scopolamine and morphine or scopolamine and narcophine for anesthesia.

128. 1899 Germany   C. L. Schleich
     Publication of *Schmerzlose Operationen,* Ed. 4. First edition published in
     1894.

128A. 1899 United States   Dudley Tait and Guido Caglieri
     First use of spinal anesthesia in the United States, October 26.

129. 1899 United States   Rudolph Matas
     First report of true spinal anesthesia for surgical operations in the
     United States.

130. 1901 France   M. F. Cathelin and M. A. Sicard
     Independent discoverers of epidural administration of cocaine by the
     caudal route.

131. 1902 United States   Charles K. Teter
     Introduction of the second machine for the administration of nitrous
     oxide and oxygen.

132. 1903 Germany   E. Fischer and J. von Mering
     Synthesis of veronal (barbital).

133. 1903 France   E. Fourneau
     Introduction of stovaine.

134. 1904 Germany   Alfred Einhorn
     Discovery of procaine (novocain).

135. 1905 Russia   N. P. Krawkow and co-workers
     Demonstration of the value of hedonal as an intravenous anesthetic agent.

136. 1906 United States
     The Clark gas machine was developed. A central valve with a slot for
     each gas was used to proportion the gases.

137. 1906 United States   Alice Magaw
     Report on production of anesthesia with ether by the drop method 14,000
     times without a death.

138. 1907 United States   E. I. McKesson
     Popularized the use of tests of blood pressure in anesthesia.

139. 1907 Germany   E. Payr
     Report on the injection of the abdominal wall with eucaine and, after
     performance of cystotomy, infiltration of the periprostatic tissues through
     the mucosa of the bladder before enucleation of the prostate gland.

140. 1907 France   Barthélemy and Dufour
     Advocate use of the insufflation principle of endotracheal anesthesia.

141. 1907 United States   C. C. Guthrie and F. H. Pike
     Excellent results in replacement of blood by plasma and serum experi-
     mentally.

142. 1908 United States   Yandell Henderson
Demonstration of the value of oxygen and carbon dioxide for the purpose of overcoming asphyxia from anesthesia as well as from other causes.

143. 1908 United States   William Crocker and Lee Irving Knight
Ethylene was the cause of losses of many carnations in Chicago. Flowers, placed in greenhouses, would "go to sleep," whereas buds already showing petals failed to open.

144. 1908 United States   G. W. Crile
First report on "anoci-association."

145. 1908 Spain   J. Goyanes
Introduction of intra-arterial anesthesia.

146. 1909 Germany   August Bier
Introduction of a method of local anesthesia by the intravenous injection of procaine.

147. 1909 United States   Arthur E. Guedel
Introduction of self-administration of nitrous oxide in obstetrics and office surgery.

148. 1909 Germany   Ludwig Burkhardt
Chloroform and ether used intravenously.

149. 1909 United States   S. J. Meltzer and John Auer
Successful use of intratracheal insufflation in animals.

150. 1909 United States   C. A. Elsberg
Successful use of intratracheal insufflation in a human being.

151. 1910 Germany   R. Kümmell
Successful anesthesia produced by the intravenous injection of hedonal.

152. 1910 United States   E. I. McKesson
Perfection of the first "intermittent flow" nitrous oxide and oxygen anesthesia apparatus with an accurate percentile control for the two gases. Introduction of fractional rebreathing.

153. 1910 United States   W. D. Gatch
Introduction of ether sight-feed apparatus.

154. 1910-11 United States   J. A. Heidbrink
Development of "timed-anesthesia," in which nitrous oxide and oxygen instead of nitrous oxide and ethyl chloride were used. Use of reducing valves as flowmeter.

155. 1911-12 United States   Karl Connell
Introduction of a gas machine.

156. 1912 United States
Ohio Monovalve anesthesia machine patented and put on the market.

157. 1912 United States   Walter M. Boothby and F. J. Cotton
Introduction of reducing valves and sight-feed apparatus.

158. 1912 United States
First Gwathmey-Woolsey gas machine was built by Langsdorf.

A Chronology of Events

159. 1912 Spain   J. Goyanes
Report of the intra-arterial use of procaine.

160. 1913 Germany   Wilhelm Graef
Ether used in combination with isopral intravenously.

161. 1913 United States   James T. Gwathmey
Introduction of successful narcosis by the rectal route by use of a mixture of ether and oil.

162. 1913 England   H. Noel and H. S. Souttar
Report on the use of paraldehyde intravenously.

163. 1913 Belgium   Danis
Introduction of transsacral anesthesia by injection of the sacral nerves individually through the posterior sacral foramina.

164. 1913 United States   Karl Connell
Demonstration with the anesthetometer that the tension of ether vapor necessary to produce narcosis in a man is about 50 mm. of mercury.

165. 1913 United States   Walter M. Boothby
Worked on ether percentages.

166. 1914 United States   J. T. Gwathmey
Published his textbook, *Anesthesia*.

167. 1914 United States   W. M. Boothby
Accurate calibration furnished for the sight-feed valves. Worked on anesthetic tension.

168. 1914 United States   Richard von Foregger
Constructed a gas-oxygen machine without a reducing valve.

169. 1914 Belgium   A. Hustin
Introduced sodium citrate for transfusion of blood.

170. 1914 Argentina   L. Agote
Introduced sodium citrate for transfusion of blood.

171. 1915 United States   Richard Lewisohn
Introduced sodium citrate for transfusion of blood.

172. 1915 United States
Gwathmey apparatus built by von Foregger without a reducing valve, but with control valves for oxygen and nitrous oxide.

173. 1915 United States
Publication of *American Yearbook of Anesthesia and Analgesia*.

174. 1915 United States   D. E. Jackson
Use of carbon dioxide absorber for general anesthesia.

175. 1916 United States   S. W. Hurwitz
First clinical use of intravenous gum saline.

176. 1916 Switzerland   Elisabeth Bredenfeld
Report on the intravenous use of morphine in connection with scopolamine.

177. 1916 United States   Peyton Rous and J. R. Turner
Transfusion with refrigerated erythrocytes.

178. 1918 United States   Frank C. Mann
Experimental studies on the use of blood substitutes in shock.

179. 1918 United States   A. B. Luckhardt and R. C. Thompson
Discovery of the anesthetic qualities of ethylene.

180. 1918 United States   Peyton Rous and G. W. Wilson
Transfusion of blood, serum, plasma, solution of acacia.

181. 1920 France   Bardet
Experimentation with the anesthetic qualities of somnifene, a derivative of barbituric acid.

182. 1920 England   I. W. Magill
Development of endotracheal anesthesia.

183. 1920 United States   Gaston Labat
Demonstration of local, regional and spinal anesthesia for most operations.

184. 1920 United States   A. E. Guedel
Publication of the *Signs of anesthesia*.

185. 1920 Spain   Fidel Pagés
Development of epidural anesthesia.

186. 1921 Japan   Koshiro Nakagawa
The use of ethyl alcohol intravenously.

187. 1922 United States   Gaston Labat
Published his *Regional anesthesia*.

188. 1922 England   A. G. Levy
Publication of *Chloroform anæsthesia*.

189. 1922 United States
Current Researches in Anesthesia and Analgesia began publication.

190. 1922 England
First meeting of the Section on Anæsthesia of the British Medical Association.

191. 1923 United States   A. B. Luckhardt, J. B. Carter and Isabella Herb
The physiologic effects of ethylene were studied and it was concluded that ethylene was a more effective anesthetic agent than nitrous oxide. First clinical use of ethylene.

192. 1923 England
British Journal of Anæsthesia began publication.

193. 1923 Germany   C. J. Gauss and H. Wieland
Report of the clinical use of narcylen.

194. 1923 Germany
Hans Finsterer's book, *Local anæsthesia*, translated into English.

195. 1923 Canada   W. E. Brown
Experimentation with ethylene as general anesthetic agent.

196. 1923 United States   Ralph M. Waters
Development of soda lime in carbon dioxide absorption.

197. 1923 United States   R. von Foregger
Construction of the Seattle model apparatus which consisted of four hanger yokes, one each for nitrous oxide, ethylene, carbon dioxide and oxygen, and an ether bottle. It was a portable model.

198. 1924 United States   J. A. Heidbrink
Construction of the Lundy-Heidbrink model machine which consisted of two hanger yokes for each of the following gases: nitrous oxide, ethylene, carbon dioxide and oxygen, and an ether bottle. It had an automatic shut-off valve which was adjustable and operated by bag pressure.

199. 1924 Canada   Wesley Bourne
Reported on the mechanism of acidosis in anesthesia.

200. 1924 United States   Albert H. Miller
Observation of thoracic (ascending respiratory) paralysis under general anesthesia.

201. 1924 France   Fredet and Perlis
Introduction of the intravenous use of somnifene.

202. 1924 Germany   L. Bogendörfer
Introduction of dial in intravenous anesthesia.

203. 1925 Switzerland   R. Feissly
Report of clinical use of blood plasma.

204. 1926 Germany   O. Butzengeiger
First clinical use of avertin in rectal anesthesia.

205. 1927 Germany   R. Bumm
Introduction of pernoston, which was the first agent to become widely used in intravenous anesthesia.

206. 1927 United States   N. F. Ockerblad and T. G. Dillon
Use of ephedrine in spinal anesthesia.

207. 1927 Canada
First meeting of the Section on Anæsthesia of the Canadian Medical Association.

208. 1928 Germany
Narkose und Anæsthesie began publication.

209. 1928 United States   Brian C. Sword
Introduction of closed circle (filter) method of anesthesia.

210. 1928 Canada   G. H. W. Lucas and V. E. Henderson
Experimental demonstration of anesthetic qualities of cyclopropane.

211. 1928 United States   Géza de Takáts
Publication of *Local anesthesia*.

212. 1929 Germany
Schmerz united with *Narkose und Anæsthesie*.

213. 1929 Mexico   M. G. Marin
Establishment of the use of ethyl alcohol as an intravenous anesthetic agent.

214. 1929 United States   L. G. Zerfas and colleagues
Report on the intravenous use of sodium amytal, which was used more frequently in the United States from 1929 to 1933 than any other intravenous anesthetic agent.

215. 1929 United States   R. E. Farr
Publication of *Practical local anesthesia*, Ed. 2. Ed. 1 published in 1923.

216. 1930 United States   J. T. Gwathmey
Report of the use of anesthesia in 20,000 obstetric cases. This report greatly stimulated the use of anesthetic agents in labor.

217. 1930 United States   R. M. Waters
Use of cyclopropane as an anesthetic agent in man.

218. 1930 United States   Chauncey D. Leake and M. Y. Chen
The use of divinyl ether as an anesthetic agent was suggested.

219. 1931 United States   J. S. Lundy
Report of the use of nembutal as a hypnotic agent administered intravenously.

220. 1932 England   C. L. Hewer
First edition of *Recent advances in anæsthesia and analgesia*.

221. 1932 Germany   H. Weese and W. Scharpff
Introduction of evipan.

222. 1932 United States
Lundy-Heidbrink kinetometer was placed on market. It was adapted for absorber use.

223. 1933 United States
Bulletin of National Association of Nurse Anesthetists began publication.

224. 1933 United States   Samuel Goldschmidt, I. S. Ravdin, et al.
Recommendation of the anesthetic use of divinyl ether.

225. 1934 United States   J. A. Stiles, R. M. Waters, W. B. Neff and E. A. Rovenstine
Cyclopropane used as an anesthetic. First clinical report.

226. 1934 United States   J. S. Lundy
Introduction of the intravenous use of pentothal sodium for anesthesia.

227. 1934 United States   G. R. Vehrs
Publication of *Spinal anesthesia*.

228. 1935 England
Diploma in anæsthetics instituted by the Royal College of Physicians and Surgeons.

229. 1935 United States   Cecil Striker, Samuel Goldblatt, I. S. Warm and D. E. Jackson
Use of trichlorethylene as an anesthetic.

230. 1935 England   M. D. Nosworthy
Publication of *The theory and practice of anæsthesia*.

231. 1935 Italy
Giornale Italiano di Anestesia e di Analgesia began publication.

A Chronology of Events

232. 1935 France
Inauguration of new journal, *Anesthésie et Analgésie*.

233. 1935 Canada   W. Bourne
Awarded Hickman medal (1st award).

234. 1935 Russia   Filatov and Kartaševskij
Report of successful transfusion of plasma to seventy-two human beings.

235. 1936 United States   A. L. Barach
Report on the therapeutic use of helium.

236. 1937 United States
Formation of the American Board of Anesthesiology, Inc.

237. 1937 United States   A. E. Guedel
Publication of *Inhalation anesthesia*.

238. 1937 United States
Publication began of *Anesthesia Abstracts*.

239. 1937 United States   A. E. Hertzler
Publication of *The technic of local anesthesia*, Ed. 6. Ed. 1 published in 1912.

240. 1938 England   I. W. Magill
Awarded Hickman medal (2nd award).

241. 1938 United States   L. H. Maxson
Publication of *Spinal anesthesia*.

242. 1938 United States   Henry K. Beecher
Publication of *Physiology of anesthesia*.

243. 1939 United States   P. D. Woodbridge, J. W. Horton and Karl Connell
Report on intercoupler.

244. 1939 United States   F. W. Clement
Publication of *Nitrous oxide-oxygen anesthesia*.

245. 1939 Argentina
Publication of *Revista Argentina de Anestesia y Analgesia*.

246. 1940 United States   W. T. Lemmon
Introduction of the continuous method of spinal anesthesia.

247. 1940 United States
Publication of *Anesthesiology* (v. 1, no. 1, July, 1940).

248. 1940 United States   Constance Black, G. E. Shannon and J. C. Krantz
Reported surgical anesthesia with cyprome ether.

249. 1940 United States   B. H. Robbins
Publication of *Cyclopropane anesthesia*.

250. 1940 United States   G. W. Jones, R. E. Kennedy and G. J. Thomas
Suggested prevention of explosions of anesthetic agents by dilution of inert gases.

251. 1941 United States
     Section of Anesthesiology of the American Medical Association held first
     meeting.

252. 1941 United States   A. E. Guedel
     Awarded Hickman medal (3rd award).

253. 1941 United States   N. A. Gillespie
     Publication of *Endotracheal anæsthesia.*

254. 1942 United States   F. M. Allen and others
     Reported on refrigeration anesthesia for amputations.

255. 1942 United States   W. B. Edwards and R. A. Hingson
     Reported on continuous caudal anesthesia in obstetrics.

256. 1942 United States   J. S. Lundy
     Publication of *Clinical anesthesia.*

257. 1942 United States   American Medical Association
     Publication of *Fundamentals of anesthesia.*

258. 1943 England   N. R. James
     Publication of *Regional analgesia for intra-abdominal surgery.*

259. 1944 United States   R. M. Waters
     Awarded Hickman medal (4th award).

260. 1944 United States   R. C. Adams
     Publication of *Intravenous anesthesia.*

261. 1944 United States   P. J. Flagg
     Publication of *The art of anæsthesia*, Ed. 7. Ed. 1 published in 1916.

Sources for a Chronology of Events
RELATING TO
Anesthesiology and Allied Subjects

1. HOLY BIBLE. Genesis II:21. King James version.

2. PRINZ, HERRMANN: Local anesthesia as applied to dentistry. In: Gwathmey, J. T.: Anesthesia. Ed. 2. New York, Macmillan Co., 1924. p. 535.

3. ARCHER, W. H.: The history of anesthesia. Typewritten MS. p. 3.

4. HUME, E. H.: Note on narcotics in ancient Greece and in ancient China. Bull. New York Acad. Med. 10:618-622 (Oct.) 1934.

5. SARTON, GEORGE: Introduction to the history of science. Vol. 1. Baltimore, Williams & Wilkins, 1927. p. 77.

6. HERODOTUS. Book 4, chapter 75.

7. HUME, op. cit., p. 619.

8. GARRISON, F. H.: An introduction to the history of medicine. Ed. 4. Philadelphia, W. B. Saunders Co., 1929. p. 110.

9. PLINY: The historie of the world. Translated by Philemon Holland. London, 1601. Vol. 1, p. 235 (Book 25, chapter 13).

10. HUME, op. cit., p. 621.

11. GARRISON, op. cit., p. 153.

12. Id.

13. KAHLE, PAUL: Anæsthesis in the Arabic medicine. MS. p. 2. Courtesy Dr. J. S. Lundy.

14. SARTON, GEORGE: Introduction to the history of science. Vol. 2, part 1. Baltimore, Published for the Carnegie Institution of Washington by Williams and Wilkins Co., 1931, p. 239.

15. [THEODORIC]: Cyrurgia Theodorici, Liber IV, Cap. VIII. In: Collectio chirurgica Veneta. Venice, 1498, Fol. 146.

16. ENCYCLOPAEDIA BRITANNICA, Ed. 9. New York, Henry G. Allen and Co., 1888, Vol. 8, p. 568.

17. GUY DE CHAULIAC: Chirurgia. Translated by E. Nicaise. Paris, F. Alcan, 1890, p. 436.

18. PARACELSUS: Opera medico-chimica sive paradoxa ... Franckfurt, 1605. p. 125.

19. TALLMADGE, G. K.: The third part of the De extractione of Valerius Cordus. Isis. 7:394-411, 1925.

20. BULLEIN, WILLIAM: Bulleins Bulwarke of defe[n]ce againste all sicknes ... London, Jhon Kyngston, [1562]. Folio 44, recto.

21. PARÉ: Les œuvres. 1575. p. 429.

22. KLEIMAN, MARCOS: Histoire de l'anesthésie. Anesth. et analg. 5:112-138 (Feb.) 1939.

23. Id.

24. GARRISON, op. cit., p. 824.

25. [OLDENBURG, HENRY]: Of a way to conveigh liquors immediatly into the mass of blood. Phil. Tr. Roy. Soc. 1:128-130 (Dec. 4) 1665. See also: [CLARCK, TIMOTHY]: A letter ... concerning some anatomical inventions ... Phil. Tr. Roy. Soc. 3:672-682 (May 18) 1668.

26. ELSHOLTZ, JOHANN SIGISMUND: Clysmatica nova. Berlin. D. Reichel, 1665. 15 pp.

27. [LOWER, RICHARD]: The method observed in transfusing the bloud ... Phil. Tr. Roy. Soc. 1:353-358 (Dec. 17) 1666.

28. DENIS, J[EAN BAPTISTE, and EMMEREZ, ———]: A letter concerning a new way of curing sundry diseases by transfusion of blood ... Phil. Tr. Roy. Soc. 2:489-504 (July 22) 1667.

29. FROBENIUS, W. G.: An account of a spiritus vini æthereus ... Phil. Tr. Roy. Soc. 36:283-289 (Mar.-Apr.) 1730.

30. FÜLÖP-MILLER, RENÉ: Triumph over pain. Translated by Eden and Cedar Paul. New York, The Literary Guild of America, Inc., 1938. p. 32.

31. GARRISON, op. cit., p. 328.

32. Id.

33. ENCYCLOPAEDIA BRITANNICA, Ed. 14. Chicago, Encyclopaedia Britannica, Inc., c1929-1944. Vol. 16. p. 469.

34. PRIESTLEY, JOSEPH: Experiments and observations relating to various branches of natural philosophy. London, 1779-1786. 3 vols. Contained in a letter from Dr. Ingenhousz. Appendix to vol. 1. pp. 474-479.

35. MOORE, JAMES: Method of preventing or diminishing pain in several operations of surgery. London, T. Cadell, 1784. 50 pp.

36. CLARK, A. J.: Aspects of the history of anæsthetics. Brit. M. J. 2:1031 (Nov. 19) 1938.

The History of Surgical Anesthesia

37. BEDDOES, THOMAS, and WATTS, JAMES: Considerations on the medicinal use and on the production of factitious airs. Bristol, 1795.

38. DAVY, HUMPHRY: Researches, chemical and philosophical. London, J. Johnson, 1800. p. 465.

39. FÜLÖP-MILLER, op. cit., p. 425.

40. WILKS, SAMUEL, and BETTANY, G. T.: A biographical history of Guy's Hospital. London, Ward, Lock, Bowden and Co., 1892. pp. 388-389.

41. RICE, N. P.: Trials of a public benefactor ... New York, Pudney and Russell, 1858. p. 82.

42. SERTÜRNER, F. W.: Darstellung der reinen Mohnsäure (Opiumsäure): nebst einer chemischen Untersuchung des Opiums, mit vorzüglicher Hinsicht auf einen darin neu entdeckten Stoff. J. d. Pharm., Leipzig. 14:47-93, 1806.

43. GWATHMEY, J. T.: Anesthesia ... Ed. 2. New York, Macmillan Co., 1924. p. 466.

44. FÜLÖP-MILLER, op. cit., pp. 35-36.

45. FARADAY, MICHAEL: Effects of inhaling the vapors of sulphuric ether. In: Quart. J. Sc. and the Arts. Miscellanea (art. XVI). 4:158-159, 1818.

46. KLEIMAN, op. cit., p. 117.

47. WELLCOME HISTORICAL MEDICAL MUSEUM, LONDON. Souvenir, Henry Hill Hickman, Centenary exhibition, 1830-1930, at the Wellcome historical medical museum. London, Wellcome Foundation, Ltd., 1930. p. 23.

48. ADAMS, R. C.: Intravenous anesthesia ... Thesis, University of Minnesota, Graduate School, 1940. p. 9.

49. GUTHRIE, SAMUEL: New mode of preparing a spirituous solution of chloric ether. Silliman J. 21:64-65, 1832.

50. SOUBEIRAN, EUGÈNE: Recherches sur quelques combinaisons du chlore. Ann. de Chim. 48:113-157, 1831.

51. VON LIEBIG, JUSTUS: Ueber die Verbindungen, welche durch die Einwirkung des Chlors auf Alcohol, Aether, ölbildenes Gas und Essiggeist entstehen. Liebig's Annalen. 1:182-230, 1832.

52. CLARK, op. cit., p. 1031.

53. BARTHOLOW, ROBERTS: Manual of hypodermic medication. Ed. 2. Philadelphia, J. B. Lippincott Co., 1873. 170 pp.

54. ELLIOTSON, JOHN: Numerous cases of surgical operations without pain in the mesmeric state. London, H. Baillière, 1843. 93 pp. Also: ESDAILE, JAMES: Mesmerism in India, and its practical application in surgery and medicine. London, Longman [and others], 1846. 287 pp.

55. LYMAN, H. M.: Artificial anæsthesia and anæsthetics. New York, William Wood and Co., 1881. p. 6.

56. TAYLOR, FRANCES L.: Crawford W. Long and the discovery of ether anesthesia. New York, Paul B. Hoeber, Inc., 1928. p. 44.

57. COLTON, G. Q.: Anæsthesia. Who made and developed this great discovery? New York, A. G. Sherwood and Co., 1886. 15 pp.

58. ARCHER, W. H.: Chronological history of Horace Wells ... Bull. Hist. Med. 7: 1140-1169 (Dec.) 1939.

59. SOIFER, M. E.: Horace Wells. Dental Items of Interest. 61:1131-1142 (Dec.) 1939.

60. HAYWARD, GEORGE: Some account of the first use of sulphuric ether. In: Warren, Edward: Some account of the Letheon. Ed. 2. Boston, Dutton and Wentworth, 1847. p. 47.

61. COCK, F. W.: The first operation under ether in Europe. University College Hospital Magazine. 1:127-144 (Feb.) 1911.

62. Same as 61.

63. CLARK, op. cit., p. 1033.

64. Id.

65. Ibid., p. 1031.

66. PIROGOFF, N. I.: Recherches pratiques et physiologiques sur l'éthérisation. St. Pétersbourg, F. Bellizard & Cie., 1847. 109 pp.

67. SNOW, JOHN: On the inhalation of the vapour of ether in surgical operations ... London, J. Churchill, 1847. 88 pp.

68. SIMPSON, J. Y.: On a new anæsthetic agent, more efficient than sulphuric ether. London M. Gaz. n.s. 5:934-937, 1847.

69. CLARK, op. cit., pp. 1029-1034.

70. REGNAULT, V., and REISET, J.: Recherches chimiques sur la respiration des animaux des diverses classes. Ann. Chim. (Phys.) 26:299-519, 1849.

70A. FLAGG, J. F. B.: Ether and chloroform; their employment in surgery, dentistry, midwifery, therapeutics ... Philadelphia, Lindsay and Blakiston, 1851. 189 pp.

71. SNOW, JOHN: On chloroform and other anæsthetics; their action and administration. Edited, with a memoir of the author, by Benjamin W. Richardson. London, John Churchill, 1858. p. xxxi.

72. ARCHER, Typewritten MS.

73. WOOD, A.: On a new method of treating neuralgia ... Edinburgh M. & S. J. 82: 265-281, 1855.

Sources for a Chronology of Events

74. PRAVAZ, C. G.: Sur un nouveau moyen d'opérer la coagulation du sang dans les artères, applicable à la guérison des anévrismes. Compt. rend. Acad. d. sc. 36: 88-90, 1853.

75. BUMPUS, H. C.: History of regional anesthesia in urology. J. A. M. A. 96:83 (Jan. 10) 1931.

76. RICE, op. cit., p. 85.

77. SNOW, On chloroform and other anæsthetics, 443 pp.

78. BUMPUS, op. cit., p. 83.

79. GWATHMEY, Anesthesia (Ed. 2), p. 23.

80, COLTON, op. cit.

81. MILLER, ALBERT: Personal communication to the author.

82. ARCHER, Typewritten MS., p. 23.

83. Id.

84. British M. J. 2:10 (July 4) 1868.

85. TRENDELENBURG, FRIEDRICH: Tamponnade der Trachea. Arch. f. klin. Chir. 12: 121-133, 1871.

86. BOWDITCH, H. P.: Ueber die Eigenthümlichkeiten der Reizbarkeit, welche die Muskelfasern des Herzens zeigen. Arb. a. d. Physiol. Anst. zu Leipzig. 6:139-176, 1871.

87. MILLER, ALBERT: Life of S. S. White. MS.

88. SPESSA, A.: Modo di rendere insensibile una parte . . . Bull. d. sc. med., Bologna, s. 5. 11:224-226, 1871.

89. ORÉ, P. C.: Des injections intra-veineuses de chloral. Paris, Bull. Soc. Chir. 1:400-412, 1872.

90. BENNETT, ALEXANDER: An experimental inquiry into the physiological actions of . . . cocaine . . . Edinburgh M. J., Pt. 1. 19:323-341 (Oct.) 1873.

90A. BERNARD, CLAUDE: Leçons sur les anesthésiques et sur l'asphyxie . . . Paris, J. B. Baillière et Fils, 1875. vii, 536 pp.

91. CLOVER, J. T.: On an apparatus for administering nitrous oxide gas and ether, singly or combined. Brit. M. J. 2:74-75 (July 15) 1876.

92. GWATHMEY, Anesthesia (Ed. 2), p. 25.

93. VON ANREP, V.: Ueber die physiologische Wirkung des Cocaïn. Arch. f. d. ges. Physiol. 21:38-77, 1880.

94. MACEWEN, WILLIAM: Clinical observations on the introduction of tracheal tubes by the mouth instead of performing tracheotomy or laryngotomy. Brit. M. J. 2: 122-124 (July 24); 163-165 (July 31), 1880.

95. FÜLÖP-MILLER, op. cit., p. 427.

96. ARCHER, Typewritten MS., p. 28.

97. MOUTARD-MARTIN, R., and RICHET, CHARLES: Recherches expérimentales sur la polyurie. Arch. de physiol. 2 s. 8:1-48, 1881.

98. ARCHER, Typewritten MS., p. 29.

99. TJOMSLAND, ANNA: Cyclopropane. Thos. A. Edison, Inc., 1937. 5 pp.

100. KOLLER, CARL: Vorläufige Mittheilung über locale Anästhesirung am Auge. Klin. Monatsb. f. Augenh. 22:Beilageheft, pp. 60-63, 1884.

101. MOLLIÈRE, DANIEL: Note sur l'éthérisation par la voie rectale. Lyon méd. 45:419-423 (Mar. 30) 1884.

102. HALSTED, W. S.: Practical comments on the use and abuse of cocaine . . . New York M. J. 42:294-295 (Sept. 12) 1885.

103. CORNING, J. L.: Spinal anæsthesia and local medication of the cord. New York M. J. 42:483-485 (Oct. 31) 1885.

104. ——: Local anæsthesia in general medicine and surgery . . . New York, D. Appleton and Co. [c1885]. 103 pp.

105. ——: A further contribution on local medication of the spinal cord . . . M. Rec. 33:291-293 (Mar. 17) 1888.

106. HEWITT, F. W.: The administration of nitrous oxide and ether . . . Brit. M. J. 2:452-454 (Aug. 27) 1887.

107. REDARD, P.: Du chlorure d'éthyle comme anesthésique local. Verhandl. d. x. internat. med. Cong. 1890, Berl. 5:14 Abth. 71-73, 1891.

108. HEWITT, F. W.: Select methods in the administration of nitrous oxide and ether; a handbook for practitioners and students. London, Baillière, Tindall and Cox [1888]. 48 pp.

109. ARCHER, Typewritten MS., p. 30.

110. GIESEL, F.: Benzollpseudotropein [tropacocaine]. Pharm. Ztg. 36:419 (July 4) 1891.

111. QUINCKE, H.: Die Lumbalpunction des Hydrocephalus. Berl. klin. Wchnschr. 28: 929-933 (Sept. 21); 965-968 (Sept. 28) 1891.

112. SCHLEICH, [C. L.]: Infiltrationsanästhesie . . . Verhandl. d. deutsch. Gesellsch. f. Chir. 21:121-127 (4 Sitzungstag 11 Juni) 1892.

113. HEWITT, F. W.: Anæsthetics and their administration. London, Charles Griffin and Co., 1893. xx, 357 pp.

114. Id.

115. GARRISON, op. cit., p. 862.

116. KLEIMAN, op. cit., p. 133.

The History of Surgical Anesthesia

117. BEECHER, H. K.: The first anesthesia records. Surg., Gynec. & Obst. 71:689-693 (Nov.) 1940.

118. KLEIMAN, op. cit., p. 134.

119. KIRSTEIN, ALFRED: Autoskopie des Larynx und der Trachea. Berl. klin. Wchnschr. 32:476-478, 1895.

120. ABEL, J. J., and CRAWFORD, A. C.: On the blood-pressure-raising constituent of the suprarenal capsule. Johns Hopkins Hosp. Bull. 8:151-157 (July) 1897.

121. BUMPUS, op. cit., p. 84.

122. MATAS, RUDOLPH: Intralaryngeal insufflation . . . J. A. M. A. 34:1468-1473 (June 9) 1900.

123. BIER, AUGUST: Versuche über Cocainisirung des Rückenmarkes. Deutsche Ztschr. f. Chir. 51:361-369 (Apr.) 1899.

124. MILLER, ALBERT: Personal communication to the author.

125. TUFFIER: Analgésie chirurgicale par l'injection sous-arachnoïdienne lombaire de cocaïne. Compt. rend. Soc. de biol. 51: 882-884, 1899.

126. ADAMS, Intravenous anesthesia . . ., p. 10.

127. FÜLÖP-MILLER, op. cit., p. 429.

128. SCHLEICH, C. L.: Schmerzlose Operationen. Vierte . . . Auflage. Berlin, Springer, 1899. 303 pp.

128A. TAIT, DUDLEY, and CAGLIERI, GUIDO: Experimental and clinical notes on the sub-arachnoid space. J. A. M. A. 35:6-10 (July 7) 1900.

129. [MATAS, RUDOLPH]: Report of sucessful spinal anesthesia. J. A. M. A. 33:1659 (Dec. 30) 1899.

130. CATHELIN, M. F.: Une nouvelle voie d'injection rachidienne. Compt. rend. Soc. de biol. 53:452-453 (April 27) 1901. Also: SICARD, M. A.: Les injections médicamenteuses extra-durales . . . Compt. rend. Soc. de biol. 53:396-398 (April 20) 1901.

131. ARCHER, Typewritten MS.

132. FISCHER, EMIL, and MERING, J.: Ueber eine neue Classe von Schlafmitteln. Therap. d. Gegenw. n.s. 5:97-101, 1903.

133. FOURNEAU, E.: Sur quelques aminoalcools à fonction alcoolique tertiare du type. Compt. rend. Acad. d. sc. Paris. 138: 766-768, 1904.

134. BUMPUS, op. cit., p. 84.

135. KRAVKOFF, N. P.: Ueber die Hedonal-Chloroform-Narkose. Arch. f. exper. Path. u. Pharmakol., Suppl. 317-326, 1908.

136. HEIDBRINK, J. A.: Personal communication to the author.

137. MAGAW, ALICE: A review of over 14,000 surgical anesthetics. Surg., Gynec. & Obst. 3:795-799, 1906.

138. McKESSON, E. I.: Blood pressure in general anesthesia. Am. J. Surg. Anesth. suppl. 30:2-5 (Jan.) 1916.

139. BUMPUS, op. cit., p. 84.

140. BARTHÉLEMY and DUFOUR: L'anesthésie dans la chirurgie de la face. Presse méd. 15:475-476 (July 27) 1907.

141. GUTHRIE, C. C., and PIKE, F. H.: The relation of the activity of the excised mammalian heart to pressure in the coronary vessels and to its nutrition. Am. J. Physiol. 18:14-38, 1907.

142. GWATHMEY, J. T.: General anesthesia. Hygeia. 14:109-112 (June) 1936.

143. CROCKER, WILLIAM, and KNIGHT, L. I.: Effect of illuminating gas and ethylene on flowering carnations. Botanical Gaz. 46: 259-276 (Oct.) 1908.

144. CRILE, G. W.: Surgical aspects of Graves' disease with reference to the psychic factor. Ann. Surg. 47:864-869 (June) 1908.

145. GOYANES, J.: Un nuevo método de anestesia regional. Rev. clin. de Madrid. 1909. p. 12.

146. ADAMS, Intravenous anesthesia . . ., p. 11.

147. GUEDEL, A. E.: Nitrous oxide air anesthesia self administered in obstetrics; a preliminary report. Indianapolis M. J. 14: 476-479 (Oct.) 1911.

148. ADAMS, Intravenous anesthesia . . ., p. 10.

149. MELTZER, S. J., and AUER, JOHN: Continuous respiration without respiratory movements. J. Exper. Med. 11:622-625 (July) 1909.

150. ELSBERG, C. A.: The value of continuous intratracheal insufflation of air (Meltzer) in thoracic surgery: with description of an apparatus. M. Rec. 77:493-495 (Mar. 19) 1910.

151. KÜMMELL, R.: Einige Erfahrungen über die Skopolamin-Morphium-Narkose. Klin. Monatsbl. f. Augenh. 48:472-476, 1910.

152. ARCHER, Typewritten MS., p. 36.

153. GATCH, W. D.: Nitrous oxid-oxygen anesthesia by the method of rebreathing: with especial reference to the prevention of surgical shock. J. A. M. A. 54:775-780 (Mar. 5) 1910.

154. ARCHER, Typewritten MS., p. 36.

155. HEIDBRINK, J. A.: Personal communication to the author.

156. OHIO CHEMICAL CO.: Letter from E. H. Cook.

157. GWATHMEY, J. T.: Personal communication to the author.

158. GWATHMEY, J. T.: Personal communication to the author.

159. ADAMS, Intravenous anesthesia..., p. 12.

160. GRAEF, WILHELM: Bericht über Erfahrungen mit den intravenösen Aether- und Isopral-Aether-Narkosen. Beitr. z. klin. Chir., Tübingen. 83:173-211 (Feb.) 1913.

161. GWATHMEY, J. T.: Oil-ether anesthesia. Lancet. 2:1756-1758 (Dec. 20) 1913.

162. NOEL, H., and SOUTTAR, H. S.: The anæsthetic effects of the intravenous injection of paraldehyde. Ann. Surg. 57:64-67 (Jan.) 1913.

163. BUMPUS, op. cit., p. 87.

164. BOOTHBY, W. M.: Ether percentages. J. A. M. A. 61:830-834 (Sept. 13) 1913.

165. Id.

166. GWATHMEY, J. T.: Anesthesia. New York, D. Appleton Co., 1914. xxxii, 945 pp.

167. BOOTHBY, W. M.: The determination of the anæsthetic tension of ether vapor in man... J. Pharmacol. & Exper. Therap. 5:379-392 (March) 1914.

168. GWATHMEY, J. T.: Personal communication to the author.

169. HUSTIN, A.: Principe d'une nouvelle méthode de transfusion muqueuse. J. de méd. de Bruxelles. 19:436-439 (Aug.) 1914.

170. AGOTE, LUIS: Un nuevo método de transfusion de sangre. An. Inst. modelo de clin. méd. 1:25-30 (Jan.) 1914-15.

171. LEWISOHN, RICHARD: A new and greatly simplified method of blood transfusion. M. Rec. 87:141-142 (Jan. 23) 1915.

172. GWATHMEY, J. T.: Personal communication to the author.

174. JACKSON, D. E.: A new method for the production of general analgesia and anesthesia with a description of the apparatus used. J. Lab. & Clin. Med. 1:1-12 (Oct.) 1915.

175. HURWITZ, S. W.: Intravenous injections of colloidal solutions of acacia in hemorrhage. J. A. M. A. 68:699-701 (Mar. 3) 1917.

176. BREDENFELD, ELISABETH: Die intravenöse Narkose mit Arzneigemischen. Ztschr. f. exper. Path. u. Therap. 18:80-90 (Apr. 4) 1916.

177. ROUS, PEYTON, and TURNER, J. R.: Preservation of living blood cells in vitro. J. Exper. Med. 23:219-237; 239-248 (Feb.) 1916.

178. MANN, F. C.: Further experimental study of surgical shock. J. A. M. A. 71:1184-1188, 1918.

179. LUCKHARDT, A. B., and CARTER, J. B.: Ethylene as a gas anesthetic; preliminary communication. J. A. M. A. 80:1440-1442 (May 19) 1923.

180. ROUS, PEYTON, and WILSON, G. W.: Fluid substances for transfusion after hemorrhage. J. A. M. A. 70:219-222, 1918.

181. KLEIMAN, op. cit., p. 137.

182. MAGILL, I. W.: Development of endotracheal anæsthesia. Proc. Roy. Soc. Med. Section of Anæsthetics. 22:83-88 (Nov. 2) 1928.

183. LUNDY, J. S.: Personal communication to the author.

184. GUEDEL, A. E.: Third stage ether anesthesia ... Nat. Anesth. Res. Soc. Bull. No. 3 (May) 1920. 4 pp.

185. PAGÉS, FIDEL: Anestesia metamérica. Rev. san. mil., Madrid. 11:351-365 (June) 385-396 (July) 1921.

186. NAKAGAWA, KOSHIRO: Experimentelle Studien über die intravenöse Infusionsnarkose mittels Alkohols. Tohoku J. Exper. Med. 2:81-126 (May 3) 1921.

187. LABAT, GASTON: Regional anesthesia; its technic and clinical application. Philadelphia, W. B. Saunders Co., 1922.

188. LEVY, A. G.: Chloroform anæsthesia. London, John Bale, Sons and Danielsson, 1922. vii, 159 pp.

191. LUCKHARDT, A. B., and CARTER, J. B.: The physiologic effects of ethylene. J. A. M. A. 80:1440-1442 (May 19) 1923. See also: HERB, ISABELLA: Ethylene: notes taken from the clinical records. Anesth. & Analg. 2:230-232 (Dec.) 1923.

193. GAUSS, C. J., and WIELAND, HERMANN: Ein neues Betäubungsverfahren. Klin. Wchnschr. 2:113 (Jan. 15); 158 (Jan. 22) 1923.

194. FINSTERER, HANS: Local anæsthesia methods and results in abdominal surgery. Translated by J. P. F. Burke. New York, Rebman, [c1923]. 349 pp.

195. BROWN, W. E.: Preliminary report; experiments with ethylene as a general anæsthetic. Canad. M. A. J. 13:210 (Mar.) 1923.

196. WATERS, R. M.: Clinical scope and utility of carbon dioxid filtration in inhalation anesthesia. Anesth. & Analg. 3:20-22; 26 (Feb.) 1924.

197. LUNDY, J. S.: Personal communication to the author.

198. HEIDBRINK, J. A.: Personal communication to the author.

199. BOURNE, WESLEY, and STEHLE, R. L.: The excretion of phosphoric acid during anesthesia. J. A. M. A. 83:117-118 (July 12) 1924.

The History of Surgical Anesthesia

200. MILLER, A. H.: Ascending respiratory paralysis under general anesthesia. J. A. M. A. 84:201-202 (Jan. 17) 1925.

201. ADAMS, Intravenous anesthesia..., p. 13.

202. BOGENDÖRFER, L.: Ueber lösliche Schlafmittel der Barbitursäurereihe (Dial löslich.) Schweiz. med. Wchnschr. 54:437-438 (May 8) 1924.

203. FEISSLY, R.: Beiträge zum Wesen und zur Therapie der Hämophilie. Jahrb. f. Kinderh. 110:297-308 (Nov.) 1925.

204. BUTZENGEIGER, O.: Klinische Erfahrungen mit Avertin (E 107). Deutsche med. Wchnschr. 53:712-713 (Apr. 22) 1927.

205. ADAMS, Intravenous anesthesia..., p. 13.

206. OCKERBLAD, N. F., and DILLON, T. G.: Use of ephedrine in spinal anesthesia. J. A. M. A. 88:1135-1136 (April 9) 1927.

209. SWORD, B. C.: The closed circle method of administration of gas anesthesia. Anesth. & Analg. 9:198-202 (Sept.-Oct.) 1930.

210. LUCAS, G. H. W., and HENDERSON, V. E.: A new anæsthetic gas: cyclopropane; a preliminary report. Canad. M. A. J. 21: 173-175 (Aug.) 1929.

211. DE TAKÁTS, GÉZA: Local anesthesia. Philadelphia, W. B. Saunders Co., 1928. 221 pp.

213. ADAMS, Intravenous anesthesia..., p. 11.

214. ZERFAS, L. G.; McCALLUM, J. T. C.; SHONLE, H. A.; SWANSON, E. E.; SCOTT, J. P., and CLOWES, G. H. A.: Induction of anesthesia in man by intravenous injection of sodium iso-amyl-ethyl barbiturate. Proc. Soc. Exper. Biol. & Med. 26:399-403 (Feb.) 1929.

215. FARR, R. E.: Practical local anesthesia and its surgical technic. Ed. 2. Philadelphia, Lea and Febiger, 1929. 611 pp.

216. GWATHMEY, J. T.: Obstetrical analgesia; a further study, based on more than twenty thousand cases. Surg., Gynec. & Obst. 51:190-195 (Aug.) 1930.

217. WATERS, R. M., and SCHMIDT, E. R.: Cyclopropane anesthesia. J. A. M. A. 103: 975-983 (Sept. 29) 1934.

218. LEAKE, C. D., and CHEN, M. Y.: The anesthetic properties of certain unsaturated ethers. Proc. Soc. Exper. Biol. & Med. 28: 151-154 (Nov.) 1930.

219. LUNDY, J. S.: Experience with sodium ethyl (1-methylbutyl) barbiturate (nembutal) in more than 2,300 cases. S. Clin. North America. 11:909-915 (Aug.) 1931.

220. HEWER, C. L.: Recent advances in anæsthesia and analgesia. London, Churchill, 1932. 187 pp.

221. WEESE, H., and SCHARPFF, W.: Evipan, ein neuartiges Einschlafmittel. Deutsche med. Wchnschr. 2:1205-1207 (July 29) 1932.

222. HEIDBRINK, J. A.: Personal communication to the author.

224. GOLDSCHMIDT, SAMUEL; RAVDIN, I. S.; LUCKÉ, BALDUIN; MULLER, G. P.; JOHNSTON, C. G., and RUIGH, W. L.: Divinyl ether; experimental and clinical studies. J. A. M. A. 102:21-26 (Jan. 6) 1934.

225. STILES, J. A.; NEFF, W. B.; ROVENSTINE, E. A., and WATERS, R. M.: Cyclopropane as an anesthetic agent: a preliminary clinical report. Anesth. & Analg. 13:56-60 (Mar.-Apr.) 1934.

226. LUNDY, J. S.: Intravenous anesthesia: preliminary report of the use of two new thiobarbiturates. Proc. Staff Meet., Mayo Clin. 10:536-543 (Aug. 21) 1935.

227. VEHRS, G. R.: Spinal anesthesia, technic and clinical application. St. Louis, C. V. Mosby Co., 1934. 269 pp.

228. GILLESPIE, N. A.: Personal communication to the author.

229. STRIKER, CECIL; GOLDBLATT, SAMUEL; WARM, I. S., and JACKSON, D. E.: Clinical experiences with the use of trichlorethylene in the production of over 300 analgesias and anesthesias. Anesth. & Analg. 14:68-71 (Mar.-Apr.) 1935.

230. NOSWORTHY, M. D.: The theory and practice of anæsthesia. London, Hutchinson, 1935. 223 pp.

234. FILATOV, A., and KARTAŠEVSKIJ, N. G.: Die Transfusion von menschlichem Blutplasma als blutstillendes Mittel. Zentralbl. f. Chir. 62:441-445 (Feb. 23) 1935.

235. BARACH, A. L.: The therapeutic use of helium. J. A. M. A. 107:1273-1280 (Oct. 17) 1936.

237. GUEDEL, A. E.: Inhalation anesthesia: a fundamental guide. New York, Macmillan Co., 1937. 172 pp.

239. HERTZLER, A. E.: The technic of local anesthesia. Ed. 6. St. Louis, C. V. Mosby Co., 1937. 284 pp.

241. MAXSON, L. H.: Spinal anesthesia. Philadelphia, J. B. Lippincott Co., 1938. xxii, 409 pp.

242. BEECHER, H. K.: The physiology of anesthesia. New York, Oxford University Press, 1938. xiv, 388 pp.

243. WOODBRIDGE, P. D.; HORTON, J. W., and CONNELL, KARL: Prevention of ignition of anesthetic gases by static spark. J. A. M. A. 113:740-744 (Aug. 26) 1939.

244. CLEMENT, F. W.: Nitrous oxide-oxygen anesthesia. Philadelphia, Lea and Febiger, 1939. 274 pp.

246. LEMMON, W. T.: A method for continuous spinal anesthesia: a preliminary report. Ann. Surg. 111:141-144 (Jan.) 1940.

248. BLACK, CONSTANCE; SHANNON, G. E., and KRANTZ, J. C., JR.: Studies with cyclopropyl methyl ether (cyprome ether) in man. Anesthesiology. 1:274-279 (Nov.) 1940.

249. ROBBINS, B. H.: Cyclopropane anesthesia. Baltimore, Williams and Wilkins, 1940. 175 pp.

250. JONES, G. W.; KENNEDY, R. E., and THOMAS, G. J.: Explosive properties of cyclopropane . . . U. S. Dept. of the Interior, Bureau of Mines. Report of Investigations. R. I. 3511 (May), 1940. 17 pp.

253. GILLESPIE, N. A.: Endotracheal anæsthesia. Madison, Wisconsin, University of Wisconsin Press, 1941. 187 pp.

254. ALLEN, F. M.; CROSSMAN, L. W.; HURLEY, VINCENT; WARDEN, C. E., and RUGGIERO, WILFRED: Refrigeration anesthesia. J. Internat. Coll. of Surgeons. 5: 125-131 (Mar.-April) 1942.

255. EDWARDS, W. B., and HINGSON, R. A.: Continuous caudal anesthesia in obstetrics. Am. J. Surg. n.s. 57:459-464 (Sept.) 1942.

256. LUNDY, J. S.: Clinical anesthesia . . . Philadelphia, W. B. Saunders Co., 1942. xxix, 771 pp.

257. NATIONAL RESEARCH COUNCIL. Subcommittee on anesthesia. Fundamentals of anesthesia, an outline. Chicago, American Medical Association, 1942. 217 pp.

258. JAMES, N. R.: Regional analgesia for intra-abdominal surgery, with special reference to amethocaine hydrochloride. London, Churchill, 1943. 57 pp.

260. ADAMS, R. C.: Intravenous anesthesia. New York, Paul B. Hoeber, Inc., c1944. xiv, 1 l., 663 pp.

261. FLAGG, P. J.: The art of anæsthesia. Ed. 7. Philadelphia, J. B. Lippincott Co., 1944. 519 pp.

III

Selected References for
A History of Surgical Anesthesia

ARRANGED BY SUBJECT

BIBLIOGRAPHY

BIBLIOTHECA OSLERIANA, a catalogue of books, illustrating the history of medicine and science, collected, arranged and annotated by Sir William Osler . . . Oxford, Clarendon Press, 1929. Anæsthesia. pp. 135-151.

CLENDENING, LOGAN: Literature and material on anæsthesia in the library of medical history of the University of Kansas Medical Department, Kansas City, Kansas. Bull. M. Library A. 33:124-138 (Jan.) 1945.

CHRONOLOGY

KEYS, T. E.: A chronology of events relating to anesthesiology and allied subjects. In: LUNDY, J. S.: Clinical anesthesia . . . Philadelphia, W. B. Saunders Co., 1942. pp. 705-717.

GENERAL REFERENCES

ANÆSTHETIC AGENTS. Tr. A. M. A. 1:176-224, 1848.

ARCHER, W. H.: The history of anesthesia. Proc. Dental Centenary Celebration. (Mar.) 1940. pp. 333-363.

BABCOCK, MYRA E.: Brief outline of the history of anesthesia. Grace Hosp. Bull. 10:16-21 (Apr.) 1926.

BAUR, MARGUERITE: Recherches sur l'histoire de l'anesthésie avant 1846. Janus. 31:24-39, 63-90, 124-137, 170-182, 213-225, 264-270, 1927. Especially good for references to early anesthetic sponges.

BEECHER, H. K.: The physiology of anesthesia. New York, Oxford University Press, 1938. xiv, 388 pp. Excellent bibliography pp. 313-358.

BETCHER, A. M.; WRIGHT, L. H.; WOOD, P. M., and CILIBERTI, B. J.: The New York State story of anesthesiology, 1807-1957. New York State J. Med. 58: 1556-1572 (May 1) 1958. Excellent.

BIGELOW, H. J.: A history of the discovery of modern anæsthesia. Am. J. M. Sc. 141:164-184 (Jan.) 1876.

——: Surgical anæsthesia; addresses and other papers. Boston, Little, Brown and Co., 1900. viii, 378 pp. Contains articles by Dr. Bigelow concerning the discovery of anesthesia.

BOURNE, WESLEY: De officiis in anæsthesia. J. Michigan M. Soc. 41:129-134 (Feb.) 1942.

Selected References Arranged by Subject

BROWN, GILBERT: The E. H. Embley Memorial lecture. The evolution of anæsthesia. M. J. Australia. 1:209-220 (Feb. 11) 1939.

BULLEIN, WILLIAM: Bulleins Bulwarke of defe[n]ce againste all sicknes, sornes, and woundes, that dooe daily assaulte mankinde . . . Doen by Williyam Bulleyn, and ended this Marche, anno salutis, 1562. London, Jhon Kyngston, [1562]. Folio consisting of 251 leaves with various foliations. The Booke of Simples (fol. 44, recto) contains, perhaps, the first mention in an English printed book of an anesthetic agent.

CLARK, A. J.: Aspects of the history of anæsthetics. Brit. M. J. 2:1029-1034 (Nov. 19) 1938.

CLAYE, A. M.: The evolution of obstetric analgesia. New York, Oxford University Press, 1939. 103 pp.

DUNCUM, B. M.: An outline of the history of anaesthesia, 1846-1900. Brit. Med. Bull. 4, no. 2:120-128, 1946.

FIGUIER: Exposition et histoire des principales découvertes scientifiques modernes. Ed. 3. Paris, 1854. 3 v. Vol. 3 contains a 120-odd page history of anesthesia, perhaps the first *general* history of the subject.

FORD, WILLIAM W.: A prelude to ether anesthesia. New England J. M. 231:219-223 (Aug. 10) 1944.

FÜLÖP-MILLER, RENÉ: Triumph over pain. Translated by Eden and Cedar Paul. New York, The Literary Guild of America, Inc., 1938. 438 pp.

FULTON, J. F., and STANTON, M. E., comps.: The centennial of surgical anesthesia, an annotated catalogue of the books and pamphlets bearing on the early history of surgical anesthesia, exhibited at the Yale Medical Library, October, 1946 . . . New York, Henry Schuman, 1946. xv, 102 pp.

GARRISON, F. H.: An introduction to the history of medicine. Ed. 4. Philadelphia, W. B. Saunders Co., 1929. 996 pp.

GUEDEL, A. E.: Inhalation anesthesia, a fundamental guide. New York, Macmillan Co., 1937. 172 pp.

GWATHMEY, J. T.: Anesthesia. Ed. 1. New York, D. Appleton Co., 1914. xxxii, 945 pp. This edition contains a list of anesthetics compiled by Dr. Charles Baskerville, pp. 688-840. (Some 400 drugs with historical data.)

——: Anesthesia . . . Ed. 2. New York, Macmillan Co., 1924. 799 pp. Chapter I, The history of anesthesia, pp. 1-29. Many other chapters have useful historical material.

HEWITT, F. W.: Anæsthetics and their administration. London, Charles Griffin and Co., 1893. xx, 357 pp. Contains reports of the work of the Hyderabad Chloroform Commission.

KEYS, T. E.: The development of anesthesia. Anesthesiology. 2:552-574 (Sept.) 1941; 3:11-23 (Jan.); 282-294 (May); 650-659 (Nov.) 1942 and 4:409-429 (July) 1943.

KLEIMAN, MARCOS: Histoire de l'anesthésie. Anesth. et analg. 5:112-138 (Feb.) 1939.

The History of Surgical Anesthesia

LAFARGUE, G. V.: Note sur les effets de quelques médicaments introduits sous l'épiderme. Compt. rend. Acad. d. sc. 3:397-398; 434 (Sept. 19) 1836. Injected morphine paste subcutaneously.

LEAKE, C. D.: The historical development of surgical anesthesia. Scient. Monthly. 20:304-328 (Mar.) 1925.

LUNDY, J. S.: Clinical anesthesia . . . Philadelphia, W. B. Saunders Co., 1942. xxix, 771 pp.

MILLER, A. H.: The origin of the word "anæsthesia." Boston M. & S. J. 197:1218-1222 (Dec. 29) 1927.

ROBINSON, VICTOR: Pathfinders of medicine. New York, Medical Life Press, 1929. 810 pp.

SERTÜRNER, F. W.: Ueber das Morphium, eine neue salzfähige Grundlage, und die Mekonsäure als Hauptbestandtheil des Opiums. Gilbert's Ann. d. Physik. 55:56-89, 1817. Discovery of morphine (1806).

SPESSA, A.: Modo di rendere insensibile una parte nella quale devesi praticare qualche atto operatorio. Bull. d. sc. med., Bologna. s. 5. 11:224-226, 1871. Injection of morphine into a fistulous tract prior to surgery.

WATERS, R. M.: The evolution of anesthesia I & II. Proc. Staff Meet., Mayo Clin. 17:428-432 (July 15); 440-445 (July 29) 1942.

WELCH, W. H.: A consideration of the introduction of surgical anæsthesia. [Boston, The Barta Press, 1908?] 24 pp. First Ether Day address. Written from memory.

ETHER

BIGELOW, H. J.: Ether and chloroform: a compendium of their history, surgical use, dangers, and discovery. Boston, David Clapp, 1848. 18 pp.

——: Insensibility during surgical operations produced by inhalation. Boston M. & S. J. 35:309-317 (Nov. 18) 1846. Excellent account of Morton's successful demonstration.

BOOTHBY, W. M.: Ether percentages. J. A. M. A. 61:830-834 (Sept. 13) 1913.

BOURNE, WESLEY: On the effects of acetaldehyde, ether peroxide, ethyl mercaptan, ethyl sulphide, and several ketones—di-methyl, ethyl-methyl, and di-ethyl—when added to anæsthetic ether. J. Pharmacol. & Exper. Therap. 28:409-432 (Sept.) 1926. Small concentrations of impurities not harmful in ether anesthesia.

CHANNING, WALTER: A treatise on etherization in childbirth. Boston, W. D. Ticknor and Co., 1848. viii, 400 pp.

FARADAY, MICHAEL: Effects of inhaling the vapors of sulphuric ether. In: Quart. J. Sc. and the Arts. Miscellanea (art. XVI). 4:158-159, 1818.

[JACKSON, C. T.]: . . . First practical use of ether in surgical operations. Boston M. & S. J. 64:229-231 (April 11) 1861. Jackson's support of Long.

——: A manual of etherization: containing directions for the ėmployment of ether, chloroform, and other anæsthetics by inhalation . . . Boston, J. B. Mansfield, 1861. 134 pp.

LEAKE, C. D.: Valerius Cordus and the discovery of ether. Isis. 7:14-24, 1925. Portrait of Valerius Cordus and three other plates.

Selected References Arranged by Subject

LONG, C. W.: An account of the first use of sulphuric ether by inhalation as an anæsthetic in surgical operations. South. M. & S. J. n.s. 5:705-713 (Dec.) 1849. Long first used ether on March 30, 1842.

LYMAN, H. M.: Artificial anæsthesia and anæsthetics. New York, William Wood and Co., 1881. p. 6. See also: LYMAN, H. M.: The discovery of anæsthesia. Virginia M. Monthly. 13:369-392 (Sept.) 1886. According to Lyman, William E. Clarke administered ether for anesthesia two months· prior to Long for a painless extraction of a tooth by Dr. Elijah Pope for Miss Hobbie. (Jan. 1842 at Rochester, New York.)

MEDICAL INTELLIGENCE: Insensibility during surgical operations produced by inhalation. Boston M. & S. J. 35:413-414 (Dec. 16) 1846.

MORTON, W. J.: The invention of anæsthetic inhalation; or, "Discovery of anæsthesia." New York, D. Appleton and Co., 1880. 48 pp.

[MORTON, W. T. G.]: Circular. Morton's Letheon. Boston, Dutton and Wentworth, [1846]. 14 pp. Morton keeps the identity of his preparation a secret.

——: The first use of ether as an anesthetic. At the Battle of the Wilderness in the Civil War. J. A. M. A. 42:1068-1073 (April 23) 1904. Written by Morton but not published until 1904.

[——]: Letter from Dr. Wm. T. G. Morton. Am. J. Dent. Sc. 8:56-77 (Oct.) 1847. Dr. Morton's story of the discovery.

——: On the physiological effects of sulphuric ether, and its superiority to chloroform. Boston, D. Clapp, 1850. 24 pp.

——: Remarks on the proper mode of administering sulphuric ether by inhalation. Boston, Dutton and Wentworth, 1847. 44 pp. Morton discloses the name of his preparation.

——: Statements, supported by evidence, of W. T. G. Morton, M.D., on his claim to the discovery of anæsthetic properties of ether . . . Washington, 1853. 582 pp. Submitted to the U. S. Senate by Mr. Davis of Massachusetts.

OSLER, WILLIAM: The first printed documents relating to modern surgical anæsthesia. Proc. Roy. Soc. Med. (Sect. Hist. Med.). 11:65-69 (May 15) 1918. Reprinted in Ann. M. Hist. 1:329-332, "1917" (1918).

RAPER, H. R.: A review of Crawford W. Long centennial anniversary celebrations. Bull. Hist. Med. 13:340-356 (March) 1943.

RICE, N. P.: Trials of a public benefactor, as illustrated in the discovery of etherization. New York, Pudney and Russell, 1858. p. 82. Morton.

SNOW, JOHN: On the inhalation of the vapour of ether in surgical operations: containing a description of the various stages of etherization, and a statement of the result of nearly eighty operations in which ether has been employed in St. George's and University College hospitals. London, J. Churchill, 1847. 88 pp.

STEHLE, R. L., and BOURNE, WESLEY: The anesthetic properties of pure ether. J. A. M. A. 79:375-376 (July 29) 1922. Conclusion: Pure ether possesses to the highest degree the anesthetic properties usually ascribed to it.

TALLMADGE, G. K.: The third part of the *De extractione* of Valerius Cordus. Isis. 7:394-411, 1925. Translation of Valerius Cordus's work on the synthesis of ether.

TAYLOR, FRANCES L.: Crawford W. Long and the discovery of ether anesthesia. New York, Paul B. Hoeber, Inc., 1928. p. 81.

THOMS, HERBERT: "Anesthésie à la Reine," a chapter in the history of anesthesia. Am. J. Obst. & Gynec. 40:340-346 (Aug.) 1940. Administration of ether between each pain in natural labor. First printed April 14, 1847 in the Boston M. & S. J.

TURNER, MATTHEW: An account of the extraordinary medicinal fluid, called aether ... London, J. Wilkie, [1743?]. 16 pp.

WARREN, EDWARD: Some account of the Letheon; or who was the discoverer. Ed. 2. Boston, Dutton and Wentworth, 1847. 79 pp. This edition was the first to contain Holmes's famous communication suggesting the terms "anæsthesia" and "anæsthetic."

WARREN, J. C.: Etherization with surgical remarks. Boston, W. D. Ticknor and Co., 1848. v, 100 pp.

——: Inhalation of ethereal vapor for the prevention of pain in surgical operations. Boston M. & S. J. 35:375-379 (Dec. 9) 1846. The surgeon's account of the first successful demonstration.

YOUNG, H. H.: Long, the discoverer of anæsthesia. Bull. Johns Hopkins Hosp. 8:174-184 (Aug.-Sept.) 1897. Documentary evidence. Contains a printing of Long's original paper read before the Georgia State Medical Society in 1852; this is an expansion of Long's paper printed in 1849.

CHLOROFORM

ANÆSTHETICS—Third interim report of the committee, consisting of Dr. A. D. Waller (chairman), Sir Frederic Hewitt (secretary), Dr. Blumfield, Mr. J. A. Gardner, and Dr. G. A. Buckmaster, appointed to acquire further knowledge, clinical and experimental, concerning anæsthetics—especially chloroform, ether, and alcohol—with special reference to deaths by or during anæsthesia and their possible diminution. Report of the British Association for the Advancement of Science. 80:154-171, 1911. (Published in 1912 by John Murray, London.)

BIGELOW, H. J.: Ether and chloroform: a compendium of their history, surgical use, dangers, and discovery. Boston, David Clapp, 1848. 18 pp.

DUMAS, J. B.: Recherches relatives à l'action du chlore sur l'alcool. L'institut. 2:106-108; 112-115, 1834. See also Liebig, Annal., 16:164-171, 1835, and Poggendorf's Annalen, 31:650-672, 1834. Describes the leading physical and chemical properties of chloroform.

FLOURENS, M. J. P.: Note touchant l'action de l'éther sur les centres nerveux. Acad. de Sci. (Paris) C. R. 24:340-344, 1847. Flourens proved that the inhalation of chloroform caused in animals the same type of temporary anesthesia as did ether.

GORDON, H. L.: Sir James Young Simpson and chloroform. London, T. Fisher Unwin, 1897. 233 pp.

Selected References Arranged by Subject

GUTHRIE, SAMUEL: New mode of preparing a spirituous solution of chloric ether. Silliman J. 21:64-65; On pure chloric ether, 22:105-106, 1832. Discovery of chloroform.

HARCOURT, A. V.: Report on experimental work done for the special chloroform committee of the British Medical Association, Oct. 1901, Jan. 1902. Brit. M. J. 2:120-122 (July 12) 1902.

HYDERABAD CHLOROFORM COMMISSION: Report of the first Hyderabad chloroform commission. Lancet. 1:421-429 (Feb. 22) 1890. Serves as appendix A to the report of the second Hyderabad chloroform commission.

———: Report of the second Hyderabad chloroform commission. Lancet. 1:149-159 (Jan. 18); 486-510 (Mar. 1); 1369-1393 (June 21) 1890.

LEVY, A. G.: Chloroform anæsthesia. London, John Bale, Sons and Danielsson, 1922. vii, 159 pp.

VON LIEBIG, JUSTUS: Ueber die Verbindungen, welche durch die Einwirkung des Chlors auf Alcohol, Aether, ölbildenes Gas und Essiggeist entstehen. Liebig's Annalen. 1:182-230, 1832. Also in Ann. de Chim., 49:146-204, 1832, and in Poggendorf's Annalen, 24:245-295, 1832. Independent discovery of chloroform.

SIMPSON, J. Y.: The obstetric memoirs and contributions of James Y. Simpson. Edited by W. O. Priestley and Horatio R. Storer. Philadelphia, J. B. Lippincott and Co., 1856. Vol. 2, 733 pp. Simpson introduced and fought for analgesia in childbirth.

———: On a new anæsthetic agent, more efficient than sulphuric ether. London M. Gaz. n.s. 5:934-937, 1847. Also Lancet, 2:549-550 (Nov. 20) 1847.

SNOW, JOHN: On chloroform and other anæsthetics; their action and administration. Edited, with a memoir of the author, by Benjamin W. Richardson. London, John Churchill, 1858. 443 pp. John Snow was the first professional anesthetist.

SOUBEIRAN, EUGÈNE: Recherches sur quelques combinaisons du chlore. Ann. de Chim. 48:113-157, 1831. Also in J. de Pharm. 17:657-672, 1831; 18:1-24, 1832. Independent discovery of chloroform.

WALLER, A. D.: The chloroform balance. A new form of apparatus for the measured delivery of chloroform vapour. Proc. Physiol. Soc. (London) 1908. Printed in the J. Physiol. 37:1908—pp. vi-viii.

NITROUS OXIDE

ANDREWS, EDMUND: Liquid nitrous oxide as an anæsthetic. Med. Exam. (Chicago). 13:34-36, 1872. Introduction of nitrous oxide in combination with oxygen.

ARCHER, W. H.: Chronological history of Horace Wells, discoverer of anesthesia. Bull. Hist. Med. 7:1140-1169 (Dec.) 1939.

———: Life and letters of Horace Wells, discoverer of anesthesia. J. Am. Coll. Dentists. 11:83-210 (June) 1944. Also issued separately as a brochure.

ARONSON, SAMUEL: Geschichte der Lachgasnarkose. In Kylos: Jahrb. f. Geschichte u. Philosophie d. Medizin. 3:183-257, 1930.

The History of Surgical Anesthesia

BERT, PAUL: Sur la possibilité d'obtenir, à l'aide du protoxyde d'azote, une insensibilité de long durée, et sur l'innocuité de cet anesthésique. Compt. Rend. Acad. d. sc. 87:728-730, 1878.

COLTON, G. Q.: Anæsthesia. Who made and developed this great discovery? New York, A. G. Sherwood and Co., 1886. 15 pp. Colton supplied Wells with nitrous oxide.

DAVY, HUMPHRY: Researches, chemical and philosophical; chiefly concerning nitrous oxide, or dephlogisticated nitrous air and its respiration. London, J. Johnson, 1800. 580 pp. Davy discovered the anesthetic qualities of nitrous oxide and suggested its use during surgical operations.

GUEDEL, A. E.: Nitrous oxide air anesthesia self administered in obstetrics; a preliminary report. Indianapolis M. J. 14:476-479 (Oct.) 1911.

HEIDBRINK, J. A.: The principles and practice of administering nitrous oxide —oxygen and ethylene oxygen. Dental Digest. 31:73-76 (Feb.); 156-158 (Mar.); 226-228 (Apr.); 296-299 (May); 382-384 (June); 457-459 (July); 545-547 (Aug.); 607-612 (Sept.); 674-677 (Oct.); 758-761 (Nov.) 1925.

McMANUS, JAMES: Notes on the history of anesthesia; the Wells memorial celebration at Hartford, 1894. Early records of dentists in Connecticut. Hartford, Clark and Smith, 1896. 116 pp.

PRIESTLEY, JOSEPH: Experiments and observations on different kinds of air. Ed. 2. London, J. Johnson, 1775. Section 6, Of nitrous air, pp. 108-128. Priestley isolated nitrous oxide in June, 1772. See his "Observations on different kinds of air." Phil. Tr. Roy. Soc. 62:147-264 (March) 1772.

SMITH, TRUMAN: An inquiry into the origin of modern anæsthesia . . . Hartford, Brown and Gross, 1867. 165 pp. The case for Horace Wells.

WATERS, R. M.: Nitrous oxide centennial. Anesthesiology. 5:551-565 (Nov.) 1944.

WELLS, HORACE: A history of the discovery of the application of nitrous oxide gas, ether and other vapors, to surgical operations. Hartford, J. G. Wells, 1847.

WILKS, SAMUEL, and BETTANY, G. T.: A biographical history of Guy's Hospital. London, Ward, Lock, Bowden and Co., 1892. pp. 388-389. Early inhalation experiments (March, 1800).

CARBON DIOXIDE

BERT, PAUL: Barometric pressure; researches in experimental physiology. Tr. by Mary A. Hitchcock and Fred A. Hitchcock. Columbus, Ohio, College Book Company, 1943, pp. 921-924. Bert noticed the anesthetic action of carbonic acid gas.

HICKMAN, H. H.: A letter on suspended animation containing experiments showing that it may be safely employed on animals, with the view of ascertaining its probable utility in surgical operations on the human subject . . . Ironbridge, W. Smith, 1824. No copy available for study.

LEAKE, C. D., and WATERS, R. M.: Anesthetic properties of carbon dioxid. Anesth. & Analg. 8:17-19 (Jan.-Feb.) 1929.

[132]

Selected References Arranged by Subject

WELLCOME HISTORICAL MEDICAL MUSEUM, LONDON. Souvenir, Henry Hill Hickman, Centenary exhibition, 1830-1930, at the Wellcome Historical Medical Museum. London, Wellcome Foundation, Ltd., 1930. 85 pp.

CARBON DIOXIDE ABSORPTION

CLOVER, J. T.: Remarks on the production of sleep during surgical operations. Brit. M. J. 1:200-203 (Feb. 14) 1874. Supplemental bag provided for rebreathing.

HEIDBRINK, J. A.: In: KEYS, T. E.: The development of anesthesia. Anesthesiology. 4:417 (July) 1943. Dr. Heidbrink's first machine (1906) provided for rebreathing.

HEWITT, F. W.: A new method of administering and economising nitrous oxide gas. Lancet. 1:840-841 (May 9) 1885. Description of face piece used for rebreathing nitrous oxide.

JACKSON, D. E.: A new method for the production of general analgesia and anæsthesia with a description of the apparatus used. J. Lab. & Clin. Med. 1:1-12 (Oct.) 1915. Classic experimental work.

KUHN, FRANZ: Perorale Tubagen mit und ohne Druck. Deutsche Ztschr. f. Chir. I. Teil, 76:148-207 (Feb.) 1905; II. Teil, 78:467-520 (July) 1905; III. Teil, 81:63-81 (Jan.) 1906. See also under endotracheal anesthesia.

SNOW, JOHN: On narcotism by the inhalation of vapours. London M. Gaz. n.s. 12:622-627 (Apr. 11) 1851. Animal experimentations to ascertain the quantity of carbon dioxide excreted while under the influence of chloroform and ether.

SWORD, B. C.: The closed circle method of administration of gas anesthesia. Anesth. & Analg. 9:198-202 (Sept.-Oct.) 1930. Circle filter.

WATERS, R. M.: Carbon dioxide absorption from anæsthetic atmospheres. Proc. Roy. Soc. Med. 30:11-22 (Nov.) 1936.

——: Clinical scope and utility of carbon dioxid filtration in inhalation anesthesia. Anesth. & Analg. 3:20-22; 26 (Feb.) 1924. Classic clinical work.

ETHYL ETHER

HAGGARD, H. W.: The absorption, distribution, and elimination of ethyl ether. J. Biol. Chem. 59:737-802 (April) 1924.

ETHYLENE

BROWN, W. E.: Preliminary report; experiments with ethylene as a general anæsthetic. Canad. M. A. J. 13:210 (Mar.) 1923. Value of ethylene as an anesthetic experimentally demonstrated without prior knowledge of the work of Luckhardt.

COTTON, J. H.: Anæsthesia from commercial ether-administration and what it is due to. Canad. M. A. J. 7:769-777 (Sept.) 1917. Anesthetic and analgesic qualities of ethylenated ether. Some of the findings here were exposed by Stehle and Bourne (1922).

[133]

CROCKER, WILLIAM, and KNIGHT, L. I.: Effect of illuminating gas and ethylene on flowering carnations. Botanical Gaz. 46:259-276 (Oct.) 1908. Ethylene was found to put flowers to sleep.

HERB, ISABELLA: Ethylene: notes taken from the clinical records. Anesth. & Analg. 2:230-232 (Dec.) 1923.

HERMANN, LUDIMAR: Ueber die physiologischen Wirkungen des Stickstoffoxydulgases. Arch. f. Anat. u. Physiol. pp. 521-536, 1864. The physiologic action of ethylene.

LEAKE, C. D.: The effect of ethylene-oxygen anesthesia on the acid-base balance of blood: a comparison with other anesthetics. J. A. M. A. 83:2062-2065 (Dec. 27) 1924.

LUCKHARDT, A. B.: Ethylene anesthesia. In: GWATHMEY, J. T.: Anesthesia. Ed. 2. New York, Macmillan Co., 1924. pp. 711-731. Luckhardt and R. C. Thompson gathered data (1918) to establish experimentally the anesthetic qualities of ethylene-oxygen.

———, and CARTER, J. B.: Ethylene as a gas anesthetic; preliminary communication. J. A. M. A. 80:1440-1442 (May 19) 1923. Clinical experience in 106 surgical operations.

———, and LEWIS, DEAN: Clinical experiences with ethylene-oxygen anesthesia. J. A. M. A. 81:1851-1857 (Dec. 1) 1923. Classic account.

LÜSSEM, FRANZ: Experimentelle Studien über die Vergiftung durch Kohlenoxyd, Methan und Aethylen. Ztschr. f. klin. Med. 9:397-428, 1885. Unsatisfactory experimental results with ethylene-oxygen.

TRICHLORETHYLENE

HEWER, C. L.: Trichlorethylene as a general analgesic and anæsthetic. Proc. Roy. Soc. Med. Section on Anæsthesia. 35:463-468 (Mar. 6) 1942.

———: Trichlorethylene as an inhalation anæsthetic. Brit. M. J. 1:924-927 (June 21) 1941.

STRIKER, CECIL; GOLDBLATT, SAMUEL; WARM, I. S., and JACKSON, D. E.: Clinical experiences with the use of trichlorethylene in the production of over 300 analgesias and anesthesias. Anesth. & Analg. 14:68-71 (Mar.-Apr.) 1935.

WATERS, R. M.; ORTH, O. S., and GILLESPIE, N. A.: Trichlorethylene anesthesia and cardiac rhythm. Anesthesiology. 4:1-5 (Jan.) 1943.

ETHYL—N—PROPYL ETHER

BROWN, W. E.: Studies with a newer anæsthetic: ethyl n. propyl ether. Canad. M. A. J. 42:370-371 (Apr.) 1940.

CYPROME ETHER

BLACK, CONSTANCE; SHANNON, G. E., and KRANTZ, J. C., JR.: Studies with cyclopropyl methyl ether (cyprome ether) in man. Anesthesiology. 1:274-279 (Nov.) 1940.

Selected References Arranged by Subject

KRANTZ, J. C., JR.; CARR, C. J.; FORMAN, S. E., and EVANS, W. E., JR.: Anesthesia. I. The anesthetic action of cyclopropyl methyl ether. J. Pharmacol. & Exper. Therap. 69:207-220 (July) 1940.

CYCLOPROPANE

FREUND, AUGUST: Über Trimethylen. Monatshefte f. Chemie. 3:625-635, 1882. Discovery of cyclopropane.

HENDERSON, V. E., and LUCAS, G. H. W.: Cyclopropane: a new anesthetic. Anesth. & Analg. 9:1-6 (Jan.-Feb.) 1930.

LUCAS, G. H. W., and HENDERSON, V. E.: A new anæsthetic gas: cyclopropane; a preliminary report. Canad. M. A. J. 21:173-175 (Aug.) 1929.

SEEVERS, M. H.; MEEK, W. J.; ROVENSTINE, E. A., and STILES, J. A.: A study of cyclopropane anesthesia with especial reference to gas concentrations, respiratory and electrocardiographic changes. J. Pharmacol. & Exper. Therap. 51:1-17 (May) 1934.

STILES, J. A.; NEFF, W. B.; ROVENSTINE, E. A., and WATERS, R. M.: Cyclopropane as an anesthetic agent: a preliminary clinical report. Anesth. & Analg. 13:56-60 (Mar.-Apr.) 1934. First clinical report.

WATERS, R. M., and SCHMIDT, E. R.: Cyclopropane anesthesia. J. A. M. A. 103:975-983 (Sept. 29) 1934.

DIVINYL OXIDE

BOURNE, WESLEY: Divinyl oxide anæsthesia in obstetrics. Lancet. 1:566-567 (Mar. 17) 1934.

GELFAN, SAMUEL, and BELL, I. R.: The anesthetic action of divinyl oxide on humans. J. Pharmacol. & Exper. Therap. 47:1-3 (Jan.) 1933.

LEAKE, C. D.: The rôle of pharmacology in the development of ideal anesthesia. J. A. M. A. 102:1-4 (Jan. 6) 1934.

——, and CHEN, M. Y.: The anesthetic properties of certain unsaturated ethers. Proc. Soc. Exper. Biol. & Med. 28:151-154 (Nov.) 1930.

——; KNOEFEL, P. K., and GUEDEL, A. E.: The anesthetic action of divinyl oxide in animals. J. Pharmacol. & Exper. Therap. 47:5-16 (Jan.) 1933.

RUIGH, W. L., and MAJOR, R. T.: The preparation and properties of pure divinyl ether. J. Am. Chem. Soc. 53:2662-2671 (July) 1931.

LOCAL ANESTHESIA

CORNING, J. L.: Local anæsthesia in general medicine and surgery . . . New York, D. Appleton and Co., [c1885]. 103 pp.

MATAS, RUDOLPH: Local and regional anesthesia; a retrospect and prospect. Am. J. Surg. 25:189-196 (July) 1934; and 25:362-379 (Aug.) 1934.

MOORE, JAMES: A method of preventing or diminishing pain in several operations of surgery. London, T. Cadell, 1784. 50 pp. Local anesthesia of a limb by compression.

The History of Surgical Anesthesia

WOOD, A.: On a new method of treating neuralgia by the direct application of opiates to the painful points. Edinburgh M. & S. J. 82:265-281, 1855. Wood invented the hollow needle in 1853.

LOCAL ANESTHESIA—COCAINE

VON ANREP, V.: Ueber die physiologische Wirkung des Cocaïn. Arch. f. d. ges. Physiol. 21:38-77, 1880. The pharmacologic properties of cocaine investigated.

BENNETT, ALEXANDER: An experimental inquiry into the physiological actions of theine, caffeine, guaranine, cocaine, and theobromine. Edinburgh M. J. Pt. 1. 19:323-341 (Oct.) 1873. Demonstration of the anesthetic properties of cocaine.

CORNING, J. L.: On the prolongation of the anæsthetic effects of the hydrochlorate of cocaine when subcutaneously injected. An experimental study. New York M. J. 42:317-319 (Sept. 19) 1885.

CRILE, G. W.: A new method of applying cocaine for producing surgical anesthesia, with the report of a case. Tr. Ohio State M. Soc. 52:90-93, 1897. Endoneural conduction anesthesia. (Halsted's method.)

CUSHING, H. W.: Cocaine anæsthesia in the treatment of certain cases of hernia and in operations for thyroid tumors. Johns Hopkins Hosp. Bull. 9:192-193 (Aug.) 1898.

——: On the avoidance of shock in major amputations by cocainization of large nerve-trunks preliminary to their division. Army Surg. 36:321-345 (Sept.) 1902.

HALL, R. J.: Hydrochlorate of cocaine. New York M. J. 40:643-644 (Dec. 6) 1884. Describes W. S. Halsted's and R. J. Hall's conduction anesthesia; direct injection of cocaine into nerve trunks.

HALSTED, W. S.: Practical comments on the use and abuse of cocaine . . . New York M. J. 42:294-295 (Sept. 12) 1885. Halsted made the first experiments on infiltration anesthesia; he also produced anesthesia by intradermal injection of water.

KOLLER, CARL: Vorläufige Mittheilung über locale Anästhesirung am Auge. Bericht 16. Versamml. d. Ophthalmologischen Gesellsch., Heidelb., 1884. In: Klin. Monatsb. f. Augenh. 22:Beilageheft, pp. 60-63, 1884. Koller developed the use of cocaine as a local anesthetic agent.

NIEMANN, ALBERT: Sur l'alcaloïde de coca. Tr. from Archiv der Pharm. 102. J. de Pharm. 37:474-475, 1860. Names cocaine (1860).

SCHLEICH, [C. L.]: Infiltrationsanästhesie (locale Anästhesie) und ihr Verhältniss zur allgemeinen Narcose (Inhalationsanästhesie). Verhandl. d. deutsch. Gesellsch. f. Chir. 21:121-127 (4 Sitzungstag 11 Juni) 1892.

LOCAL ANESTHESIA—EPIDURAL

CORNING, J. L.: Spinal anæsthesia and local medication of the cord. New York M. J. 42:483-485 (Oct. 31) 1885.

DOGLIOTTI, A. M.: Eine neue Methode der regionären Anästhesie: die peridurale segmentäre Anästhesie. Zentralbl. f. Chir. 58:3141-3145 (Dec. 12) 1931.

Selected References Arranged by Subject

ODOM, C. B.: Epidural anesthesia. Am. J. Surg. 34:547-558 (Dec.) 1936.

PAGÉS, FIDEL: Anestesia metamérica. Rev. san. mil., Madrid. 11:351-365 (June); 385-396 (July) 1921.

LOCAL ANESTHESIA—NOVOCAINE

BRAUN, H.: Ueber einige neue örtliche Anæsthetica. (Stovain, Alypin, Novocain.) Deutsche med. Wchnschr. 31:1667-1671 (Oct. 19) 1905. Einhorn prepares novocain, 1904. Introduced by Braun.

LOCAL ANESTHESIA—STOVAINE

FOURNEAU, E.: Sur quelques aminoalcools à fonction alcoolique tertiaire du type. Compt. rend. Acad. d. sc. Paris. 138:766-768 (Mar. 21) 1904. Preparation of stovaine, 1903. See also: Fourneau, E.: Stovaine, anesthésique locale. Bull. Soc. Pharmacol. 10:141-148, 1904.

LOCAL ANESTHESIA—TROPACOCAINE

GIESEL, F.: Benzollpseudotropein [tropacocaine]. Pharm. Ztg. 36:419 (July 4) 1891. Discovery of tropacocaine.

INTRAVENOUS ANESTHESIA

ADAMS, R. C.: Intravenous anesthesia. New York, Paul B. Hoeber, Inc., c1944. xiv, 1 l., 663 pp. Well documented with references.

——: Intravenous anesthesia: chemical, pharmacologic and clinical consideration of the anesthetic agents including the barbiturates. Thesis, University of Minnesota, Graduate School, 1940. H. Dresser introduces methylpropylcarbinol urethane (hedonal), 1899. N. P. Krawkow demonstrates intravenous use of hedonal, 1905. Bier develops regional intravenous anesthesia with novocain, 1909. L. Burkhardt reports on the intravenous use of chloroform and ether, 1909. J. Goyanes reports on the intra-arterial use of procaine hydrochloride, 1912. M. G. Marin of Mexico introduces clinical intravenous use of ethyl alcohol, 1929.

BOURNE, WESLEY; BRUGER, MAURICE, and DREYER, N. B.: The effects of sodium amytal on liver function; the rate of secretion and composition of the urine; the reaction, alkali reserve, and concentration of the blood; and the body temperature. Surg., Gynec. & Obst. 51:356-360 (Sept.) 1930.

BREDENFELD, ELISABETH: Die intravenöse Narkose mit Arzneigemischen. Ztschr. f. exper. Path. u. Therap. 18:80-90 (Apr. 4) 1916. Morphine in combination with scopolamine.

BULLARD, O. K.: Intravenous anesthesia in office practice . . . Anesth. & Analg. 19:26-30 (Jan.-Feb.) 1940.

[CLARCK, TIMOTHY]: A letter, written to the publisher by the learned and experienced Dr. Timothy Clarck, one of his majesties physicians in ordinary, concerning some anatomical inventions and observations, particularly the origin of the injection into veins, the transfusion of bloud, and the parts of generation. Phil. Tr. Roy. Soc. 3:672-682 (May 18) 1668. Reporting Sir Christopher Wren's experiments begun "towards the end of 1656."

The History of Surgical Anesthesia

[DENIS, JEAN BAPTISTE]: An extract of a letter written by J. Denis, Doctor of Physick, and Professor of Philosophy and the Mathematicks at Paris, touching a late cure of an inveterate phrensy by the transfusion of bloud. Phil. Tr. Roy. Soc. 2:617-624 (Feb. 10) 1667/8 (i.e., 1668).

DENIS, J[EAN BAPTISTE, and EMMEREZ, ——]: A letter concerning a new way of curing sundry diseases by transfusion of blood . . . Phil. Tr. Roy. Soc. 2:489-504 (July 22) 1667. Reports first transfusion of animal blood (lamb's) to man, June 15, 1667.

ELSHOLTZ, JOHANN SIGISMUND: Clysmatica nova. Berlin, D. Reichel, 1665. 15 pp.

HUBBELL, A. O.: Intravenous anesthesia in dentistry. Ann. Dent. 3:84-93 (Dec.) 1944.

——, and ADAMS, R. C.: Intravenous anesthesia for dental surgery . . . J. Am. Dent. A. 27:1186-1191 (Aug.) 1940.

JARMAN, RONALD: History of intravenous anæsthesia with six years' experience in the use of pentothal sodium. Post-Grad. M. J. 17:70-80 (May) 1941. Sigismund Elzholtz injected an opiate intravenously to obtain insensibility, 1665.

KIRSCHNER, M.: Eine psycheschonende und steuerbare Form der Allgemein-betäubung. Chirurg. 1:673-682 (June 15) 1929. Intravenous use of tri-bromethyl alcohol in amylene hydrate (avertin).

[LOWER, RICHARD]: The method observed in transfusing the bloud out of one animal into another. Phil. Tr. Roy. Soc. 1:353-358 (Dec. 17) 1666. Robert Boyle communicated this account of Lower's experiments. (First known transfusion of blood to animals.)

[——, and KING, EDMUND]: An account of the experiment of transfusion, practised upon a man in London. Phil. Tr. Roy. Soc. 2:557-559 (Dec. 9) 1667.

LUNDY, J. S.; TUOHY, E. B.; ADAMS, R. C., and MOUSEL, L. H.: Clinical use of local and intravenous anesthetic agents: general anesthesia from the standpoint of hepatic function. Proc. Staff Meet., Mayo Clin. 16:78-80 (Jan. 29) 1941. Simultaneous use of oxygen or oxygen-nitrous oxide as a precautionary measure.

MOUSEL, L. H.: Modern trends in anesthesia. Kansas M. Soc. J. 41:279-287 (July) 1940. Intravenous anesthesia recommended as a safety measure in cases in which diathermy or cautery is to be used.

NAKAGAWA, KOSHIRO: Experimentelle Studien über die intravenöse Infusionsnarkose mittels Alkohols. Tohoku J. Exper. Med. 2:81-126 (May 3) 1921.

NOEL, H., and SOUTTAR, H. S.: The anæsthetic effects of the intravenous injection of paraldehyde. Ann. Surg. 57:64-67 (Jan.) 1913.

[OLDENBURG, HENRY]: An account of the rise and attempts, of a way to conveigh liquors immediatly into the mass of blood. Phil. Tr. Roy. Soc. 1:128-130 (Dec. 4) 1665. Sir Christopher Wren's experiments.

Selected References Arranged by Subject

Oré, P. C.: Etudes cliniques sur l'anesthésie chirurgicale par la méthode des injections de chloral dans les veines. Paris, J. B. Baillière et Fils, 1875. 154 pp. First monograph on intravenous anesthesia.

———: Des injections intra-veineuses de chloral. Paris, Bull. Soc. Chir. 1:400-412, 1872. Preliminary report.

Peck, C. H., and Meltzer, S. J.: Anesthesia in human beings by intravenous injection of magnesium sulphate. J. A. M. A. 67:1131-1133 (Oct. 14) 1916.

Wycoff, B. S.: Intravenous anesthesia in oral surgery. Am. J. Orthodontics. 24:875-877 (Sept.) 1938.

BARBITURATES

Lundy, J. S.: Intravenous anesthesia: particularly hypnotic, anesthesia and toxic effects of certain new derivatives of barbituric acid. Anesth. & Analg. 9:210-217 (Sept.-Oct.) 1930.

BARBITURATES—BARBITAL

Fischer, Emil, and Mering, J.: Ueber eine neue Classe von Schlafmitteln. Therap. d. Gegenw. n.s. 5:97-101, 1903. Barbital (veronal) synthesized in 1902 by Emil Fischer.

BARBITURATES—DIAL

Bogendörfer, L.: Ueber lösliche Schlafmittel der Barbitursäurereihe (Dial löslich). Schweiz. med. Wchnschr. 54:437-438 (May 8) 1924. Dial (diallyl-barbituric acid).

BARBITURATES—EUNARCON

Gandow, Otto: Erfahrungen mit "Eunarcon." Zentralbl. f. Gynäk. 60:1701-1719 (July 18) 1936.

BARBITURATES—EVIPAN

Jarman, Ronald, and Abel, A. Lawrence: Evipan: an intravenous anæsthetic. Lancet. 2:18-20 (July 1) 1933.

Weese, H.: Pharmakologie des intravenösen Kurznarkotikums Evipan-Natrium. Deutsche med. Wchnschr. 1:47-48 (Jan. 13) 1933. Evipan.

———, and Scharpff, W.: Evipan, ein neuartiges Einschlafmittel. Deutsche med. Wchnschr. 2:1205-1207 (July 29) 1932. Evipan.

BARBITURATES—NEMBUTAL

Fitch, R. H.; Waters, R. M., and Tatum, A. J.: The intravenous use of the barbituric acid hypnotics in surgery. Am. J. Surg. 9:110-114 (July) 1930. Pentobarbital sodium (nembutal).

Lundy, J. S.: Experience with sodium ethyl (1-methylbutyl) barbiturate (nembutal) in more than 2,300 cases. S. Clin. North America. 11:909-915 (Aug.) 1931. Pentobarbital sodium (nembutal).

[139]

The History of Surgical Anesthesia

BARBITURATES—PENTOTHAL SODIUM

E. M. S. MEMORANDUM: Local treatment of burns. Brit. M. J. 1:489 (Mar. 29) 1941. Lancet. 1:425-426 (Mar. 29) 1941. Use of pentothal sodium as well as gas and oxygen prior to local treatment of severe burns.

FULTON, J. R.: Anesthesia in naval practice. S. Clin. North America. 21: 1545-1558 (Dec.) 1941. Pentothal sodium recommended for wartime conditions.

LUNDY, J. S.: Intravenous anesthesia: preliminary report of the use of two new thiobarbiturates. Proc. Staff Meet., Mayo Clin. 10:536-543 (Aug. 21) 1935. Pentothal sodium found better than sodium allyl secondary butyl thiobarbituric acid.

BARBITURATES—SODIUM AMYTAL

LUNDY, J. S.: The barbiturates as anesthetics, hypnotics and antispasmodics: their use in more than 1000 surgical and non-surgical clinical cases and in operations on animals. Anesth. & Analg. 8:360-365 (Nov.-Dec.) 1929. Sodium amytal.

ZERFAS, L. G., and McCALLUM, J. T. C.: The analgesic and anesthetic properties of sodium isoamylethyl barbiturate: preliminary report. Indiana State M. A. J. 22:47-50 (Feb.) 1929. Sodium amytal.

——; McCALLUM, J. T. C.; SHONLE, H. A.; SWANSON, E. E.; SCOTT, J. P., and CLOWES, G. H. A.: Induction of anesthesia in man by intravenous injection of sodium iso-amyl-ethyl barbiturate. Proc. Soc. Exper. Biol. & Med. 26:399-403 (Feb.) 1929. Sodium amytal.

BARBITURATES—SODIUM ISO-AMYL

CULLEN, S. C., and ROVENSTINE, E. A.: Sodium thio-ethylamyl anesthesia: preliminary report of observations during its clinical use. Anesth. & Analg. 17:201-205 (July-Aug.) 1938. Sodium iso-amyl ethyl thio-barbiturate.

BARBITURATES—SOMNIFENE

GEYER, GUIDO: Zur Geschichte der intravenösen Narkose. Med. Klin. 37: 497-499 (May 9) 1941. Somnifene (dieth-diallyl-barbiturate of diethylamine) injected intramuscularly for production of anesthesia.

SPINAL ANESTHESIA

BABCOCK, W. W.: Spinal anesthesia, an experience of twenty-four years. Am. J. Surg. 5:571-576 (Dec.) 1928.

——: Spinal anesthesia with especial reference to the use of stovaine. Therap. Gaz. 30:239-244 (Apr. 15) 1906.

BIER, AUGUST: Versuche über Cocainisirung des Rückenmarkes. Deutsche Ztschr. f. Chir. 51:361-369 (Apr.) 1899. Production of true spinal anesthesia.

BOURNE, WESLEY; LEIGH, M. D.; INGLIS, A. N., and HOWELL, G. R.: Spinal

Selected References Arranged by Subject

anesthesia for thoracic surgery. Anesthesiology. 3:272-281 (May) 1942. Employment of Etherington-Wilson's technic.

CORNING, J. L.: A further contribution on local medication of the spinal cord, with cases. M. Rec. 33:291-293 (Mar. 17) 1888. Corning obtains regional anesthesia.

——: Spinal anæsthesia and local medication of the cord. New York M. J. 42:483-485 (Oct. 31) 1885. First experiments with spinal anesthesia. Corning obtained epidural anesthesia.

ETHERINGTON-WILSON, W.: Intrathecal nerve root block. Some contributions and a new technique. Proc. Roy. Soc. Med. Section of Anæsthetics. 27, part one. 323-331 (Dec. 1) 1933.

HOWARD-JONES, W.: Spinal analgesia—a new method and a new drug—percaine. Brit. J. Surg. 7:99-113 (April) 1930 and 146-156 (July) 1930.

[MATAS, RUDOLPH]: Report of successful spinal anesthesia. J. A. M. A. 33: 1659 (Dec. 30) 1899. Used by Matas on a Negro patient Nov. 10, 1899. First report on the use of spinal anesthesia in the U. S.

——: Local and regional anesthesia with cocain and other analgesic drugs, including the subarachnoid method, as applied in general surgical practice. Philadelphia M. J. 6:820-843 (Nov. 3) 1900.

MAXSON, L. H.: Spinal anesthesia. Philadelphia, J. B. Lippincott Co., 1938. xxii, 409 pp.

NEWTON, H. F.: Spinal anesthesia in thoracoplastic operations for pulmonary tuberculosis. J. Thorac. Surg. 4:414-428 (April) 1935.

PITKIN, G. P.: Controllable spinal anesthesia. Am. J. Surg. 5:537-553 (Dec.) 1928.

QUINCKE, H.: Die Lumbalpunction des Hydrocephalus. Berl. klin. Wchnschr. 28:929-933 (Sept. 21); 965-968 (Sept. 28) 1891. Development of spinal puncture.

SEBRECHTS, J.: Note au sujet de la rachianesthésie. Bull. Acad. Roy. de Méd. de Belgique. 10:543-638, 1930.

SHIELDS H. J.: Spinal anesthesia in thoracic surgery. Anes. and Analg. 14: 193-198 (Sept.-Oct.) 1935.

TAIT, DUDLEY, and CAGLIERI, GUIDO: Experimental and clinical notes on the subarachnoid space. Tr. Med. Soc. California. Abstracted J. A. M. A. 35:6-10 (July 7) 1900. First patient Oct. 26, 1899. Earliest use of spinal anesthesia in the U. S.

TUFFIER: Analgésie chirurgicale par l'injection sous-arachnoïdienne lombaire de cocaïne. Compt. rend. Soc. de biol. 51:882-884,1899. Spinal anesthesia demonstrated independent of Bier.

SPINAL ANESTHESIA—CONTINUOUS

LEMMON, W. T.: A method for continuous spinal anesthesia: a preliminary report. Ann. Surg. 111:141-144 (Jan.) 1940.

The History of Surgical Anesthesia

CONTINUOUS CAUDAL ANESTHESIA

CATHELIN, M. F.: Une nouvelle voie d'injection rachidienne. Méthodes des injections épidurales par le procédé du canal sacré. Applications à l' homme. Compt. rend. Soc. de biol. 53:452-453 (April 27) 1901. Classical account.

EDWARDS, W. B., and HINGSON, R. A.: Continuous caudal anesthesia in obstetrics. Am. J. Surg. n.s. 57:459-464 (Sept.) 1942.

LULL, C. B., and HINGSON, R. A.: The control of pain in childbirth: anesthesia, analgesia, amnesia . . . with an introduction by Norris W. Vaux. Philadelphia, J. B. Lippincott Co., 1944. xii, 356 pp.

SICARD, M. A.: Les injections médicamenteuses extra-durales par voie sacrococcygienne. Compt. rend. Soc. de biol. 53:396-398 (April 20) 1901. Classical account.

SCOPOLAMINE MORPHINE IN OBSTETRICS

VON STEINBÜCHEL (GRAZ): Die Scopolamin-Morphium-Halbnarkose in der Geburtshülfe. Beitr. z. Geburtsh. u. Gynäk. Rudolf Chrobak . . . 60. Geburtst. 1:294-326, 1903. Introduction of "twilight sleep."

RECTAL ANESTHESIA

BOURNE, WESLEY: Avertin anæsthesia for crippled children. Canad. M. A. J. 35:278-281 (Sept.) 1936.

BUTZENGEIGER, O.: Klinische Erfahrungen mit Avertin (E 107). Deutsche med. Wchnschr. 53:712-713 (Apr. 22) 1927. First clinical use of avertin.

CUNNINGHAM, J. H., and LAHEY, F. H.: A method of producing ether narcosis by rectum, with the report of forty-one cases. Boston M. & S. J. 152:450-457 (Apr. 20) 1905. Air used to transport ether vapor into the intestine.

DUPUY, MARC: Note sur les effets de l'injection de l'éther dans le rectum. L'Union Médicale 1:34 (Mar. 23) 1847.

EICHHOLTZ, FRITZ: Ueber rektale Narkose mit Avertin (E 107). Pharmakologischer Teil. Deutsche med. Wchnschr. 53:710-712 (Apr. 22) 1927. Eichholtz's experimental studies.

GWATHMEY, J. T.: Obstetrical analgesia; a further study, based on more than twenty thousand cases. Surg., Gynec. & Obst. 51:190-195 (Aug.) 1930. Successful use of oil-ether colonic anesthesia in obstetrics.

———: Oil-ether anesthesia. Lancet. 2:1756-1758 (Dec. 20) 1913. By adding carron oil to ether, Gwathmey overcame irritation of the mucosa.

———: The story of oil-ether colonic anesthesia. Anesthesiology. 3:171-175 (March) 1942.

MADDOX, J. K.: An introduction to "avertin" rectal anæsthesia. Sydney, Australia, Angus and Robertson, 1931. viii, 2 l., 124 pp.

MOLLIÈRE, DANIEL: Note sur l'éthérisation par la voie rectale. Lyon méd. 45:419-423 (Mar. 30) 1884. Reintroduction of rectal ether anesthesia.

Selected References Arranged by Subject

PIROGOFF, N. I.: Recherches pratiques et physiologiques sur l'éthérisation. St. Pétersbourg, F. Bellizard & Cie, 1847. 109 pp. First description of rectal anesthesia.

PROSKAUER, CURT: The simultaneous discovery of rectal anesthesia by Marc Dupuy and Nikolai Ivanovich Pirogoff. J. Hist. Med. and Allied Sciences 2:379-384 (Summer) 1947.

SHIPWAY, FRANCIS: The selection of cases for avertin anæsthesia. Brit. J. Anæsth. 7:114-120 (April) 1930.

SUTTON, W. S.: Anæsthesia by colonic absorption of ether. Ann. Surg. 51: 457-479 (April) 1910. Improvement over Dr. John H. Cunningham's technique.

——: Anesthesia by colonic absorption of ether and oil-ether colonic anesthesia. Part I. Anesthesia by colonic absorption of ether. In: GWATHMEY, J. T.: Anesthesia. Ed. 2. New York, Macmillan Co., 1924. pp. 433-438. Includes historical survey.

WOOD, P. M., and BICKLEY, R. S.: Observations on the use of tribromethanol (avertin). Am. J. Surg. 34:598-605 (Dec.) 1936.

ANOCI-ASSOCIATION

CRILE, G. W.: Nitrous oxide anæsthesia and a note on anoci-association, a new principle in operative surgery. Surg., Gynec. & Obst. 13:170-173 (Aug.) 1911. Use of morphine and scopolamine as adjuncts to ether or nitrous oxide anesthesia reported in over 3000 operations.

——: Surgical aspects of Graves' disease with reference to the psychic factor. Ann. Surg. 47:864-869 (June) 1908. First published report on "anociation."

REFRIGERATION ANESTHESIA

ALLEN, F. M.; CROSSMAN, L. W.; HURLEY, VINCENT; WARDEN, C. E., and RUGGIERO, WILFRED: Refrigeration anesthesia. J. Internat. Coll. of Surgeons. 5:125-131 (Mar.-April) 1942. Classic account of refrigeration anesthesia in amputations.

BLUNDELL, WALTER: Painless tooth extraction without chloroform; with observations on local anæsthesia by congelation in general surgery. London, Churchill, 1854. 64 pp. See other references in Index Catalogue, Ser. I, v. 3, "Ch-Dz," p. 258, under Cold as an anæsthetic.

LARREY, D. J.: No pain in amputations at very low temperatures (1807). In: Gwathmey, J. T.: Anesthesia . . . Ed. 2. New York, Macmillan Co., 1924. p. 466.

MOCK, H. E., and MOCK, H. E., JR.: Refrigeration anesthesia in amputations. J. A. M. A. 123:13-17 (Sept. 4) 1943.

NUNN, T. W.: Application of cold as an anæsthetic agent in operations for removing warty excrescences. Lancet. 2·262 (Aug. 31) 1850.

The History of Surgical Anesthesia

Perrin, Maurice, and Lallemand, Ludger: Traité d'anesthésie chirurgicale. Paris, Chamerot, 1863. p. 16. John Hunter's experiments, Larrey's amputations in cold weather, and recent experiences of Arnott and Velpeau.

Richardson, B. W.: Reports and lectures on original researches in scientific practical medicine. I. On a new mode of producing local anæsthesia. M. Times & Gaz. 1:115-117 (Feb. 3) 1866. Introduction of ether spray.

Rottenstein, J. B.: Traité d'anesthésie chirurgicale. Paris, 1880. p. 299. Anesthesia by means of refrigeration with ethyl chloride.

Severino, M. A.: Use of snow and ice for surgical anesthesia (1646). In: Garrison, op. cit. p. 824.

ENDOTRACHEAL ANESTHESIA

Barthélemy and Dufour: L'anesthésie dans la chirurgie de la face. Presse méd. 15:475-476 (July 27) 1907. Advocated use of insufflation principle in endotracheal anesthesia.

Cotton, F. J., and Boothby, W. M.: Anæsthesia by intratracheal insufflation. Advances in technique; a practicable tube-introducer; nitrous oxide-oxygen as the anæsthetic. Surg., Gynec. & Obst. 13:572-573 (Nov.) 1911. Advocated endotracheal insufflation of mixture of oxygen and nitrous oxide.

Eisenmenger, Victor: Zur Tamponnade des Larynx nach Prof. Maydl. Wien. med. Wchnschr. 43:199-201 (Jan. 28) 1893. Eisenmenger's apparatus with semirigid tracheal tube and inflatable cuff.

Elsberg, C. A.: The value of continuous intratracheal insufflation of air (Meltzer) in thoracic surgery: with description of an apparatus. M. Rec. 77:493-495 (Mar. 19) 1910. Clinical application.

Gale, J. W., and Waters, R. M.: Closed endobronchial anesthesia in thoracic surgery: preliminary report. Anesth. & Analg. 11:283-287 (Nov.-Dec.) 1932.

Gillespie, N. A.: Endotracheal anæsthesia. Madison, Wisconsin, University of Wisconsin Press, 1941. 187 pp. Introductory chapter historical.

Guedel, A. E., and Waters, R. M.: A new intratracheal catheter. Anesth. & Analg. 7:238-239 (July-Aug.) 1928. Inflatable cuff.

[Hook, Robert]: An account of an experiment made by M. Hook, of preserving animals alive by blowing through their lungs with bellows. Phil. Tr. Roy. Soc. 2:539-540 (Oct. 21) 1667.

Kirstein, Alfred: Autoskopie des Larynx und der Trachea. Berliner Klin. Wchnschr. 32:476-478, 1895. Introduction of intratracheal tubes via the first direct-vision laryngoscope.

Kuhn, Franz: Perorale Tubagen mit und ohne Druck. Deutsche Ztschr. f. Chir. I. Teil, 76:148-207 (Feb.) 1905; II. Teil, 78:467-520 (July) 1905; III. Teil, 81:63-81 (Jan.) 1906. See also Kuhn's book, Die Perorale Intubation. Berlin, Karger, 1911. 162 pp.

Selected References Arranged by Subject

MACEWEN, WILLIAM: Clinical observations on the introduction of tracheal tubes by the mouth instead of performing tracheotomy or laryngotomy. Brit. M. J. 2:122-124 (July 24); 163-165 (July 31) 1880. First clinical use by introduction of tracheal tubes instead of preliminary tracheotomy.

MAGILL, I. E.: Endotracheal anæsthesia. Proc. Roy. Soc. Med. (Sec. Anæsthetics) 22:1-6 (Dec.) 1928.

———: Technique in endotracheal anæsthesia. Anesth. & Analg. 10:164-168 (July-Aug.) 1931.

MATAS, RUDOLPH: Intralaryngeal insufflation for the relief of acute surgical pneumothorax. Its history and methods with a description of the latest devices for this purpose. J. A. M. A. 34:1468-1473 (June 9) 1900. Matas modified the Fell-O'Dwyer apparatus for maintenance of anesthesia.

———: On the management of acute traumatic pneumothorax. Ann. Surg. 29:409-434, 1899. Recommends use of the Fell-O'Dwyer apparatus in thoracic surgery.

MAYDL, K.: Ueber die Intubation des Larynx als Mittel gegen das Einfliessen von Blut in die Respirationsorgane bei Operationen. Wien. med. Wchnschr. 43:57-59 (Jan. 7); 102-106 (Jan. 14) 1893. Maydl's apparatus a modification of O'Dwyer's.

MELTZER, S. J., and AUER, JOHN: Continuous respiration without respiratory movements. J. Exper. Med. 11:622-625 (July) 1909. Classic account.

O'DWYER, JOSEPH: Fifty cases of croup in private practice treated by intubation of the larynx, with a description of the method and of the dangers incident thereto. M. Rec. 32:557-561 (Oct. 29) 1887. O'Dwyer's original apparatus.

PARHAM, F. W.: Thoracic resection for tumors growing from the bony wall of the chest. Tr. South. S. A. 11:223-363, 1898. First use of Fell-O'Dwyer apparatus in thoracic surgery.

PECK, C. H.: Intratracheal insufflation anæsthesia (Meltzer-Auer). Observations on a series of 216 anæsthesias with the Elsberg apparatus. Ann. Surg. 56:192-200 (July) 1912. Clinical application demonstrated by Peck.

ROWBOTHAM, E. S., and MAGILL, I. W.: Anæsthetics in the plastic surgery of the face and jaws. Proc. Roy. Soc. Med. Section of Anæsthetics. 14:17-27 (Feb. 4) 1921. Based upon nearly 3000 anesthesias—all war injuries.

TRENDELENBURG, FRIEDRICH: Beiträge zur den Operationen an den Luftwegen. 2. Tamponnade der Trachea. Arch. f. klin. Chir. 12:121-133, 1871. First clinical use with preliminary tracheotomy.

TUFFIER and HALLION: Opérations intrathoraciques avec respiration artificielle par insufflation. Compt. rend. Soc. de biol. 48:951-953 (Nov. 21) 1896. Experimental studies.

VESALIUS, ANDREAS: De humani corporis fabrica libri septem. Basel, Oporinus, 1543. pp. 661-663 (misnumbered 661, 658, 659) tell of insufflation experiment. Large "Q" on folio *2 recto illustrates this experiment.

WATERS, R. M.; ROVENSTINE, E. A., and GUEDEL, A. E.: Endotracheal anesthesia and its historical development. Anesth. & Analg. 12:196-203 (Sept.-Oct.) 1933.

[145]

The History of Surgical Anesthesia

ACIDOSIS IN ANESTHESIA

BOURNE, WESLEY: On an attempt to alleviate the acidosis of anesthesia. Proc. Roy. Soc. Med. Section of Anæsthetics. 19:49-51 (July) 1926.

——, and STEHLE, R. L.: The excretion of phosphoric acid during anesthesia. J. A. M. A. 83:117-118 (July 12) 1924.

LEAKE, C. D.: Anæsthesia and blood reaction. Brit. J. Anæsth. 2:56-71 (Oct.) 1924.

——, and HERTZMAN, A. B.: Blood reaction in ethylene and nitrous oxid anesthesia. J. A. M. A. 82:1162-1165 (Apr. 12) 1924.

STEHLE, R. L., and BOURNE, WESLEY: Concerning the mechanism of acidosis in anæsthesia. J. Biol. Chem. 60:17-29 (May) 1924.

STEHLE, R. L.; BOURNE, WESLEY, and BARBOUR, H. G.: Effects of ether anæsthesia alone or preceded by morphine upon the alkali metabolism of the dog. J. Biol. Chem. 53:341-348 (Aug.) 1922.

SAFETY FEATURES

JONES, G. W.; KENNEDY, R. E., and THOMAS, G. J.: Explosive properties of cyclopropane: prevention of explosions by dilution with inert gases. U. S. Dept. of the Interior, Bureau of Mines. Report of Investigations. R. I. 3511 (May), 1940. 17 pp.

WOODBRIDGE, P. D.; HORTON, J. W., and CONNELL, KARL: Prevention of ignition of anesthetic gases by static spark. J. A. M. A. 113:740-744 (Aug. 26) 1939.

BALANCED ANESTHESIA

LUNDY, J. S.: Balanced anesthesia. Minnesota Med. 9:399-404 (July) 1926.

ANESTHETIC TENSION

BOOTHBY, W. M.: The determination of the anæsthetic tension of ether vapor in man, with some theoretical deductions therefrom, as to the mode of action of the common volatile anæsthetics. J. Pharmacol. & Exper. Therap. 5:379-392 (March) 1914.

——: Ether anesthesia. In: KEEN, W. W.: Surgery, its principles and practice by various authors. Philadelphia, W. B. Saunders Co., 1921. Vol. 8, pp. 824-835. Clinical study.

CONNELL, KARL: An apparatus—anæsthetometer—for measuring and mixing anæsthetic and other vapors and gases. Surg., Gynec. & Obst. 17:245-255 (Aug.) 1913. The anesthetometer—Connell apparatus.

MANN, F. C.: Some bodily changes during anesthesia; an experimental study. J. A. M. A. 67:172-175 (July 15) 1916. Experimental study.

——: Vascular reflexes with various tensions of ether vapor. Am. J. Surg. Anesth. suppl. 31:107-112 (Oct.) 1917. Experimental study.

ANESTHETICS AND KIDNEY FUNCTION

STEHLE, R. L., and BOURNE, WESLEY: The effects of morphine and ether on the function of the kidneys. Arch. Int. Med. 42:248-255 (Aug.) 1928.

Selected References Arranged by Subject

ANESTHESIA IN WAR

PENDER, J. W., and LUNDY, J. S.: Anesthesia in war surgery. War Med. 2:193-212 (Mar.) 1942. Historical review, 169 references.

ANESTHETICS AND LIVER FUNCTION

BOURNE, WESLEY: Anesthetics and liver function. Am. J. Surg. 34:486-495 (Dec.) 1936.

——; BRUGER, M., and DREYER, N. B.: The effects of sodium amytal on liver function; the rate of secretion and composition of the urine; the reaction, alkali reserve, and concentration of the blood; and the body temperature. Surg., Gynec. & Obst. 51:356-360 (Sept.) 1930.

——, and RAGINSKY, B. B.: The effects of avertin upon the normal and impaired liver. Am. J. Surg. 14:653-656 (Dec.) 1931.

BRUGER, MAURICE; BOURNE, WESLEY, and DREYER, N. B.: The effects of avertin on liver function: the rate of secretion and composition of the urine, the reaction, alkali reserve and concentration of the blood and the body temperature. Am. J. Surg. 9:82-87 (July) 1930.

ROSENTHAL, S. M., and BOURNE, WESLEY: The effect of anesthetics on hepatic function. J. A. M. A. 90:377-379 (Feb. 4) 1928.

ANALEPTICS IN ANESTHESIA

BOURNE, WESLEY; LEIGH, M. D.; INGLIS, A. N., and HOWELL, G. R.: Spinal anesthesia for thoracic surgery. Anesthesiology. 3:272-281 (May) 1942. See also under "Spinal anesthesia."

RAGINSKY, B. B., and BOURNE, WESLEY: The action of ephedrine in avertin anesthesia. J. Pharmacol. & Exper. Therap. 43:209-218 (Sept.) 1931.

ANESTHETICS AND THE NERVOUS SYSTEM

DWORKIN, SIMON; BOURNE, WESLEY, and RAGINSKY, B. B.: Changes in conditioned responses brought about by anesthetics and sedatives. Canad. M. A. J. 37:136-139 (Aug.) 1937.

——; RAGINSKY, B. B., and BOURNE, WESLEY: Action of anesthetics and sedatives upon the inhibited nervous system. Anesth. & Analg, 16:238-240 (July-Aug.) 1937.

APPARATUS

BEDDOES, THOMAS, and WATTS, JAMES: Considerations on the medicinal use and on the production of factitious airs. Bristol, 1795.

BOOTHBY, W. M.: Nitrous oxide-oxygen anesthesia, with a description of a new apparatus. M. Communicat. Massachusetts M. Soc. 22:126-138, 1911. Boston M. & S. J. 146:86-90 (Jan. 18) 1912.

CLOVER, T. J.: On an apparatus for administering nitrous oxide gas and ether, singly or combined. Brit. M. J. 2:74-75 (July 15) 1876.

COTTON, F. J., and BOOTHBY, W. M.: Nitrous oxide-oxygen-ether anæsthesia: notes on administration; a perfected apparatus. Surg., Gynec. & Obst. 15:281-289 (Sept.) 1912.

GATCH, W. D.: Nitrous oxid-oxygen anesthesia by the method of rebreathing: with especial reference to the prevention of surgical shock. J. A. M. A. 54:775-780 (Mar. 5) 1910.

GWATHMEY, J. T., and WOOLSEY, W. C.: The Gwathmey-Woolsey nitrous oxide-oxygen apparatus. New York M. J. 96:943-946 (Nov. 9) 1912. Takes note of the Hewitt, Teter, Coburn, Gatch, Ohio mono-valve, Boothby-Cotton, and Guedel apparatus also.

HEWITT, F. W.: The administration of nitrous oxide and ether in combination or succession. Brit. M. J. 2:452-454 (Aug. 27) 1887. Modification of Clover apparatus fitted with a bag for nitrous oxide.

——: Anæsthetics and their administration. London, Charles Griffin and Co., 1893. xx, 357 pp. Contains descriptions and illustrations of the better known apparatus. See also under "General references."

JUNKER, F. E.: Description of a new apparatus for administering narcotic vapours. Med. Times & Gaz. 2:590 (Nov. 30) 1867.

KAYE, GEOFFREY: Scope and utility of the absorption and pressure techniques in gas anesthesia. Anesth. & Analg. 18:5-9 (Jan.-Feb.) 1939.

McKESSON, E. I.: Fractional rebreathing in anesthesia; its physiologic basis, technic and conclusions. Am. J. Surg. Anesth. suppl. 29:51-57 (Jan.) 1915.

——: Nitrous oxid oxygen anæsthesia. With a description of a new apparatus. Surg., Gynec. & Obst. 13:456-462 (Oct.) 1911. In 1910 McKesson perfected the first intermittent flow nitrous oxide and oxygen anesthesia apparatus.

MILLER, A. H.: Technical development of gas anesthesia. Anesthesiology. 2:398-409 (July) 1941.

SIGNS AND STAGES OF ANESTHESIA

GILLESPIE, N. A.: The signs of anæsthesia. Anesth. & Analg. 22:275-282 (Sept.-Oct.) 1943. Includes historical survey.

GUEDEL, A. E.: Inhalation anesthesia: a fundamental guide. New York, Macmillan Co., 1937. 172 pp. Includes Guedel's classification of the signs of anesthesia and its four stages.

——: Third stage ether anesthesia: a sub-classification regarding the significance of the position and movements of the eyeball. Nat. Anesth. Res. Soc. Bull. No. 3 (May) 1920. 4 pp. Guedel's first paper on "signs."

MILLER, A. H.: Ascending respiratory paralysis under general anesthesia. J. A. M. A. 84:201-202 (Jan. 17) 1925. Miller described intercostal paralysis in anesthesia. Guedel placed this phenomenon in the third plane of the third stage.

SNOW, JOHN: On the inhalation of the vapour of ether in surgical operations. London, Churchill, 1847, pp. 1-4. Snow defined the "five degrees of narcotism."

Selected References Arranged by Subject

CURARE

CULLEN, S. C.: The use of curare for improvement of abdominal muscle relaxation during inhalation anesthesia; report on 131 cases. Surgery. 14:261-266 (Aug.) 1943.

DITTRICK, HOWARD: From the jungle to the operating room. Anesth. & Analg. 23:132 (May-June) 1944.

GRIFFITH, H. R., and JOHNSON, G. E.: The use of curare in general anesthesia. Anesthesiology. 3:418-420 (July) 1942.

WELLS, T. S.: Three cases of tetanus in which "woorara" was used. Proc. Roy. Med. Chir. Soc. London. 3:142-157 (Nov. 22) 1859.

RECORDS AND STATISTICS

BEECHER, H. K.: The first anesthesia records (Codman, Cushing). Surg., Gynec. & Obst. 71:689-693 (Nov.) 1940.

BROWN, GILBERT: Notes on 300 cases of general anæsthesia combined with narcotics. Lancet. 1:1005-1006 (Apr. 15) 1911.

LUNDY, J. S.: Keeping anesthetic records and what they show. Am. J. Surg. (Quart. Suppl. Anes. and Analg.) 38:16-25 (Jan.) 1924.

McKESSON, E. I.: Blood pressure in general anesthesia. Am. J. Surg. Anesth. suppl. 30:2-5 (Jan.) 1916.

NOSWORTHY, M. D.: A method of keeping anæsthetic records and assessing results. Brit. J. Anæsth. 18:160-179 (July) 1943.

——: The value of anæsthetic records. St. Thomas's Hosp. Rep. 2:54-66, 1937.

ROVENSTINE, E. A.: A method of combining anesthetic and surgical records for statistical purposes. Anesth. & Analg. 13:122-128 (May-June) 1934.

SAKLAD, MEYER; GILLESPIE, NOEL, and ROVENSTINE, E. A.: Inhalation therapy, a method for the collection and analysis of statistics. Anesthesiology. 5:359-369 (July) 1944.

WANGEMAN, C. P.: An experiment in the recording of surgical and anesthetic data in military service. Anesthesiology 2:179-185 (March) 1941.

——, and MARTIN, S. J.: The recording of surgical and anesthetic data in two Army general hospitals. Anesthesiology 6:64-80 (Jan.) 1945.

MUSIC AS AN AID TO ANESTHESIA

GATEWOOD, E. L.: The psychology of music in relation to anesthesia. Am. J. Surg. Anesth. suppl. 35:47-50 (April) 1921.

KIRSCHNER, M.: Musik und Operation. Chirurg. 8:249-431 (June 1) 1936.

McGLINN, J. A.: Music in the operating room. Am. J. Obst. & Gynec. 20:678-683 (Nov.) 1930. Also published in Tr. Am. Gynec. Soc. 55:126-131, 1930.

PODOLSKY, EDWARD: Music as an anæsthetic. Etude. 57:707 (Nov.) 1939.

RUSCA: Rachianæsthesie mit Tutocain und Percain, psychische Beeinflussung der Patienten durch Musik während der Operation. Schweiz. med. Wchnschr. 65:637-638 (July 13) 1935.

IV

Selected References for
A History of Surgical Anesthesia

ARRANGED BY AUTHOR

ABEL, A. LAWRENCE. See No. 145.

1. ADAMS, R. C.: Intravenous anesthesia. New York, Paul B. Hoeber, Inc., c1944. xiv, 1 l., 663 pp.

2. ——: Intravenous anesthesia: chemical, pharmacologic and clinical consideration of the anesthetic agents including the barbiturates. Thesis, University of Minnesota, Graduate School, 1940.

ADAMS, R. C. See also Nos. 138B, 183.

3. ALLEN, F. M.; CROSSMAN, L. W.; HURLEY, VINCENT; WARDEN, C. E., and RUGGIERO, WILFRED: Refrigeration anesthesia. J. Internat. Coll. of Surgeons. 5:125-131 (Mar.-April) 1942.

4. ANÆSTHETIC AGENTS. Tr. A. M. A. 1:176-224, 1848.

5. ANÆSTHETICS—Third interim report of the committee, consisting of Dr. A. D. Waller (chairman), Sir Frederic Hewitt (secretary), Dr. Blumfield, Mr. J. A. Gardner, and Dr. G. A. Buckmaster, appointed to acquire further knowledge, clinical and experimental, concerning anæsthetics— especially chloroform, ether, and alcohol—with special reference to deaths by or during anæsthesia and their possible diminution. Report of the British Association for the Advancement of Science. 80:154-171, 1911. (Published in 1912 by John Murray, London.)

6. ANDREWS, EDMUND: Liquid nitrous oxide as an anæsthetic. Med. Exam. (Chicago). 13:34-36, 1872.

7. VON ANREP, V.: Ueber die physiologische Wirkung des Cocaïn. Arch. f. d. ges. Physiol. 21:38-77, 1880.

8. ARCHER, W. H.: Chronological history of Horace Wells, discoverer of anesthesia. Bull. Hist. Med. 7:1140-1169 (Dec.) 1939.

9. ——: The history of anesthesia. Proc. Dental Centenary Celebration. (Mar.) 1940. pp. 333-363.

10. ——: Life and letters of Horace Wells, discoverer of anesthesia. J. Am. Coll. Dentists. 11:83-210 (June) 1944.

10A. ARONSON, SAMUEL: Geschichte der Lachgasnarkose. In Kylos: Jahrb. f. Geschichte u. Philosophie d. Medizin. 3:183-257, 1930.

AUER, JOHN. See No. 203.

11. BABCOCK, MYRA E.: Brief outline of the history of anesthesia. Grace Hosp. Bull. 10:16-21 (Apr.) 1926.

12. BABCOCK, W. W.: Spinal anesthesia, an experience of twenty-four years. Am. J. Surg. 5:571-576 (Dec.) 1928.

13. ——: Spinal anesthesia with especial reference to the use of stovaine. Therap. Gaz. 30:239-244 (Apr. 15) 1906.

Selected References Arranged by Author

BARBOUR, H. G. See No. 267.

14. BARTHÉLEMY and DUFOUR: L'anesthésie dans la chirurgie de la face. Presse méd. 15:475-476 (July 27) 1907.

15. BAUR, MARGUERITE: Recherches sur l'histoire de l'anesthésie avant 1846. Janus. 31:24-39, 63-90, 124-137, 170-182, 213-225, 264-270, 1927.

16. BEDDOES, THOMAS, and WATTS, JAMES: Considerations on the medicinal use and on the production of factitious airs. Bristol, 1795.

17. BEECHER, H. K.: The first anesthesia records (Codman, Cushing). Surg., Gynec. & Obst. 71:689-693 (Nov.) 1940.

18. ———: The physiology of anesthesia. New York, Oxford University Press, 1938. xiv, 388 pp.

BELL, I. R. See No. 104.

19. BENNETT, ALEXANDER: An experimental inquiry into the physiological actions of theine, caffeine, guaranine, cocaine, and theobromine. Edinburgh M. J. Pt. 1. 19:323-341 (Oct.) 1873.

19A. BERT, PAUL: Barometric pressure: researches in experimental physiology. Tr. by Mary A. Hitchcock and Fred A. Hitchcock. Columbus, Ohio, College Book Company, 1943. pp. 921-924.

19B. ———: Sur la possibilité d'obtenir, à l'aide du protoxyde d'azote, une insensibilité de long durée, et sur l'innocuité de cet anesthésique. Compt. Rend. Acad. d. sc. 87:728-730, 1878.

19C. BETCHER, A. M., and others: The New York State story of anesthesiology. New York State J. Med. 58:1556-1572 (May 1) 1958.

BETTANY, G. T. See No. 297.

20. BIBLIOTHECA OSLERIANA, a catalogue of books illustrating the history of medicine and science collected, arranged and annotated by Sir William Osler . . . Oxford, Clarendon Press, 1929. Anæsthesia. pp. 135-151.

BICKLEY, R. S. See No. 299.

21. BIER, AUGUST: Versuche über Cocainisirung des Rückenmarkes. Deutsche Ztschr. f. Chir. 51:361-369 (Apr.) 1899.

22. BIGELOW, H. J.: Ether and chloroform: a compendium of their history, surgical use, dangers, and discovery. Boston, David Clapp, 1848. 18 pp.

23. ———: A history of the discovery of modern anæsthesia. Am. J. M. Sc. 141:164-184 (Jan.) 1876.

24. ———: Insensibility during surgical operations produced by inhalation. Boston M. & S. J. 35:309-317 (Nov. 18) 1846.

25. ———: Surgical anæsthesia; addresses and other papers. Boston, Little, Brown and Co., 1900. viii, 378 pp.

26. BLACK, CONSTANCE; SHANNON, G. E., and KRANTZ, J. C., JR.: Studies with cyclopropyl methyl ether (cyprome ether) in man. Anesthesiology. 1:274-279 (Nov.) 1940.

27. BLUNDELL, WALTER: Painless tooth extraction without chloroform; with observations on local anæsthesia by congelation in general surgery. London, Churchill, 1854. 64 pp.

28. BOGENDÖRFER, L.: Ueber lösliche Schlafmittel der Barbitursäurereihe (Dial löslich). Schweiz. med. Wchnschr. 54:437-438 (May 8) 1924.

29. BOOTHBY W. M.: The determination of the anæsthetic tension of ether vapor in man, with some theoretical deductions therefrom, as to the mode of action of the common volatile anæsthetics. J. Pharmacol. & Exper. Therap. 5:379-392 (March) 1914.

30. ———: Ether anesthesia. In: Keen, W. W.: Surgery, its principles and practice by various authors. Philadelphia, W. B. Saunders Co., 1921. Vol. 8, pp. 824-835.

31. ———: Ether percentages. J. A. M. A. 61:830-834 (Sept. 13) 1913.

32. ———: Nitrous oxide-oxygen anesthesia, with a description of a new apparatus. M. Communicat. Massachusetts M. Soc. 22:126-138, 1911. Boston M. & S. J. 146:86-90 (Jan. 18) 1912.

BOOTHBY, W. M. See also Nos. 63, 64.

33. BOURNE, WESLEY: Anesthetics and liver function. Am. J. Surg. 34:486-495 (Dec.) 1936.

34. ———: Avertin anæsthesia for crippled children. Canad. M. A. J. 35:278-281 (Sept.) 1936.

35. ———: *De officiis* in anæsthesia. J. Michigan M. Soc. 41:129-134 (Feb.) 1942.

36. ———: Divinyl oxide anæsthesia in obstetrics. Lancet. 1:566-567 (Mar. 17) 1934.

37. ———: On an attempt to alleviate the acidosis of anesthesia. Proc. Roy. Soc. Med. Section of Anæsthetics. 19:49-51 (July) 1926.

38. ———: On the effects of acetaldehyde, ether peroxide, ethyl mercaptan, ethyl sulphide, and several ketones—di-methyl, ethyl-methyl, and di-ethyl —when added to anæsthetic ether. J. Pharmacol. & Exper. Therap. 28:409-432 (Sept.) 1926.

39. ———; BRUGER, M., and DREYER, N. B.: The effects of sodium amytal on liver function; the rate of secretion and composition of the urine; the reaction, alkali reserve, and concentration of the blood; and the body temperature. Surg., Gynec. & Obst. 51:356-360 (Sept.) 1930.

40. ———; LEIGH, M. D.; INGLIS, A. N., and HOWELL, G. R.: Spinal anesthesia for thoracic surgery. Anesthesiology. 3:272-281 (May) 1942.

41. ———, and RAGINSKY, B. B.: The effects of avertin upon the normal and impaired liver. Am. J. Surg. 14:653-656 (Dec.) 1931.

42. ———, and STEHLE, R. L.: The excretion of phosphoric acid during anesthesia. J. A. M. A. 83:117-118 (July 12) 1924.

BOURNE, WESLEY. See also Nos. 47, 81, 82, 238, 243, 264, 265, 266, 267.

43. BRAUN, H.: Ueber einige neue örtliche Anæsthetica. (Stovain, Alypin, Novocain.) Deutsche med. Wchnschr. 31:1667-1671 (Oct. 19) 1905.

44. BREDENFELD, ELISABETH: Die intravenöse Narkose mit Arzneigemischen. Ztschr. f. exper. Path. u. Therap. 18:80-90 (Apr. 4) 1916.

44A. BROWN, GILBERT: Notes on 300 cases of general anæsthesia combined with narcotics. Lancet. 1:1005-1006 (Apr. 15) 1911.

Selected References Arranged by Author

44B. ——: The E. H. Embley Memorial lecture. The evolution of anæsthesia. M. J. Australia. 1:209-220 (Feb. 11) 1939.

45. BROWN, W. E.: Preliminary report; experiments with ethylene as a general anæsthetic. Canad. M. A. J. 13:210 (Mar.) 1923.

46. ——: Studies with a newer anæsthetic: ethyl n. propyl ether. Canad. M. A. J. 42:370-371 (Apr.) 1940.

47. BRUGER, MAURICE; BOURNE, WESLEY, and DREYER, N. B.: The effects of avertin on liver function: the rate of secretion and composition of the urine, the reaction, alkali reserve and concentration of the blood and the body temperature. Am. J. Surg. 9:82-87 (July) 1930.

BRUGER, MAURICE. See also No. 39.

47A. BULLARD, O. K.: Intravenous anesthesia in office practice . . . Anesth. & Analg. 19:26-30 (Jan.-Feb.) 1940.

48. BULLEIN, WILLIAM: Bulleins Bulwarke of defe[n]ce againste all sicknes, sornes, and woundes, that dooe daily assaulte mankinde . . . Doen by Williyam Bulleyn, and ended this Marche, anno salutis, 1562. London, Jhon Kyngston, [1562]. Folio consisting of 251 leaves with various foliations.

49. BUTZENGEIGER, O.: Klinische Erfahrungen mit Avertin (E 107). Deutsche med. Wchnschr. 53:712-713 (Apr. 22) 1927.

CAGLIERI, GUIDO. See No. 274.

CARR, C. J. See No. 155.

CARTER, J. B. See No. 175.

50. CATHELIN, M. F.: Une nouvelle voie d'injection rachidienne. Méthodes des injections épidurales par le procédé du canal sacré. Applications à l'homme. Compt. rend. Soc. de biol. 53:452-453 (April 27) 1901.

51. CHANNING, WALTER: A treatise on etherization in childbirth. Boston, W. D. Ticknor and Co., 1848. viii, 400 pp.

CHEN, M. Y. See No. 163.

52. [CLARCK, TIMOTHY]: A letter, written to the publisher by the learned and experienced Dr. Timothy Clarck, one of his majesties physicians in ordinary, concerning some anatomical inventions and observations, particularly the origin of the injection into veins, the transfusion of bloud, and the parts of generation. Phil. Tr. Roy. Soc. 3:672-682 (May 18) 1668.

53. CLARK, A. J.: Aspects of the history of anæsthetics. Brit. M. J. 2:1029-1034 (Nov. 19) 1938.

54. CLAYE, A. M.: The evolution of obstetric analgesia. New York, Oxford University Press, 1939. 103 pp.

54A. CLENDENING, LOGAN: Literature and material on anæsthesia in the library of medical history of the University of Kansas Medical Department, Kansas City, Kansas. Bull. M. Library A. 33:124-138 (Jan.) 1945.

55. CLOVER, J. T.: On an apparatus for administering nitrous oxide gas and ether, singly or combined. Brit. M. J. 2:74-75 (July 15) 1876.

56. ——: Remarks on the production of sleep during surgical operations. Brit. M. J. 1:200-203 (Feb. 14) 1874.

CLOWES, G. H. A. See No. 303.

57. COLTON, G. Q.: Anæsthesia. Who made and developed this great discovery? New York, A. G. Sherwood and Co., 1886. 15 pp.

58. CONNELL, KARL: An apparatus—anæsthetometer—for measuring and mixing anæsthetic and other vapors and gases. Surg., Gynec. & Obst. 17:245-255 (Aug.) 1913.

CONNELL, KARL. See also No. 300.

59. CORNING, J. L.: A further contribution on local medication of the spinal cord, with cases. M. Rec. 33:291-293 (Mar. 17) 1888.

60. ——: Local anæsthesia in general medicine and surgery . . . New York, D. Appleton and Co., [c1885]. 103 pp.

61. ——: On the prolongation of the anæsthetic effects of the hydrochlorate of cocaine when subcutaneously injected. An experimental study. New York M. J. 42:317-319 (Sept. 19) 1885.

62. ——: Spinal anæsthesia and local medication of the cord. New York M. J. 42:483-485 (Oct. 31) 1885.

63. COTTON, F. J., and BOOTHBY, W. M.: Anæsthesia by intratracheal insufflation. Advances in technique; a practicable tube-introducer; nitrous oxide-oxygen as the anæsthetic. Surg., Gynec. & Obst. 13:572-573 (Nov.) 1911.

64. ——, and BOOTHBY, W. M.: Nitrous oxide-oxygen-ether anæsthesia: notes on administration; a perfected apparatus. Surg., Gynec. & Obst. 15:281-289 (Sept.) 1912.

65. COTTON, J. H.: Anæsthesia from commercial ether-administration and what it is due to. Canad. M. A. J. 7:769-777 (Sept.) 1917.

66. CRILE, G. W.: A new method of applying cocaine for producing surgical anesthesia, with the report of a case. Tr. Ohio State M. Soc. 52:90-93, 1897.

67. ——: Nitrous oxide anæsthesia and a note on anociassociation, a new principle in operative surgery. Surg., Gynec. & Obst. 13:170-173 (Aug.) 1911.

68. ——: Surgical aspects of Graves' disease with reference to the psychic factor. Ann. Surg. 47:864-869 (June) 1908.

69. CROCKER, WILLIAM, and KNIGHT, L. I.: Effect of illuminating gas and ethylene on flowering carnations. Botanical Gaz. 46:259-276 (Oct.) 1908.

CROSSMAN, L. W. See No. 3.

70. CULLEN, S. C.: The use of curare for improvement of abdominal muscle relaxation during inhalation anesthesia; report on 131 cases. Surgery. 14:261-266 (Aug.) 1943.

71. ——, and ROVENSTINE, E. A.: Sodium thio-ethylamyl anesthesia: preliminary report of observations during its clinical use. Anesth. & Analg. 17:201-205 (July-Aug.) 1938.

72. CUNNINGHAM, J. H., and LAHEY, F. H.: A method of producing ether narcosis by rectum, with the report of forty-one cases. Boston M. & S. J. 152:450-457 (Apr. 20) 1905.

Selected References Arranged by Author

73. CUSHING, H. W.: Cocaine anæsthesia in the treatment of certain cases of hernia and in operations for thyroid tumors. Johns Hopkins Hosp. Bull. 9:192-193 (Aug.) 1898.

74. ——: On the avoidance of shock in major amputations by cocainization of large nerve-trunks preliminary to their division. Army Surg. 36:321-345 (Sept.) 1902.

75. DAVY, HUMPHRY: Researches, chemical and philosophical; chiefly concerning nitrous oxide, or dephlogisticated nitrous air and its respiration. London, J. Johnson, 1800. 580 pp.

76. [DENIS, JEAN BAPTISTE]: An extract of a letter written by J. Denis, Doctor of Physick, and Professor of Philosophy and the Mathematicks at Paris, touching a late cure of an inveterate phrensy by the transfusion of bloud. Phil. Tr. Roy. Soc. 2:617-624 (Feb. 10) 1667/8 (i.e. 1668).

77. DENIS, J[EAN BAPTISTE, and EMMEREZ, ——]: A letter concerning a new way of curing sundry diseases by transfusion of blood . . . Phil. Tr. Roy. Soc. 2:489-504 (July 22) 1667.

78. DITTRICK, HOWARD: From the jungle to the operating room. Anesth. & Analg. 23:132 (May-June) 1944.

79. DOGLIOTTI, A. M.: Eine neue Methode der regionären Anästhesie: die peridurale segmentäre Anästhesie. Zentralbl. f. Chir. 58:3141-3145 (Dec. 12) 1931.

DREYER, N. B. See Nos. 39, 47.

DUFOUR. See No. 14.

80. DUMAS, J. B.: Recherches relatives à l'action du chlore sur l'alcool. L'institut. 2:106-108; 112-115, 1834. See also Liebig, Annal., 16:164-171, 1835, and Poggendorf's Annalen, 31:650-672, 1834.

80A. DUNCUM, B. M.: An outline of the history of anaesthesia, 1846-1900. Brit. Med. Bull. 4, no. 2:120-128, 1946.

80B. DUPUY, MARC: Note sur les effets de l'injection de l'éther dans le rectum. L'Union Médicale 1:34 (Mar. 23) 1847.

81. DWORKIN, SIMON; BOURNE, WESLEY, and RAGINSKY, B. B.: Changes in conditioned responses brought about by anesthetics and sedatives. Canad. M. A. J. 37:136-139 (Aug.) 1937.

82. ——; RAGINSKY, B. B., and BOURNE, WESLEY: Action of anesthetics and sedatives upon the inhibited nervous system. Anesth. & Analg. 16:238-240 (July-Aug.) 1937.

83. E. M. S. MEMORANDUM: Local treatment of burns. Brit. M. J. 1:489 (Mar. 29) 1941. Lancet. 1:425-426 (Mar. 29) 1941.

84. EDWARDS, W. B., and HINGSON, R. A.: Continuous caudal anesthesia in obstetrics. Am. J. Surg. n.s. 57:459-464 (Sept.) 1942.

85. EICHHOLTZ, FRITZ: Ueber rektale Narkose mit Avertin (E 107). Pharmakologischer Teil. Deutsche med. Wchnschr. 53:710-712 (Apr. 22) 1927.

86. EISENMENGER, VICTOR: Zur Tamponnade des Larynx nach Prof. Maydl. Wien. med. Wchnschr. 43:199-201 (Jan. 28) 1893.

87. ELSBERG, C. A.: The value of continuous intratracheal insufflation of air (Meltzer) in thoracic surgery: with description of an apparatus. M. Rec. 77:493-495 (Mar. 19) 1910.

87A. ELSHOLTZ, J. S.: Clysmatica nova. Berlin, D. Reichel, 1665. 15 pp. EMMEREZ. See No. 77.

88. ETHERINGTON-WILSON, W.: Intrathecal nerve root block. Some contributions and a new technique. Proc. Roy. Soc. Med. Section of Anæsthetics. 27, part 1. 323-331 (Dec. 1) 1933.

EVANS, W. E., JR. See No. 155.

89. FARADAY, MICHAEL: Effects of inhaling the vapors of sulphuric ether. In: Quart. J. Sc. and the Arts. Miscellanea (art. XVI). 4:158-159, 1818.

90. FIGUIER: Exposition et histoire des principales découvertes scientifiques modernes. Ed. 3. Paris, 1854. 3 v.

91. FISCHER, EMIL, and MERING, J.: Ueber eine neue Classe von Schlafmitteln. Therap. d. Gegenw. n.s. 5:97-101, 1903.

92. FITCH, R. H.; WATERS, R. M., and TATUM, A. J.: The intravenous use of the barbituric acid hypnotics in surgery. Am. J. Surg. 9:110-114 (July) 1930.

93. FLOURENS, M. J. P.: Note touchant l'action de l'éther sur les centres nerveux. Acad. de Sci. (Paris) C. R. 24:340-344, 1847.

94. FORD, WILLIAM W.: A prelude to ether anesthesia. New England J. M. 231:219-223 (Aug. 10) 1944.

FORMAN, S. E. See No. 155.

95. FOURNEAU, E.: Sur quelques aminoalcools à fonction alcoolique tertiaire du type. Compt. rend. Acad. d. sc. Paris. 138:766-768 (Mar. 21) 1904.

96. FREUND, AUGUST: Ueber Trimethylen. Monatshefte f. Chemie. 3:625-635, 1882.

97. FÜLÖP-MILLER, RENÉ: Triumph over pain. Translated by Eden and Cedar Paul. New York, The Literary Guild of America, Inc., 1938. 438 pp.

97A. FULTON, J. F., and STANTON, M. E., comps.: The centennial of surgical anesthesia, an annotated catalogue of books and pamphlets bearing on the early history of surgical anesthesia, exhibited at the Yale Medical Library, October, 1946 . . . New York, Henry Schuman, 1946. xv, 102 pp.

98. FULTON, J. R.: Anesthesia in naval practice. S. Clin. North America. 21:1545-1558 (Dec.) 1941.

99. GALE, J. W., and WATERS, R. M.: Closed endobronchial anesthesia in thoracic surgery: preliminary report. Anesth. & Analg. 11:283-287 (Nov.-Dec.) 1932.

100. GANDOW, OTTO: Erfahrungen mit "Eunarcon." Zentralbl. f. Gynäk. 60:1701-1719 (July 18) 1936.

101. GARRISON, F. H.: An introduction to the history of medicine. Ed. 4. Philadelphia, W. B. Saunders Co., 1929. 996 pp.

102. GATCH, W. D.: Nitrous oxid-oxygen anesthesia by the method of re-

breathing: with especial reference to the prevention of surgical shock. J. A. M. A. 54:775-780 (Mar. 5) 1910.

103. GATEWOOD, E. L.: The psychology of music in relation to anesthesia. Am. J. Surg. Anesth. suppl. 35:47-50 (April) 1921.

104. GELFAN, SAMUEL, and BELL, I. R.: The anesthetic action of divinyl oxide on humans. J. Pharmacol. & Exper. Therap. 47:1-3 (Jan.) 1933.

105. GEYER, GUIDO: Zur Geschichte der intravenösen Narkose. Med. Klin. 37:497-499 (May 9) 1941.

106. GIESEL, F.: Benzollpseudotropein [tropacocaine]. Pharm. Ztg. 36:419 (July 4) 1891.

107. GILLESPIE, N. A.: Endotracheal anæsthesia. Madison, Wisconsin, University of Wisconsin Press, 1941. 187 pp.

108. ———: The signs of anæsthesia. Anesth. & Analg. 22:275-282 (Sept.-Oct.) 1943.

GILLESPIE, N. A. See also Nos. 249, 288.

GOLDBLATT, SAMUEL. See No. 270.

109. GORDON, H. L.: Sir James Young Simpson and chloroform. London, T. Fisher Unwin, 1897. 233 pp.

110. GRIFFITH, H. R., and JOHNSON, G. E.: The use of curare in general anesthesia. Anesthesiology. 3:418-420 (July) 1942.

111. GUEDEL, A. E.: Inhalation anesthesia: a fundamental guide. New York, Macmillan Co., 1937. 172 pp.

112. ———: Nitrous oxide air anesthesia self administered in obstetrics; a preliminary report. Indianapolis M. J. 14:476-479 (Oct.) 1911.

113. ———: Third stage ether anesthesia: a sub-classification regarding the significance of the position and movements of the eyeball. Nat. Anesth. Res. Soc. Bull. No. 3 (May) 1920. 4 pp.

114. ———, and WATERS, R. M.: A new intratracheal catheter. Anesth. & Analg. 7:238-239 (July-Aug.) 1928.

GUEDEL, A. E. See also Nos. 165, 289.

115. GUTHRIE, SAMUEL: New mode of preparing a spirituous solution of chloric ether. Silliman J. 21:64-65; On pure chloric ether, 22:105-106, 1832.

116. GWATHMEY, J. T.: Anesthesia. Ed. 1. New York, D. Appleton Co., 1914. xxxii, 945 pp.

117. ———: Anesthesia . . . Ed. 2. New York, Macmillan Co., 1924. 799 pp.

118. ———: Obstetrical analgesia; a further study, based on more than twenty thousand cases. Surg., Gynec. & Obst. 51:190-195 (Aug.) 1930.

119. ———: Oil-ether anesthesia. Lancet. 2:1756-1758 (Dec. 20) 1913.

120. ———: The story of oil-ether colonic anesthesia. Anesthesiology. 3:171-175 (March) 1942.

121. ———, and WOOLSEY, W. C.: The Gwathmey-Woolsey nitrous oxide-oxygen apparatus. New York M. J. 96:943-946 (Nov. 9) 1912.

122. HAGGARD, H. W.: The absorption, distribution, and elimination of ethyl ether. J. Biol. Chem. 59:737-802 (April) 1924.

123. HALL, R. J.: Hydrochlorate of cocaine. New York M. J. 40:643-644 (Dec. 6) 1884.

HALLION. See No. 280.

124. HALSTED, W. S.: Practical comments on the use and abuse of cocaine . . . New York M. J. 42:294-295 (Sept. 12) 1885.

125. HARCOURT, A. V.: Report on experimental work done for the special chloroform committee of the British Medical Association, Oct. 1901, Jan. 1902. Brit. M. J. 2:120-122 (July 12) 1902.

126. HEIDBRINK, J. A.: In: Keys, T. E.: The development of anesthesia. Anesthesiology. 4:417 (July) 1943.

127. ———: The principles and practice of administering nitrous oxide-oxygen and ethylene oxygen. Dental Digest. 31:73-76 (Feb.); 156-158 (Mar.); 226-228 (Apr.); 296-299 (May); 382-384 (June); 457-459 (July); 545-547 (Aug.); 607-612 (Sept.); 674-677 (Oct.); 758-761 (Nov.) 1925.

128. HENDERSON, V. E., and LUCAS, G. H. W.: Cyclopropane: a new anesthetic. Anesth. & Analg. 9:1-6 (Jan.-Feb.) 1930.

HENDERSON, V. E. See also No. 173.

129. HERB, ISABELLA: Ethylene: notes taken from the clinical records. Anesth. & Analg. 2:230-232 (Dec.) 1923.

130. HERMANN, LUDIMAR: Ueber die physiologischen Wirkungen des Stickstoffoxydulgases. Arch. f. Anat. u. Physiol. pp. 521-536, 1864.

HERTZMAN, A. B. See No. 164.

131. HEWER, C. L.: Trichlorethylene as a general analgesic and anæsthetic. Proc. Roy. Soc. Med. Sect. on Anæsthesia. 35:463-468 (Mar. 6) 1942.

132. ———: Trichlorethylene as an inhalation anæsthetic. Brit. M. J. 1:924-927 (June 21) 1941.

133. HEWITT, F. W.: The administration of nitrous oxide and ether in combination or succession. Brit. M. J. 2:452-454 (Aug. 27) 1887.

134. ———: Anæsthetics and their administration. London, Charles Griffin and Co., 1893. xx, 357 pp.

135. ———: A new method of administering and economising nitrous oxide gas. Lancet. 1:840-841 (May 9) 1885.

136. HICKMAN, H. H.: A letter on suspended animation containing experiments showing that it may be safely employed on animals, with the view of ascertaining its probable utility in surgical operations on the human subject . . . Ironbridge, W. Smith, 1824.

HINGSON, R. A. See No. 84, 176A.

137. [HOOK, ROBERT]: An account of an experiment made by M. Hook, of preserving animals alive by blowing through their lungs with bellows. Phil. Tr. Roy. Soc. 2:539-540 (Oct. 21) 1667.

HORTON, J. W. See No. 300.

138. HOWARD-JONES, W.: Spinal analgesia—a new method and a new drug —percaine. Brit. J. Surg. 7:99-113 (April) 1930 and 146-156 (July) 1930.

HOWELL, G. R. See No. 40.

Selected References Arranged by Author

138A. HUBBELL, A. O.: Intravenous anesthesia in dentistry. Ann. Dent. 3:84-93 (Dec.) 1944.

138B. ——, and ADAMS, R. C.: Intravenous anesthesia for dental surgery . . . J. Am. Dent. A. 27:1186-1191 (Aug.) 1940.

HURLEY, VINCENT. See No. 3.

139. HYDERABAD CHLOROFORM COMMISSION: Report of the first Hyderabad chloroform commission. Lancet. 1:421-429 (Feb. 22) 1890.

140. ——: Report of the second Hyderabad chloroform commission. Lancet. 1:149-159 (Jan. 18); 486-510 (Mar. 1); 1369-1393 (June 21) 1890.

INGLIS, A. N. See No. 40.

141. [JACKSON, C. T.]: . . . First practical use of ether in surgical operations. Boston M. & S. J. 64:229-231 (April 11) 1861.

142. ——: A manual of etherization: containing directions for the employment of ether, chloroform, and other anæsthetics by inhalation . . . Boston, J. B. Mansfield, 1861. 134 pp.

143. JACKSON, D. E.: A new method for the production of general analgesia and anæsthesia with a description of the apparatus used. J. Lab. & Clin. Med. 1:1-12 (Oct.) 1915.

JACKSON, D. E. See also No. 270.

144. JARMAN, RONALD: History of intravenous anæsthesia with six years' experience in the use of pentothal sodium. Post-Grad. M. J. 17:70-80 (May) 1941.

145. ——, and ABEL, A. LAWRENCE: Evipan: an intravenous anæsthetic. Lancet. 2:18-20 (July 1) 1933.

JOHNSON, G. E. See No. 110.

146. JONES, G. W.; KENNEDY, R. E., and THOMAS, G. J.: Explosive properties of cyclopropane: prevention of explosions by dilution with inert gases. U. S. Dept. of the Interior, Bureau of Mines, Report of Investigations. R. I. 3511 (May) 1940. 17 pp.

147. JUNKER, F. E.: Description of a new apparatus for administering narcotic vapours. Med. Times & Gaz. 2:590 (Nov. 30) 1867.

148. KAYE, GEOFFREY: Scope and utility of the absorption and pressure techniques in gas anesthesia. Anesth. & Analg. 18:5-9 (Jan.-Feb.) 1939.

KENNEDY, R. E. See No. 146.

149. KEYS, T. E.: A chronology of events relating to anesthesiology and allied subjects. In: Lundy, J. S.: Clinical anesthesia . . . Philadelphia, W. B. Saunders Co., 1942. pp. 705-717.

150. ——: The development of anesthesia. Anesthesiology. 2:552-574 (Sept.) 1941; 3:11-23 (Jan.); 282-294 (May); 650-659 (Nov.) 1942 and 4:409-429 (July) 1943.

KING, EDMUND. See No. 172.

151. KIRSCHNER, M.: Musik und Operation. Chirurg. 8:429-431 (June 1) 1936.

152. ——: Eine psycheschonende und steuerbare Form der Allgemein-betäubung. Chirurg. 1:673-682 (June 15) 1929.

152A. KIRSTEIN, ALFRED: Autoskopie des Larynx und der Trachea. Berliner Klin. Wchnschr. 32:476-478, 1895.

153. KLEIMAN, MARCOS: Histoire de l'anesthésie. Anesth. et analg. 5:112-138 (Feb.) 1939.

KNIGHT, L. I. See No. 69.

KNOEFEL, P. K. See No. 165.

154. KOLLER, CARL: Vorläufige Mittheilung über locale Anästhesirung am Auge. Bericht 16. Versamml. d. Ophthalmologischen Gesellsch., Heidelb., 1884. In: Klin. Monatsb. f. Augenh. 22:Beilageheft, pp. 60-63, 1884.

155. KRANTZ, J. C., JR.; CARR, C. J.; FORMAN, S. E., and EVANS, W. E., JR.: Anesthesia. I. The anesthetic action of cyclopropyl methyl ether. J. Pharmacol. & Exper. Therap. 69:207-220 (July) 1940.

KRANTZ, J. C., JR. See also No. 26.

156. KUHN, FRANZ: Perorale Tubagen mit und ohne Druck. Deutsche Ztschr. f. Chir. I. Teil, 76:148-207 (Feb.) 1905; II. Teil, 78:467-520 (July) 1905; III. Teil, 81:63-81 (Jan.) 1906. See also Kuhn's book, Die Perorale Intubation. Berlin, Karger, 1911. 162 pp.

157. LAFARGUE, G. V.: Note sur les effets de quelques médicaments intro-ducts sous l'épiderme. Compt. rend. Acad. d. sc. 3:397-398; 434 (Sept. 19) 1836.

LAHEY, F. H. See No. 72.

LALLEMAND, LUDGER. See No. 232.

157A. LARREY, D. J.: No pain in amputations at very low temperatures (1807). In: Gwathmey, J. T.: Anesthesia ... Ed. 2. New York, Macmillan Co., 1924. p. 466.

158. LEAKE, C. D.: Anæsthesia and blood reaction. Brit. J. Anæsth. 2:56-71 (Oct.) 1924.

159. ——: The effect of ethylene-oxygen anesthesia on the acid-base balance of blood: a comparison with other anesthetics. J. A. M. A. 83:2062-2065 (Dec. 27) 1924.

160. ——: The historical development of surgical anesthesia. Scient. Mthly. 20:304-328 (Mar.) 1925.

161. ——: The rôle of pharmacology in the development of ideal anesthesia. J. A. M. A. 102:1-4 (Jan. 6) 1934.

162. ——: Valerius Cordus and the discovery of ether. Isis. 7:14-24, 1925.

163. ——, and CHEN, M. Y.: The anesthetic properties of certain unsaturated ethers. Proc. Soc. Exper. Biol. & Med. 28:151-154 (Nov.) 1930.

164. ——, and HERTZMAN, A. B.: Blood reaction in ethylene and nitrous oxid anesthesia. J. A. M. A. 82:1162-1165 (Apr. 12) 1924.

165. ——; KNOEFEL, P. K., and GUEDEL, A. E.: The anesthetic action of divinyl oxide in animals. J. Pharmacol. & Exper. Therap. 47:5-16 (Jan.) 1933.

166. ——, and WATERS, R. M.: Anesthetic properties of carbon dioxid. Anesth. & Analg. 8:17-19 (Jan.-Feb.) 1929.

LEIGH, M. D. See No. 40.

167. LEMMON, W. T.: A method for continuous spinal anesthesia: a preliminary report. Ann. Surg. 111:141-144 (Jan.) 1940.

168. LEVY, A. G.: Chloroform anæsthesia. London, John Bale, Sons and Danielsson, 1922. vii, 159 pp.

LEWIS, DEAN. See No. 176.

169. VON LIEBIG, JUSTUS: Ueber die Verbindungen, welche durch die Einwirkung des Chlors auf Alcohol, Aether, ölbildenes Gas und Essiggeist entstehen. Liebig's Annalen. 1:182-230, 1832. Also in Ann. de Chim., 49:146-204, 1832, and in Poggendorf's Annalen, 24:245-295, 1832.

170. LONG, C. W.: An account of the first use of sulphuric ether by inhalation as an anæsthetic in surgical operations. South. M. & S. J. n.s. 5:705-713 (Dec.) 1849.

171. [LOWER, RICHARD]: The method observed in transfusing the bloud out of one animal into another. Phil. Tr. Roy. Soc. 1:353-358 (Dec. 17) 1666.

172. [——, and KING, EDMUND]: An account of the experiment of transfusion, practised upon a man in London. Phil. Tr. Roy. Soc. 2:557-559 (Dec. 9) 1667.

173. LUCAS, G. H. W., and HENDERSON, V. E.: A new anæsthetic gas: cyclopropane; a preliminary report. Canad. M. A. J. 21:173-175 (Aug.) 1929.

LUCAS, G. H. W. See also No. 128.

174. LUCKHARDT, A. B.: Ethylene anesthesia. In: Gwathmey, J. T.: Anesthesia. Ed. 2. New York, Macmillan Co., 1924. pp. 711-731.

175. ——, and CARTER, J. B.: Ethylene as a gas anesthetic; preliminary communication. J. A. M. A. 80:1440-1442 (May 19) 1923.

176. ——, and LEWIS, DEAN: Clinical experiences with ethylene-oxygen anesthesia. J. A. M. A. 81:1851-1857 (Dec. 1) 1923.

176A. LULL, C. B., and HINGSON, R. A.: The control of pain in childbirth: anesthesia, analgesia, amnesia . . . with an introduction by Norris W. Vaux. Philadelphia, J. B. Lippincott Co., 1944. xii, 356 pp.

177. LUNDY, J. S.: Balanced anesthesia. Minnesota Med. 9:399-404 (July) 1926.

178. ——: The barbiturates as anesthetics, hypnotics and antispasmodics: their use in more than 1000 surgical and non-surgical clinical cases and in operations on animals. Anesth. & Analg. 8:360-365 (Nov.-Dec.) 1929.

179. ——: Clinical anesthesia . . . Philadelphia, W. B. Saunders Co., 1942. xxix, 771 pp.

180. ——: Experience with sodium ethyl (1-methylbutyl) barbiturate (nembutal) in more than 2,300 cases. S. Clin. North America. 11:909-915 (Aug.) 1931.

181. ——: Intravenous anesthesia: particularly hypnotic, anesthesia and toxic effects of certain new derivatives of barbituric acid. Anesth. & Analg. 9:210-217 (Sept.-Oct.) 1930.

182. ——: Intravenous anesthesia: preliminary report of the use of two new thiobarbiturates. Proc. Staff Meet., Mayo Clin. 10:536-543 (Aug. 21) 1935.

182A. ——: Keeping anesthetic records and what they show. Am. J. Surg. (Quart. Suppl. Anes. and Analg.) 38:16-25 (Jan.) 1924.

183. ——; TUOHY, E. B.; ADAMS, R. C., and MOUSEL, L. H.: Clinical use of local and intravenous anesthetic agents: general anesthesia from the standpoint of hepatic function. Proc. Staff Meet., Mayo Clin. 16:78-80 (Jan. 29) 1941.

LUNDY, J. S. See also No. 231.

184. LÜSSEM, FRANZ: Experimentelle Studien über die Vergiftung durch Kohlenoxyd, Methan und Aethylen. Ztschr. f. klin. Med. 9:397-428, 1885.

185. LYMAN, H. M.: Artificial anæsthesia and anæsthetics. New York, William Wood and Co., 1881. p. 6. See also: Lyman, H. M.: The discovery of anæsthesia. Virginia M. Monthly. 13:369-392 (Sept.) 1886.

MCCALLUM, J. T. C. See Nos. 302, 303.

186. MACEWEN, WILLIAM: Clinical observations on the introduction of tracheal tubes by the mouth instead of performing tracheotomy or laryngotomy. Brit. M. J. 2:122-124 (July 24); 163-165 (July 31) 1880.

187. McGLINN, J. A.: Music in the operating room. Am. J. Obst. & Gynec. 20:678-683 (Nov.) 1930. Also published in Tr. Am. Gynec. Soc. 55:126-131, 1930.

188. McKESSON, E. I.: Blood pressure in general anesthesia. Am. J. Surg. Anesth. suppl. 30:2-5 (Jan.) 1916.

189. ——: Fractional rebreathing in anesthesia; its physiologic basis, technic, and conclusions. Am. J. Surg. Anesth. suppl. 29:51-57 (Jan.) 1915.

190. ——: Nitrous oxid-oxygen anæsthesia. With a description of a new apparatus. Surg., Gynec. & Obst. 13:456-462 (Oct.) 1911.

191. McMANUS, JAMES: Notes on the history of anesthesia; the Wells memorial celebration at Hartford, 1894. Early records of dentists in Connecticut. Hartford, Clark and Smith, 1896. 116 pp.

192. MADDOX, J. K.: An introduction to "avertin" rectal anæsthesia. Sydney, Australia, Angus and Robertson, 1931. viii, 2 l., 124 pp.

192A. MAGILL, I. W.: Endotracheal anesthesia. Proc. Roy. Soc. Med. (Sect. Anesthetics) 22:1-6 (Dec.) 1928.

192B. ——: Technique in endotracheal anesthesia. Anesth. & Analg. 10:164-168 (July-Aug.) 1931.

MAGILL, I. W. See also No. 246.

MAJOR, R. T. See No. 247.

193. MANN, F. C.: Some bodily changes during anesthesia; an experimental study. J. A. M. A. 67:172-175 (July 15) 1916.

194. ——: Vascular reflexes with various tensions of ether vapor. Am. J. Surg. Anesth. suppl. 31:107-112 (Oct.) 1917.

195. MATAS, RUDOLPH: Intralaryngeal insufflation for the relief of acute surgical pneumothorax. Its history and methods with a description of the

Selected References Arranged by Author

latest devices for this purpose. J. A. M. A. 34:1468-1473 (June 9) 1900.

196. ——: Local and regional anesthesia; a retrospect and prospect. Am. J. Surg. 25:189-196 (July) 1934; and 25:362-379 (Aug.) 1934.

197. ——: Local and regional anesthesia with cocain and other analgesic drugs, including the subarachnoid method, as applied in general surgical practice. Philadelphia M. J. 6:820-843 (Nov. 3) 1900.

198. ——: On the management of acute traumatic pneumothorax. Ann. Surg. 29:409-434, 1899.

199. [——]: Report of successful spinal anesthesia. J. A. M. A. 33:1659 (Dec. 30) 1899.

200. MAXSON, L. H.: Spinal anesthesia. Philadelphia, J. B. Lippincott Co., 1938. xxii, 409 pp.

201. MAYDL, K.: Ueber die Intubation des Larynx als Mittel gegen das Einfliessen von Blut in die Respirationsorgane bei Operationen. Wien. med. Wchnschr. 43:57-59 (Jan. 7) ; 102-106 (Jan. 14) 1893.

202. MEDICAL INTELLIGENCE: Insensibility during surgical operations produced by inhalation. Boston M. & S. J. 35:413-414 (Dec. 16) 1846.

MEEK, W. J. See No. 252.

203. MELTZER, S. J., and AUER, JOHN: Continuous respiration without respiratory movements. J. Exper. Med. 11:622-625 (July) 1909.

MELTZER, S. J. See also No. 230.

MERING, J. See No. 91.

204. MILLER, A. H.: Ascending respiratory paralysis under general anesthesia. J. A. M. A. 84:201-202 (Jan. 17) 1925.

205. ——: The origin of the word "anæsthesia." Boston M. & S. J. 197:1218-1222 (Dec. 29) 1927.

206. ——: Technical development of gas anesthesia. Anesthesiology. 2:398-409 (July) 1941.

207. MOCK, H. E., and MOCK, H. E., JR.: Refrigeration anesthesia in amputations. J. A. M. A. 123:13-17 (Sept. 4) 1943.

MOCK, H. E., JR. See No. 207.

208. MOLLIÈRE, DANIEL: Note sur l'éthérisation par la voie rectale. Lyon méd. 45:419-423 (Mar. 30) 1884.

209. MOORE, JAMES: A method of preventing or diminishing pain in several operations of surgery. London, T. Cadell, 1784. 50 pp.

210. MORTON, W. J.: The invention of anæsthetic inhalation; or, "Discovery of anæsthesia." New York, D. Appleton and Co., 1880. 48 pp.

211. [MORTON, W. T. G.]: Circular. Morton's Letheon. Boston, Dutton and Wentworth, [1846]. 14 pp.

211A. ——: The first use of ether as an anesthetic. At the Battle of the Wilderness in the Civil War. J. A. M. A. 42:1068-1073 (April 23) 1904.

212. [——]: Letter from Dr. Wm. T. G. Morton. Am. J. Dent. Sc. 8:56-77 (Oct.) 1847.

212A. ——: On the physiological effects of sulphuric ether, and its superiority to chloroform. Boston, D. Clapp, 1850. 24 pp.

[163]

213. ———: Remarks on the proper mode of administering sulphuric ether by inhalation. Boston, Dutton and Wentworth, 1847. 44 pp.

214. ———: Statements, supported by evidence, of W. T. G. Morton, M.D., on his claim to the discovery of anæsthetic properties of ether . . . Washington, 1853. 582 pp.

215. MOUSEL, L. H.: Modern trends in anesthesia. Kansas M. Soc. J. 41:279-287 (July) 1940.

MOUSEL, L. H. See also No. 183.

216. NAKAGAWA, KOSHIRO: Experimentelle Studien über die intravenöse Infusionsnarkose mittels Alkohols. Tohoku J. Exper. Med. 2:81-126 (May 3) 1921.

NEFF, W. B. See No. 269.

216A. NEWTON, H. F.: Spinal anesthesia in thoracoplastic operations for pulmonary tuberculosis. J. Thorac. Surg. 4:414-428 (April 1935).

217. NIEMANN, ALBERT: Sur l'alcaloïde de coca. Tr. from Archiv der Pharm. 102. J. de Pharm. 37:474-475, 1860.

218. NOEL, H., and SOUTTAR, H. S.: The anæsthetic effects of the intravenous injection of paraldehyde. Ann. Surg. 57:64-67 (Jan.) 1913.

218A. NOSWORTHY, M. D.: A method of keeping anesthetic records and assessing results. Brit. J. Anæsth. 18:160-179 (July) 1943.

219. ———: The value of anæsthetic records. St. Thomas's Hosp. Rep. 2:54-66, 1937.

220. NUNN, T. W.: Application of cold as an anæsthetic agent in operations for removing warty excrescences. Lancet. 2:262 (Aug. 31) 1850.

221. ODOM, C. B.: Epidural anesthesia. Am. J. Surg. 34:547-558 (Dec.) 1936.

222. O'DWYER, JOSEPH: Fifty cases of croup in private practice treated by intubation of the larynx, with a description of the method and of the dangers incident thereto. M. Rec. 32:557-561 (Oct. 29) 1887.

223. [OLDENBURG, HENRY]: An account of the rise and attempts, of a way to conveigh liquors immediatly into the mass of blood. Phil. Tr. Roy. Soc. 1:128-130 (Dec. 4) 1665.

224. ORÉ, P. C.: Des injections intra-veineuses de chloral. Paris, Bull. Soc. Chir. 1:400-412, 1872.

225. ———: Etudes cliniques sur l'anesthésie chirurgicale par la méthode des injections de chloral dans les veines. Paris, J. B. Baillière et Fils, 1875. 154 pp.

ORTH, O. S. See No. 288.

226. OSLER, WILLIAM: The first printed documents relating to modern surgical anæsthesia. Proc. Roy. Soc. Med. (Sect. Hist. Med.) 11:65-69 (May 15) 1918. Reprinted in Ann. M. Hist. 1:329-332, "1917" (1918).

227. PAGÉS, FIDEL: Anestesia metamérica. Rev. san. mil., Madrid. 11:351-365 (June); 385-396 (July) 1921.

228. PARHAM, F. W.: Thoracic resection for tumors growing from the bony wall of the chest. Tr. South S. A. 11:223-363, 1898.

229. PECK, C. H.: Intratracheal insufflation anæsthesia (Meltzer-Auer).

Selected References Arranged by Author

Observations on a series of 216 anæsthesias with the Elsberg apparatus. Ann. Surg. 56:192-200 (July) 1912.

230. ——, and MELTZER, S. J.: Anesthesia in human beings by intravenous injection of magnesium sulphate. J. A. M. A. 67:1131-1133 (Oct. 14) 1916.

231. PENDER, J. W., and LUNDY, J. S.: Anesthesia in war surgery. War Med. 2:193-212 (Mar.) 1942.

232. PERRIN, MAURICE, and LALLEMAND, LUDGER: Traité d'anesthésie chirurgicale. Paris, Chamerot, 1863. p. 16.

233. PIROGOFF, N. I.: Recherches pratiques et physiologiques sur l'éthérisation. St. Pétersbourg, F. Bellizard & Cie, 1847. 109 pp.

234. PITKIN, G. P.: Controllable spinal anesthesia. Am. J. Surg. 5:537-553 (Dec.) 1928.

235. PODOLSKY, EDWARD: Music as an anæsthetic. Etude. 57:707 (Nov.) 1939.

236. PRIESTLEY, JOSEPH: Experiments and observations on different kinds of air. Ed. 2. London, J. Johnson, 1775. For original description see his "Observations on different kinds of air." Phil. Tr. Roy. Soc. 62:147-264 (March) 1772.

236A. PROSKAUER, CURT: The simultaneous discovery of rectal anesthesia by Marc Dupuy and Nikolai Ivanovich Pirogoff. J. Hist. Med. and Allied Sciences 2:379-384 (Summer) 1947.

237. QUINCKE, H.: Die Lumbalpunction des Hydrocephalus. Berl. klin. Wchnschr. 28:929-933 (Sept. 21); 965-968 (Sept. 28) 1891.

238. RAGINSKY, B. B., and BOURNE, WESLEY: The action of ephedrine in avertin anesthesia. J. Pharmacol. & Exper. Therap. 43:209-218 (Sept.) 1931.

RAGINSKY, B. B. See also Nos. 41, 81, 82.

239. RAPER, H. R.: A review of Crawford W. Long centennial anniversary celebrations. Bull. Hist. Med. 13:340-356 (March) 1943.

240. RICE, N. P.: Trials of a public benefactor, as illustrated in the discovery of etherization. New York, Pudney and Russell, 1858. xx, 460 pp.

241. RICHARDSON, B. W.: Reports and lectures on original researches in scientific practical medicine. I. On a new mode of producing local anæsthesia. M. Times and Gaz. 1:115-117 (Feb. 3) 1866.

242. ROBINSON, VICTOR: Pathfinders of medicine. New York, Medical Life Press, 1929. 810 pp.

243. ROSENTHAL, S. M., and BOURNE, WESLEY: The effect of anesthetics on hepatic function. J. A. M. A. 90:377-379 (Feb. 4) 1928.

244. ROTTENSTEIN, J. B.: Refrigeration anesthesia. In: Traité d'anesthésie chirurgicale. Paris, 1880. p. 299.

245. ROVENSTINE, E. A.: A method of combining anesthetic and surgical records for statistical purposes. Anesth. & Analg. 13:122-128 (May-June) 1934.

ROVENSTINE, E. A. See also Nos. 71, 249, 252, 269, 289.

246. ROWBOTHAM, E. S., and MAGILL, I. W.: Anæsthetics in the plastic surgery of the face and jaws. Proc. Roy. Soc. Med. Section of Anæsthetics. 14:17-27 (Feb. 4) 1921.

RUGGIERO, WILFRED. See No. 3.

247. RUIGH, W. L., and MAJOR, R. T.: The preparation and properties of pure divinyl ether. J. Am. Chem. Soc. 53:2662-2671 (July) 1931.

248. RUSCA: Rachianæsthesie mit Tutocain und Percain, psychische Beeinflussung der Patienten durch Musik während der Operation. Schweiz. med. Wchnschr. 65:637-638 (July 13) 1935.

249. SAKLAD, MEYER; GILLESPIE, NOEL, and ROVENSTINE, E. A.: Inhalation therapy, a method for the collection and analysis of statistics. Anesthesiology. 5:359-369 (July) 1944.

SCHARPFF, W. See No. 292.

250. SCHLEICH, [C. L.]: Infiltrationsanästhesie (locale Anästhesie) und ihr Verhältniss zur allgemeinen Narcose (Inhalationsanästhesie). Verhandl. d. deutsch. Gesellsch. f. Chir. 21:121-127 (4 Sitzungstag 11 Juni) 1892.

SCHMIDT, E. R. See No. 290.

SCOTT, J. P. See No. 303.

251. SEBRECHTS, J.: Note au sujet de la rachianesthésie. Bull. Acad. Roy. de Méd. de Belgique. 10:543-638, 1930.

252. SEEVERS, M. H.; MEEK, W. J.; ROVENSTINE, E. A., and STILES, J. A.: A study of cyclopropane anesthesia with especial reference to gas concentrations, respiratory and electrocardiographic changes. J. Pharmacol. & Exper. Therap. 51:1-17 (May) 1934.

253. SERTÜRNER, F. W.: Ueber das Morphium, eine neue salzfähige Grundlage, und die Mekonsäure als Hauptbestandtheil des Opiums. Gilbert's Ann. d. Physik. 55:56-89, 1817.

253A. SEVERINO, M. A.: Use of snow and ice for surgical anesthesia (1646). In: Garrison, op. cit., p. 824.

SHANNON, G. E. See No. 26.

253B. SHIELDS, H. J.: Spinal anesthesia in thoracic surgery. Anesth. and Analg. 14:193-198 (Sept.-Oct.) 1935.

254. SHIPWAY, FRANCIS: The selection of cases for avertin anæsthesia. Brit. J. Anæsth. 7:114-120 (April) 1930.

SHONLE, H. A. See No. 303.

255. SICARD, M. A.: Les injections médicamenteuses extradurales par voie sacro-coccygienne. Compt. rend. Soc. de biol. 53:396-398 (April 20) 1901.

256. SIMPSON, J. Y.: The obstetric memoirs and contributions of James Y. Simpson. Edited by W. O. Priestley and Horatio R. Storer. Philadelphia, J. B. Lippincott and Co., 1856. Vol. 2, 733 pp.

257. ——: On a new anæsthetic agent, more efficient than sulphuric ether. London M. Gaz. n.s. 5:934-937, 1847. Also Lancet, 2:549-550 (Nov. 20) 1847.

258. SMITH, TRUMAN: An inquiry into the origin of modern anæsthesia . . . Hartford, Brown and Gross, 1867. 165 pp.

Selected References Arranged by Author

259. SNOW, JOHN: On chloroform and other anæsthetics; their action and administration. Edited, with a memoir of the author, by Benjamin W. Richardson. London, John Churchill, 1858. 443 pp.

260. ——: On narcotism by the inhalation of vapours. London M. Gaz. n.s. 12:622-627 (Apr. 11) 1851.

261. ——: On the inhalation of the vapour of ether in surgical operations: containing a description of the various stages of etherization, and a statement of the result of nearly eighty operations in which ether has been employed in St. George's and University College hospitals. London, J. Churchill, 1847. 88 pp.

262. SOUBEIRAN, EUGÈNE: Recherches sur quelques combinaisons du chlore. Ann. de Chim. 48:113-157, 1831. Also in J. de Pharm. 17:657-672, 1831; 18:1-24, 1832.

SOUTTAR, H. S. See No. 218.

263. SPESSA, A.: Modo di rendere insensibile una parte nella quale devesi praticare qualche atto operatorio. Bull. d. sc. med., Bologna. s. 5. 11:224-226, 1871.

264. STEHLE, R. L., and BOURNE, WESLEY: The anesthetic properties of pure ether. J. A. M. A. 79:375-376 (July 29) 1922.

265. ——, and BOURNE, WESLEY: Concerning the mechanism of acidosis in anæsthesia. J. Biol. Chem. 60:17-29 (May) 1924.

266. ——, and BOURNE, WESLEY: The effects of morphine and ether on the function of the kidneys. Arch. Int. Med. 42:248-255 (Aug.) 1928.

267. ——; BOURNE, WESLEY, and BARBOUR, H. G.: Effects of ether anæsthesia alone or preceded by morphine upon the alkali metabolism of the dog. J. Biol. Chem. 53:341-348 (Aug.) 1922.

STEHLE, R. L. See also No. 42.

268. VON STEINBÜCHEL (GRAZ): Die Scopolamin-Morphium-Halbnarkose in der Geburtshülfe. Beitr. z. Geburtsh. u. Gynäk. Rudolf Chrobak . . .60. Geburtst. 1:294-326, 1903.

269. STILES, J. A.; NEFF, W. B.; ROVENSTINE, E. A., and WATERS, R. M.: Cyclopropane as an anesthetic agent: a preliminary clinical report. Anesth. & Analg. 13:56-60 (Mar.-Apr.) 1934.

STILES, J. A. See also No. 252.

270. STRIKER, CECIL; GOLDBLATT, SAMUEL; WARM, I. S., and JACKSON, D. E.: Clinical experiences with the use of trichlorethylene in the production of over 300 analgesias and anesthesias. Anesth. & Analg. 14:68-71 (Mar.-Apr.) 1935.

271. SUTTON, W. S.: Anæsthesia by colonic absorption of ether. Ann. Surg. 51:457-479 (April) 1910.

272. ——: Anesthesia by colonic absorption of ether and oil-ether colonic anesthesia. Part I. Anesthesia by colonic absorption of ether. In: Gwathmey, J. T.: Anesthesia. Ed. 2. New York, Macmillan Co., 1924. pp. 433-438.

SWANSON, E. E. See No. 303.

273. SWORD, B. C.: The closed circle method of administration of gas anesthesia. Anesth. & Analg. 9:198-202 (Sept.-Oct.) 1930.

274. TAIT, DUDLEY, and CAGLIERI, GUIDO: Experimental and clinical notes on the subarachnoid space. Tr. Med. Soc. California. Abstracted J. A. M. A. 35:6-10 (July 7) 1900.

275. TALLMADGE, G. K.: The third part of the *De extractione* of Valerius Cordus. Isis. 7:394-411, 1925.

TATUM, A. J. See No. 92.

276. TAYLOR, FRANCES L.: Crawford W. Long and the discovery of ether anesthesia. New York, Paul B. Hoeber, Inc., 1928. p. 81.

THOMAS, G. J. See No. 146.

277. THOMS, HERBERT: "Anesthésie à la Reine," a chapter in the history of anesthesia. Am. J. Obst. & Gynec. 40:340-346 (Aug.) 1940.

278. TRENDELENBURG, FRIEDRICH: Beiträge zur den Operationen an den Luftwegen. 2. Tamponnade der Trachea. Arch. f. klin. Chir. 12:121-133, 1871.

279. TUFFIER: Analgésie chirurgicale par l'injection sous-arachnoïdienne lombaire de cocaïne. Compt. rend. Soc. de biol. 51:882-884, 1899.

280. ———, and HALLION: Opérations intrathoraciques avec respiration artificielle par insufflation. Compt. rend. Soc. de biol. 48:951-953 (Nov. 21) 1896.

TUOHY, E. B. See No. 183.

280A. TURNER, MATTHEW: An account of the extraordinary medicinal fluid, called aether . . . London, J. Wilkie, [1743?]. 16 pp.

281. VESALIUS, ANDREAS: De humani corporis fabrica libri septem. Basel, Oporinus, 1543.

282. WALLER, A. D.: The chloroform balance. A new form of apparatus for the measured delivery of chloroform vapour. Proc. Physiol. Soc. (London) 1908. Printed in the J. Physiol. 37:1908—pp. vi-viii.

282A. WANGEMAN, C. P.: An experiment in the recording of surgical and anesthetic data in military service. Anesthesiology, 2:179-185 (March) 1941.

282B. ———, and MARTIN, S. J.: The recording of surgical and anesthetic data in two Army general hospitals. Anesthesiology, 6:64-80 (Jan.) 1945.

WARDEN, C. E. See No. 3.

WARM, I. S. See No. 270.

283. WARREN, EDWARD: Some account of the Letheon; or who was the discoverer. Ed. 2. Boston, Dutton and Wentworth, 1847. 79 pp.

284. WARREN, J. C.: Etherization with surgical remarks. Boston, W. D. Ticknor and Co., 1848. v, 100 pp.

285. ———: Inhalation of ethereal vapor for the prevention of pain in surgical operations. Boston M. & S. J. 35:375-379 (Dec. 9) 1846.

285A. WATERS, R. M.: Carbon dioxide absorption from anæsthetic atmospheres. Proc. Roy. Soc. Med. 30:11-22 (Nov.) 1936.

286. ——: Clinical scope and utility of carbon dioxid filtration in inhalation anesthesia. Anesth. & Analg. 3:20-22; 26 (Feb.) 1924.

287. ——: The evolution of anesthesia I & II. Proc. Staff Meet., Mayo Clin. 17:428-432 (July 15); 440-445 (July 29) 1942.

287A. ——: Nitrous oxide centennial. Anesthesiology. 5:551-565 (Nov.) 1944.

288. ——; ORTH, O. S., and GILLESPIE, N. A.: Trichlorethylene anesthesia and cardiac rhythm. Anesthesiology. 4:1-5 (Jan.) 1943.

289. ——; ROVENSTINE, E. A., and GUEDEL, A. E.: Endotracheal anesthesia and its historical development. Anesth. & Analg. 12:196-203 (Sept.-Oct.) 1933.

290. ——, and SCHMIDT, E. R.: Cyclopropane anesthesia. J. A. M. A. 103: 975-983 (Sept. 29) 1934.

WATERS, R. M. See also Nos. 92, 99, 114, 166, 269.

WATTS, JAMES. See No. 16.

291. WEESE, H.: Pharmakologie des intravenösen Kurznarkotikums Evipan-Natrium. Deutsche med. Wchnschr. 1:47-48 (Jan. 13) 1933.

292. ——, and SCHARPFF, W.: Evipan, ein neuartiges Einschlafmittel. Deutsche med. Wchnschr. 2:1205-1207 (July 29) 1932.

293. WELCH, W. H.: A consideration of the introduction of surgical anæsthesia. [Boston, The Barta Press, 1908?] 24 pp.

294. WELLCOME HISTORICAL MEDICAL MUSEUM, LONDON. Souvenir, Henry Hill Hickman, Centenary exhibition, 1830-1930, at the Wellcome Historical Medical Museum. London, Wellcome Foundation, Ltd., 1930. 85 pp.

295. WELLS, HORACE: A history of the discovery of the application of nitrous oxide gas, ether and other vapors, to surgical operations. Hartford, J. G. Wells, 1847.

296. WELLS, T. S.: Three cases of tetanus in which "woorara" was used. Proc. Roy. Med. Chir. Soc. London. 3:142-157 (Nov. 22) 1859.

297. WILKS, SAMUEL, and BETTANY, G. T.: A biographical history of Guy's Hospital. London, Ward, Lock, Bowden and Co., 1892. pp. 388-389.

298. WOOD, A.: On a new method of treating neuralgia by the direct application of opiates to the painful points. Edinburgh M. & S. J. 82:265-281, 1855.

299. WOOD, P. M., and BICKLEY, R. S.: Observations on the use of tribromethanol (avertin). Am. J. Surg. 34:598-605 (Dec.) 1936.

300. WOODBRIDGE, P. D.; HORTON, J. W., and CONNELL, KARL: Prevention of ignition of anesthetic gases by static spark. J. A. M. A. 113:740-744 (Aug. 26) 1939.

WOOLSEY, W. C. See No. 121.

300A. WYCOFF, B. S.: Intravenous anesthesia in oral surgery. Am. J. Orthodontics. 24:875-877 (Sept.) 1938.

301. YOUNG, H. H.: Long, the discoverer of anæsthesia. Bull. Johns Hopkins Hosp. 8:174-184 (Aug.-Sept.) 1897.

302. ZERFAS, L. G., and McCALLUM, J. T. C.: The analgesic and anesthetic properties of sodium isoamylethyl barbiturate: preliminary report. Indiana State M. A. J. 22:47-50 (Feb.) 1929.

303. ——; McCALLUM, J. T. C.; SHONLE, H. A.; SWANSON, E. E.; SCOTT, J. P., and CLOWES, G. H. A.: Induction of anesthesia in man by intravenous injection of sodium iso-amyl-ethyl barbiturate. Proc. Soc. Exper. Biol. & Med. 26:399-403 (Feb.) 1929.

The Future of Anaesthesia

BY

NOEL A. GILLESPIE

"RESPICE, aspice, prospice," said the ancients. The earlier chapters of this monograph have complied with the first two parts of this exhortation. Any attempt to apply the third is tempered with the reflection that the events of the last five years have shown the folly of pretending to the gift of prophecy. Nevertheless an attempt to forecast the outcome of the events of the past which have been related is too alluring to be omitted. Surgical anæsthesia has now been known to us for a century, and more advances have been made in the last thirty years than in the first seventy. From the general trend of these advances it should be possible to deduce what the future holds in store for the subject.

The outstanding advance in anæsthesia in this century is something more fundamental than the introduction of new drugs or of methods for their administration. It is that an increasing number of medical men are learning to apply their knowledge of physiology, pharmacology, pathology, and clinical diagnosis to the art of anæsthesia. It was this characteristic that gave John Snow his position as the pioneer among clinical anæsthetists. Since his day far too many persons who lacked the knowledge, ability, or enterprise to do this have been associated with the specialty. The result has been that the position of anæsthetist came to be regarded as a menial one, and the contribution that he had to make to the well-being of the patient as a purely mechanical one. Indeed this view has been so widely held that in many cases administrations of anæsthesia have been confided to persons without a medical training and therefore with a minimal knowledge of how the human body works, or of the processes of disease and the modifications of function which they produce.

The History of Surgical Anesthesia

In recent years the specialty of anæsthesia has been taken up by men of sound medical training prepared to devote their lives to the study of the alterations of function induced in the human body by the effects of disease, of drugs which produce unconsciousness, and of surgical manipulation. They found that the condition of the anæsthetized human being could be observed as carefully as that of an experimental animal and that accurate records could be kept of his behaviour at the time. They also learned the importance of written records of his physical condition before operation and of the complications which occurred after operation. They evolved mechanical systems so that these facts could be correlated reasonably rapidly and be compared statistically.

Surgeons soon found that their work was facilitated and their responsibility was lessened when they secured the assistance of a medical anæsthetist who "thought in physiological terms." Anæsthesia itself was of higher quality so that they were provided with better conditions under which to operate. They felt free to concentrate their attention entirely on the site of operation because they knew that a diagnostician of skill was devoting his attention to the general condition of the patient. He, they knew from experience, was competent to recognize and treat effectively any emergency which might arise. Indeed, on occasion, his observations of the effects produced by some action of the surgeon's could be of assistance to the latter.

In the last ten years the professional anæsthetist has shown that his services as a consultant can be of value in places other than the operating room. Since he is intimately concerned with both normal and abnormal respiration, and is skilled in the treatment of respiratory obstruction or depression, his opinion or help is of value in the recognition and management of respiratory complications after operation. It is also his daily practice to administer gases by inhalation, and therefore he is the person best qualified to apply inhalational therapy. He is adept at producing analgesia by "blocking" nerves in various parts of the body and this procedure is as useful for therapeutic or diagnostic purposes as for the performance of operations. Daily he observes the great variability of response of individuals to a given dose of an hypnotic or analgesic drug, and he is often in a position to advise the least harmful means of procuring the comfort of a patient. He is accustomed to diagnose and treat emergencies which may arise in either of the two systems which are vital: the respiratory or the circulatory, and such cases are seen in the casualty room and the ward as well as in the operating room.

The efficient discharge of these duties demands the services of a person of sound clinical judgment as well as manual skill. The technician, no matter how experienced, lacks the training in physiology, pharmacology, pathology and clinical diagnosis which is essential to these functions. The administration of anæsthesia by technicians, therefore, will progressively disappear in the future.

The task, however, of training enough professional anæsthetists to make this possible is of considerable magnitude. The American Medical Association enumerates some six thousand four hundred hospitals in the United States, whereas the membership of the American Society of Anæsthetists does not greatly exceed fifteen hundred. Our primary aim must be to provide at least one efficient professional anæsthetist for every hospital in the country. To do this the teaching of the subject must undergo drastic reform. There are still medical schools from which a student can graduate without any instruction in anæsthesia; and in far too many the "teaching" is reminiscent of "the blind leading the blind." It seems safe to forecast, therefore, that before long every medical school in the country will possess a Department of Anæsthesia staffed exclusively by medical men of sound training and proved skill of judgment.

These Departments will have a sufficient staff to undertake research as well as the effective teaching of students, interns, and residents. The staff should be employed "whole-time." In the past careful work has often been made impossible because an individual who was a "part-time" teacher was forced to wear himself out by rushing from one hospital to another in an effort to earn a living. Although many still believe that the lure of personal gain is the only motive for which men will put forth their best endeavour I believe that the best work of the future will be produced by departments manned by "full-time" personnel. Few can produce good work when driven by the prospect of want and uncertainty; and the possibility of personal gain is subversive of conscience and scruple. On the other hand the man whose heart is in his work will use the freedom provided by economic security to its best advantage, and will justify the ideal conditions provided by the employment of the whole of his energy. If he is found lacking in this respect he should be discharged. In such a professional department there will probably be a tendency towards specialization of interest: for instance one member of the permanent staff is likely to undertake the leadership of a sub-department of inhalational therapy, another will be responsible for diagnostic and therapeutic procedures, and so forth.

In the past, as a study of the outstanding events clearly shows, far too much importance has been attached to the particular drug or to the method by which it is administered. Even today the literature is full of controversy between the proponents of rival drugs and methods. There is, however, no ideal agent or method: none which is equally well suited to every purpose, for any patient and in any hands. It has been wisely said that no anæsthetic agent is safer than its worst administrator. The few who have cultivated the art of "thinking physiologically" are perfectly aware that the agent and the method by which it is administered are unimportant. What is vital is the clinical judgment with which the anæsthetist selects the ones to be used for a particular operation in a given patient and under specific circumstances. Thus, as the number of skilled professional anæsthetists increases, we shall develop more balance of judgment and we shall realize more clearly that our lack is not of new agents and methods, but of skill in the use of those we already possess.

The individual is more important to the future than the

machinery. Anæsthesia has shown of recent years that it makes greater claims upon a man, and offers more intellectual exercise, than the mere unthinking repetition of a manual process. It has become evident that it offers to men of the highest intellectual and personal qualities a life full of interest, value, and utility. As this fact becomes more widely appreciated so will a supply of men of the highest ability come forward to adopt anæsthesia as a career. It is this contribution of which the subject stands in the greatest need today. No prophetic powers are needed, however, to point out that if such men are to be attracted to the specialty it must be able to offer candidates of ability proper financial remuneration as well as some assistance in the pursuit of their studies. In the past there has been little, if any, endowment destined to promote training in anæsthesia. The munificent foundation by Lord Nuffield of a Chair in the University of Oxford represents a new departure. Already, in several countries, there are signs that other, if lesser, foundations for the same purpose will shortly come into being.

Anæsthesia is a young specialty, and it is still possible for one person to be personally acquainted with the majority of full-time workers in other countries. But few bonds of international friendship and understanding are closer than those formed by professional interests in common, and this is especially true of the medical profession. The human body is subject to similar lesions which respond to the same treatment the world over; and a passionate interest in the succor of the ills of mankind transcends national boundaries. If we are not to "lose the peace" there must be a more brotherly feeling between nations. In the interest of the world of the future a representative International Society of Anæsthetists is greatly to be desired. I will hazard the prophecy that ere long we shall see its foundation.

Hickman died prematurely, ridiculed and disillusioned; Wells, having been laughed to scorn, took his own life: in this century Howard-Jones and Ivor Lewis, who had both made outstanding contributions to anæsthesia, died by their own hands. Thus did medicine reward pioneers in anæsthesia. We hope that this era is past. Isolated tragedies caused by lack of understanding there still will be, but in the main the medical profession is beginning to appreciate the anæsthetist. The future lies in the hands of the generation which strives to build the phœnix of a new world that is to arise from the ashes of this war. We have had enough of mediocrity; we now need the best—those who will not hesitate "to give, and not to count the cost; to fight, and not to heed the wounds; to toil, and not to seek for rest; to labor, and not to seek for any reward." If but a few members of the younger generation of the highest integrity and competence can but see the opportunity and decide to spend their lives and efforts in the service of anæsthesia, the future is bright indeed.

Appendix

The Morton and Warren Tracts on Ether (Letheon)

BY JOHN F. FULTON

W HEN WILLIAM MORTON decided to take out a patent on his anesthetic he found it essential to print directions concerning his new agent and its use. Sir William Osler drew attention to these printed circulars and expressed the hope that they might one day be collected and studied bibliographically.[1] During the past year we have attempted to do this and we are glad to make such

[FIG. 43a] Verso of the folded leaf of Morton's notice carrying the postmark and the address of Dr. J. Mason Warren, Boston.

information as we have gleaned available for Major Keys' timely volume. A full bibliographical description of the tracts will follow later in a catalogue of an exhibit on the history of surgical anesthesia displayed at the Yale Medical Library during December 1944.

In the little-known biography of Morton published by Benjamin P. Poore in 1856[2] one finds the following statement:

"The medium through which Dr. Morton communicated the results of experiments on etherization to the public, was a 'circular' which he had printed, at his own expense, almost every week. It was at first, as its name imports, a mere letter of advice;

TO SURGEONS AND PHYSICIANS.

The subscriber is prepared to furnish a person fully competent to administer his compound to patients who are to have surgical operations performed, and when it is desired by the Operator that the patient should be rendered insensible to pain. Personal or written application may be made to

W. T. G. MORTON,

Dentist,

No. 19, Tremont Row, Boston.

[FIG. 43b] Morton's first printed notice relating to surgical anesthesia; a folded leaf conjugate with Figure 43a.

[178]

but, as it became the receptacle of newspaper articles, and correspondence from every portion of the Union, announcing the success of etherization, it was necessarily enlarged into a large and closely-printed sheet of four pages. Soon this 'circular' became a pamphlet, and of this five different editions were published, under Dr. Morton's immediate supervision, embodying a digest of all the authentic information, both from Europe and America, on anesthesia. This was a perfect magazine of arguments against the opponents of etherization, and its preparation naturally gave Dr. Morton a good deal of care and anxiety, as he was considered responsible for the contents.

"When the news of the European success of Dr. Morton's discovery came back across the Atlantic, he changed the form of his publication, although he retained its simple title, adding to it 'A Voice from Europe.' This last edition of this valuable work, which was of nearly one hundred closely-printed pages, embodies much of great interest, and it conquered the prejudices of many who had previously had such imperfect sources of authentic information on the discovery, that their minds had remained warped by prejudice, or they had been unable to form a candid opinion on the subject.

"This 'Voice from Europe,' as the fifth edition of Dr. Morton's circular was also called, acted like sunlight upon the skeptical among the American medical fraternity, and before its bright rays of truth, the darkness of prejudice was soon dissolved."

It is curious that exactly the same passage occurs in the other contemporary biography of Morton published in 1858 by Nathan P. Rice.[3] Rice makes no reference to Poore's biography, but a comparison of the two texts indicates that Rice lifted the greater part of his text directly from Poore without a shadow of acknowledgment—and despite Poore's note on the title-page which contains the statement: "A few copies of this compilation have been published, for such revisions, additions or alterations as Dr. Morton's friends may seem [*sic*] fit. The re-publication of any portion or of all of it, should a copy find its way into public hands, (which is not intended,) is positively forbidden."

[179]

The first printed document issued by Morton is a single-page folded sheet addressed "To Surgeons and Physicians" stating that the "Subscriber" is prepared to furnish "a person fully competent to administer his compounds." The copy (see figs. 43a and 43b) preserved in the Library of the Massachusetts Historical Society, addressed to Dr. J. Mason Warren, bears a postmark dated November 20 [1846]. The same day Morton also published a notice in the *Boston Evening Transcript*. The *Boston Medical and Surgical Journal* for December 2nd also carried a notice in its advertising sheet headed "General Circular—Public Caution." It is probable that this General Circular was also issued separately, and we have reason to believe that this separate Circular, copies of which are still unlocated, was regarded by Morton as the first edition of the Letheon circular. We have also been unable to locate the closely printed four-page circular mentioned by Rice.

The tracts and notices by Morton may thus be listed as follows:

THE WRITINGS OF W. T. G. MORTON

Notice "To Surgeons and Physicians"

1. The folded, single-page notice headed "To Surgeons and Physicians" was printed sometime prior to November 20, 1846, and since it represents Morton's earliest public statement on the subject we list it first. It is folded once and is intended for mailing without envelope (see figs. 43a and 43b). Two copies have been traced, one in the Massachusetts Historical Society addressed to Dr. J. Mason Warren, the other at the Essex Institute, Salem, Mass., addressed to Dr. Henry Wheatland, Salem, Mass., postmarked "Boston, Nov. 23".

Notices in Public Press

2. *Boston Evening Transcript*, Nov. 20, 1846, headed "To the Public", stating that he has applied for Letters Patent.

3. *Boston Medical and Surgical Journal*, Nov. 25, 1846. Notice headed "To Surgeons and Physicians"; on back Advertising Sheet. The text is the same as No. 1 above, but Morton adds in a postscript: "Surgeons and Physicians who may wish to witness this effect of the new agent, are respectfully invited to call at my rooms. In the next No. of the Journal a name for this new operation will be given." There is also a second notice by Morton on this page offering instruction in Dentistry.

Appendix

4. *Boston Medical and Surgical Journal*, Dec. 2, 1846, headed "General Circular . . . Public Caution" on Advertising Sheet. The same notice reappears in the *Journal* for Dec. 9, 16, 23, 30, 1846, and Jan. 13, 1847.

Circular. Morton's Letheon

5. 1ST EDITION, 1 PAGE   *Boston*, Nov. 26, 1846

   Probably the 1-page sheet headed "General Circular . . . Public Caution" with text identical with that of No. 3 above. No copy found.

6. 2ND EDITION, 4 PAGES   *Boston*, Dec. 1846

   Probably the four-page Circular mentioned by Poore and Rice in their biographies of Morton. No copy traced.

7. 3RD EDITION, 14 PAGES   *Boston*, ? Dec. 1846

   The Circular is now expanded by inclusion of letters and excerpts from journals up to the middle of December. Copies in the Army Medical Library and Treadwell Library of the Massachusetts General Hospital.

8. 4TH EDITION, 42 PAGES   *Boston*, Jan. 1847

   This edition of the Circular, now expanded to 42 pages, contains dated excerpts through Dec. 30, 1846. One copy found, in the Library of the College of Physicians, Philadelphia.

9. 5TH EDITION, 88 PAGES   *Boston*, May 1847

   This, the final edition of the Circular, which carries the additional title "Voice from Europe", must have been printed in large numbers since many copies have been preserved. It occurs in wrappers of three colors: yellow, green, and blue.

Morton's Other Writings on Ether

10. Remarks on the proper mode of administering sulphuric ether by inhalation. Boston: Dutton and Wentworth, Printers, 1847. 44 pp. [Light-grey cardboard covers with petit-point design, gold edges.]

11. Mémoire sur la découverte du nouvel emploi de l'éther sulfurique, suivi des pièces justificatives. Paris, Imprimerie d'Edouard Bautruche, 1847. 60 pp. [Copy in Boston Athenaeum.]

12. On the loss of the teeth, and the modern way of restoring them, as practised by W. T. G. Morton and Francis Whitman. Boston: Printed by Damrell & Moore, 1847. 32°. 23 pp., 2 illus. [Appendix pp. 18-23 "Great Discovery", letters and excerpts describing the success of the new anesthetic agent; latest date, Paris, Aug. 16, 1847.]

13. Rapport des administrateurs de l'Hôpital Général de Massachusetts; suivi de l'histoire de la découverte de l'éther; et du mémoire addressé par

le Docteur Morton, à l'Académie française. R. H. Dana, Jr., Editeur. Cambridge: Imprimerie de Metcalf et Compagnie, 1848. 144 pp., 2 *ll.*

14. On the loss of the teeth, and the modern way of restoring them, as practised by W. T. G. Morton. Second edition of ten thousand copies. Boston: Printed by William A. Hall, 1848. 32°. 2 *p.l.*, 32 pp. [Although 10,000 copies are said to have been printed, only two have been traced, one at the Essex Institute in Salem, Mass., the other at the Army Medical Library. The Appendix which now runs from p. 17 to p. 31 is augmented by a series of quotations headed "Opinions of the Press". Dr. Whitman, the co-author of the first edition, had died early in 1848.]

15. On the physiological effects of sulphuric ether, and its superiority to chloroform. Boston: Printed by David Clapp. Medical and Surgical Journal Office. 1850. 24 pp. [Light cream-colored paper covers.]

16. Comparative value of sulphuric ether and chloroform. *Boston med. surg. J.*, Sept. 11, 1850, *43*, 109-119. [Signed 19 Tremont Row, Boston, Sept. 3, 1850.]

17. Remarks on the comparative value of ether and chloroform, with hints upon natural and artificial teeth. Boston: Printed by William A. Hall, 1850. 16°, 2 *ll.*, 48 pp. [The preliminary two leaves consist of an illustration labelled "Morton's Tooth Manufactory", followed by half-title, "Morton"; pp. 37-48 are made up of testimonial letters bearing on the virtues of Morton's artificial teeth. The first pages of text reprint the paper listed above as No. 16 from the *Boston Medical and Surgical Journal.*]

18. The use of ether as an anesthetic at the Battle of the Wilderness in the Civil War. *J. Amer. med. Ass.*, April 23, 1904, *42*, 1068-1073. Reprint: 15 pp. [in grey wrappers.]

EDWARD WARREN ON THE LETHEON

Morton had employed as a legal agent one Edward Warren of Palmyra, Maine, who aided him in negotiations for his patent. Warren, who was untrained in medicine and dentistry, collected letters and relevant excerpts from journals in support of the patent claim and issued them periodically in a pamphlet which bore the title, *Some Account of the Letheon*. The testimonial technique which Morton had used in his Circular Warren also employed, and his Letheon pamphlets contain in consequence a wealth of source material which has an important bearing on the ether controversy. The celebrated letter to Morton from Oliver Wendell Holmes appears in the second issue of the second edition of Warren's tract. This in consequence has become one of the great collector's items both for those who pursue the literature of anesthesia and for those who collect the Autocrat. As with Morton's Circular, Edward Warren's tract passed through five issues but technically there were only three "editions."

Some Account of the Letheon

19. 1ST EDITION, 38 PAGES   *Boston*, March 1847

Inserted following the title-page is an engraved lithographed portrait of Morton signed "W. Judson Jr. pinxt. On Stone, by J. H. Peirce." Only the first edition contains the portrait.

20. 2ND EDITION, 49 PAGES   *Boston*, April 1847

This, a little-known issue of the Warren pamphlet, contains several letters not included in the first edition, the latest of which is Dr. George Hayward's communication read to the Boston Society for Medical Improvement, April 12, 1847. Five copies have been traced.

21. 2ND EDITION, 2ND ISSUE, 2 + 79 PAGES   *Boston*, May 1847

The second issue of the second edition of Warren's tract contains on page 79 the memorable letter to Morton from Oliver Wendell Holmes, dated November 21, 1846, in which Holmes proposed the term "anæsthesia" to describe the state of insensibility produced by ether vapor; and he also suggested the adjective "anæsthetic". Eight copies of this issue have been traced.

22. 3RD EDITION, 1ST ISSUE, 88 PAGES   *Boston*, June 1847

In this edition Warren's tract has been considerably expanded, with type completely reset. The Holmes letter appears in the Appendix on pp. 84-85 and much in the way of testimonial material has been added. Copies are bound in salmon or in blue covers. Twelve copies have been traced.

23. 3RD EDITION, 2ND ISSUE, 90 PAGES   *Boston*, July 1847

This issue is identical with the first issue of the third edition save for the addition of "Dr. Jacob Bigelow and the Ether Question" on pp. 89-90. One copy in the original state, inscribed to Dr. John Homans, is in green covers. Twelve copies have been traced.

---

[1] OSLER, W. The first printed documents relating to modern surgical anæsthesia. *Proc. roy. Soc. Med.*, 1918, *11* (Section Hist. Med.), 65-69.

[2] POORE, B. P. Historical materials for the biography of W. T. G. Morton, discoverer of etherization, with an account of anæsthesia. Washington, 1856.

[3] RICE, N. P. Trials of a public benefactor, as illustrated in the discovery of etherization. New York, 1858.

Index

A. C. E. mixture, 49, 50
Abbot, Gilbert, 27
Abel, A., 61
Abel, John, 110
Abreu, Benjamin, xxx
Abū Bekr Hamidb, Samajūn, 104
Academy of Sciences (France), 13
Acetone, 33
Acetylcholine, xvii
Acidosis in anesthesia, xxix, 81, 146
Adams, R. C., 55, 60, 63, 118
Adrenalin, 76
Adrenin, 82
Adsorption, xviii
Aesculapius, 6, 103
Agamede, 4
Agote, Luis, 56, 113
Alcohol, xiii, xvii, xxx, 5, 9, 14, 48, 50, 59, 81
Aliphatic cyclopropyl ethers, 53
Allen, Frederick M., 45, 118
Allen, William, 17, 105
Alles, Gordon, xxviii
Alurate, see Barbital and barbital derivatives
American Association of Anesthetists, 89
American Board of Anesthesiology, 92, 117
American Dental Association, 41
American Medical Association, 34, 36, 43, 69, 92, 118, 173
American Society for Pharmacology and Experimental Therapeutics, xxii
American Society of Anesthetists, xxi, 47, 88, 89, 173
American Society of Heating and Ventilating Engineers, 91
Ammonia, 38
Ampère, 26
Amphetamine, xxviii
Amyl nitrite, 44
Analeptic measures, 81, 147
Anderson, Hamilton, xxviii
Andral, Gabriel, 29
Andrews, Edmund W., 72, 73, 84, 108
Anesthesia Abstracts, 117
Anesthesia Collections, xix-xxi
Anesthesia in war, 146
Anesthésie à la reine, 32
Anesthésie et Analgesie, 117
Anesthesiology, x, xix, 117
Anesthetic apparatus, 83-86
Anesthetic narcotism, 44
Anesthetic tension, 78, 79, 146
Anesthetometer, 79
Animal magnetism, 12, 13
Anoci-association, xvii, 44, 143
Anociation, see Anoci-association
Anrep, Vasili Konstantinovich von, 40, 109
Anticoagulants, 56
Antony and Cleopatra, 11
Arabians, 7

Archer, Harry, xx, 3, 6, 39
Area of swallowing, 78
Area of vomiting, 78
Army, 70
Army General Hospitals, 89
Army Medical Library, ix, xi, xix, xx, 46, 57
Arterial pressure, 88
Artificial respiration, 63, 66
Ascending respiratory paralysis, 78
Asphyxia, xviii, 37, 49, 64, 72, 73, 74, 75
Association for Research in Nervous and Mental Diseases, xvi
Assyrians, 6, 11
Asthma, 15
Atkinson, A. S., 82
Auer, John, 67, 68, 112
Avertin, see Tribromethyl alcohol
Babcock, Myra E., 8
Babcock, Wayne, 43
Bacon, Sir Francis, 3
Bailey, N., 30
Baillie, Matthew, 29
Bailly, 13
Balanced anesthesia, 78, 146
Bamberg Antidotarium, 7
Bancroft, W. D., 72
Barach, A. L., 117
Barbital and Barbital Derivatives, xvii, xxiii, xxviii, xxx, 58, 59, 60, 61, 62, 63, 81, 82, 139-140
Barbiturates, see Barbital and barbital derivatives
Bardet, 59, 114
Barthélemy, 67, 111
Bartlett, Willard, 69, 70
Bay, Jens C., xi
Beattie, John, 59
Becker, 49
Beddoes, Thomas, 17, 21, 83
Beecher, H. K., 86, 87, 117
Beer, 54
Behan, R. J., xv, xvi
Bell, I. R., 52
Bell, Jacob, 107
Bennett, Alexander, 40, 108
Bentley, Y., 23
Benzedrine, see Amphetamine
Benzine, 33
Berkshire Medical College, 21
Bernard, Claude, xviii, 39, 71, 72, 73, 82, 108
Bert, Paul, 19, 72, 73
Bert's apparatus, 75
Bettany, G. T., 17
Bevan, Arthur Dean, 51
Bier, August, 42, 58, 110, 112
Bigelow, 22, 28, 29
Bischoff, Theodor, 55
Black, Constance, 53, 117
Blake, xxx

Blood bank, 56
Blood serum, 56
Blood transfusion, 54-56
Blood types, 56
Blundell, James, 55
Boccaccio, 8
Bogendörfer, L., 59, 61, 115
Boothby, Walter, 68, 79, 86, 112, 113
Boothby-Cotton sight-feed apparatus, 86
Borderan, 40
Boston Society of Medical Improvement, 29
Botsford, Mary, xxix
Bourne, Wesley, xxix, 43, 76, 80, 81, 82, 115, 117
Bowditch, Henry Pickering, 108
Boyle, H. E. G., 68, 86
Boyle machine, 86
Bradley, 17
Braid, James, 13
Braun, Heinrich, 39, 40, 42, 110
Braxton-Hicks, John, 55
Bredenfeld, Elisabeth, 58, 82, 113
Briffault, Robert, 4
British Army Plastic Unit, 68
British Journal of Anaesthesia, 114
British Medical Association, 74, 114
Brooke, Arthur, 10
Broussais, François, 29
Brown, Gilbert, 88
Brown, William E., 51, 114
Brunton, Lauder, 75
Bull, 47
Bullard, O. K., 63
Bullein, William, 9, 104
Bulletin of National Association of Nurse Anesthetists, 116
Bumm, R., 60, 115
Bumpus, 39, 41
Burkhardt, Ludwig, 58, 112
Butylene, 18
Butzengeiger, O., 48, 115
Buxton, 19
Caglieri, Guido, 42, 111
Calcium hydrate, 69
Canadian Medical Association, 51, 115
Cannabis indica, 7
Capillary activity, xviii
Carbon dioxide, xiii, xxix, 6, 14, 19, 21, 69, 86, 132-133
Carbon dioxide absorption, 69-71, 133
Carbon monoxide, 50
Carbonic acid gas, *see* Carbon dioxide
Cardiac damage, 52
Carlson, H. J., 110
Carnations, 50, 51
Carr, C. Jelleff, 53
Carron oil, 47, 48
Carter, J. B., 51, 114
Cartwright prize, 88
Cathelin, M. F., 90, 111
Cautery, 62
Cerebral cortex, xvii
Cerebral excitement, 37

Charles X of France, 20
Chemical Warfare Service, xxiv
Chen, Mei-Yu, *see* Mei-Yu Chen
Chinese, 6
Chloral hydrate, 56, 58
Chloroform, xvii, 33, 35, 37, 48, 50, 57, 58, 64, 65, 69, 72, 73, 74, 75, 76, 82, 83, 84, 130-131
Chloroform commission in Paris, 74
Chloroform percentages, 83
Circle filter, 70
Circulatory collapse, 19
Circumcision, 6
Clarck, Timothy, 54
Clark, Sir James, 35
Clark machine, 85
Clarke, William E., 21, 22, 106
Claye, A. M., 48
Clement, F. W., 117
Clendening, Logan, xi, xx, 22
Clendening, Mrs. Logan, xi
Clendening's library on anesthesia, xi, xii, 30
Cleveland Clinic, 79
Cleveland Dental Manufacturing Company, 84
Cleveland Medical Library Association, xi, xix
Clover, Joseph T., 83, 84, 108, 109
Coal gas, 49
Coburn, 86
Coca, xiii, 39, 40
Cocaine, 39, 40, 41, 42, 43, 82, 136
Codman, E. A., 87, 88, 110
Coga, Arthur, 54
Cold, xviii, 44
Colish, A., xii
College of Physicians and Surgeons, New York City, 88
Collins, K. H., 82
Colloids, 44
Colonic anesthesia, *see* Rectal anesthesia
Colt, Samuel, 21
Colton, Gardner Q., 23, 24, 83, 108
Compatibility of the blood, 56
Conditioned reflexes, 81
Conduction anesthesia, 41, 43
Connell, Karl A., x, 79, 85, 91, 112, 113, 117
Continuous caudal analgesia, 90, 142
Continuous spinal anesthesia, 90, 141
Convulsions, 37
Cooley, Samuel A., 23
Cooper, Astley, 17, 105
Corneal reflex, 40
Cornell University, 72
Corning, J. Leonard, 41, 42, 44, 109, 110
Cotton, F. J., 68, 79, 112
Cotton, J. H., 51
Cotton-Boothby apparatus, 79
Coupart, 40
Crile, George W., x, xvii, 43, 49, 82, 87, 88, 112
Crocker, William, 50, 112
Crocus metallorum, 54

Index

Crombil, Alexander, 109
Cullen, 30
Cullen, S. C., 62, 89
Cunningham, J. H., 47, 86
Curare, 89, 149
Current Researches in Anesthesia and Analgesia, ix,
    x, 90, 114
Cushing, Harvey, 43, 87, 88
Cushing Laboratory, 44
Cuvier, Baron, 29
Cyanosis, 66
Cyclopropane, 49, 52, 53, 77, 89, 91, 135
Cyclopropyl methyl ether, 49, 53, 134–135
Cyprome ether, *see* Cyclopropyl methyl ether
Dale, Sir Henry, 80
Dana, F., Jr., 29
Danis, 113
David, N., xxx
Davy, 50
Davy, Humphry, xiv, 15, 16, 17, 18, 21, 105
Death, 8, 47, 54, 55, 74, 76
DeBory, 13
Decameron, 8
De Castello, 56
Dehydration, xviii
Delirium, xiii, 39
Dementia praecox, xxix
Denis, Jean-Baptiste, 54, 55, 105
Dental operations, Intravenous anesthesia, 63
Deslon, Charles, 13
Di-allyl-barbituric acid, *see* Barbital and
    barbital derivatives
Dial, *see* Barbital and barbital derivatives
Diathermy, 62
Dillon, T. G., 115
Dinitrophenylmorphine, xxviii
Dioneo, 8
Dioscorides, 6, 9, 10, 30, 103
Dittrick, Howard, ix, xxi, 89, 90
Divine right of kings, 5
Divinyl ether, *see* Divinyl oxide
Divinyl oxide, xviii, xxvi, xxvii, xxviii, xxx,
    49, 52, 77, 135
Dogliotti, A. M., 44
Dresser, H., 58, 111
"Drowsy" syrups, 11
Du Bartas, Guillaume de Saluste, 35
Du Bois, R., xviii
Duc de Bordeaux, 54
Ducros, 71
Dufour, 67, 111
Duke of Bourbon, 12
Dumas, Jean Baptiste, 33, 106
Duncan, 33
Duncum, Barbara, 83
Dupuy, Marc, 46
Eckman, James, xii
Edinburgh, Medico-Chirurgical Society of, 33
Edward III, 5
Edwards, W. B., 90, 118
Egyptians, 6, 7
Ehrenfried, Albert, 79
Eichholz, 48

Einhorn, Alfred, 42, 111
Eisenhart, C., 89
Eisenmenger, Victor, 65
Elliotson, John, 13, 29, 106
Elsberg, Charles A., 68, 112
Elsholtz, Sigismund, 38, 54, 105
Embley, Edward Henry, 75, 76
Emerson, George, xxviii, xxx
Emmerez, 54
Endotracheal anesthesia, 59, 63–69, 144–145
Enzyme chain reactions, xvii
Ephedrine, 81
Epidural anesthesia, 41, 43, 44, 136–137
Epinephrine, 42, 110
Erlanger, Joseph, xvi
Erythroxylin, 39
Esdaile, James, 13, 14, 106
Ether, xiv, xvii, xxv, 3, 9, 18, 25, 26, 27, 29,
    31, 32, 33, 35, 36, 37, 45, 46, 47, 48, 50, 53,
    57, 58, 69, 71, 79, 80, 82, 83, 84, 87, 89,
    128–130, 177–183
Ether frolics, 21, 22
Ether percentages, 78, 79
Ether spray, 45
Ethyl alcohol, *see* Alcohol
Ethyl bromide, 69
Ethyl chlorate, 110
Ethyl chloride, 45, 69
Ethyl ether, 52, 53, 133
Ethyl-N-Propyl ether, 134
Ethylene, xxv, 18, 49, 50, 51, 52, 86, 133-134
Ethylene dichloride, 49
Ethylene-oxygen anesthesia, 50, 81
Eulenberg, 50
Eunarcon, *see* Barbital, barbital derivatives
Evans, Herbert, xxvi
Evans, William E., Jr., 53
Everett, 30
Evipal sodium, *see* Barbital and barbital
    derivatives
Evipan, *see* Barbital and barbital derivatives
Explosiometer, xxx
Explosion hazards, 62
Explosions, xxx, 90, 91
Eye, 40
Eyelid reflex, 78
Eyster, J. A. E., xxiv
Fabrica, 62, 63, 64
Face mask, 66
Faculty of Paris, 13
Failure of respiration, 67, 75
Failure of the circulation, 74
Faraday, Michael, 18, 106
Farr, R. E., 116
Farrington, Benjamin, 64
Fauvel, 40
Federated Societies for Experimental Medi-
    cine, xxiii
Fedorow, 58
Feissly, R., 115
Fell, George H., 65, 66
Fell-O'Dwyer apparatus, 65, 67
Fibrillation of the heart, 76

Filatov, 117
Finsterer, Hans, 114
Fisch, Max H., xi
Fischer, Emil, 59, 111
Fitch, R. H., 60
Flagg, J. F. B., 107
Flagg, P. J., 86, 118
Flourens, Marie-Jean-Pierre, 31, 33, 74, 107
Flowmeter apparatus, xxx
Floyd, Ada, xi
Foregger, Richard V., 70, 71, 85, 86, 113, 114
Forman, Sylvan E., 53
Fourneau, E., 42, 111
Fox, 17
Fractional rebreathing, 85
Fraenkel, Sigmund, xxvi, 40
Francis, W. W., xx
Franklin, Benjamin, 12, 13, 26
Fredet, 59, 115
French Academy of Medicine, 20, 32
French Academy of Sciences, 57
French Revolution, 14
Freud, Sigmund, xxii, 40
Freund, August, 52, 109
Frobenius, 9, 105
Frost, Eben H., 26, 27
Fuller, 32
Fülöp-Miller, 3, 12, 14, 39
Fulton, J. R., 61
Fulton, John F., x, xx, 14, 30, 59, 60, 176–182
Future of anæsthesia, 171–176
Gaedicke, 39, 108
Gale, Joseph W., 68
Gandow, Otto, 61
Garrison, F. H., 7, 28
Gärtner tonometer, 88
Gas-ether sequence, 84
Gasser, Herbert, xvi, xxiv
Gatch, Willis D., 85, 112
Gauss, C. J., 48, 114
Gelfan, Samuel, xxvi, 52
Geyer, Guido, 61
Giesel, 42, 110
Gillespie, Noel, x, 62, 67, 77, 86, 89, 118, 171–176
Giornale Italiano di Anestesia e di Analgesia, 116
Glasgow committee, 75
Goldblatt, Samuel, 116
Goldenweiser, A. A., 4
Goldschmidt, Samuel, 116
Good, 30
Goodell, H., xvi
Goodwille's patented inhaler, 83
Goyanes, J., 58, 112, 113
Graef, Wilhelm, 113
Greeks, 5, 6
Greene, B. A., 58, 59, 60, 63
Greene, W. W., 39, 108
Griffith, H. R., 35, 89
Guedel, Arthur E., xxi, xxviii, xxix, xxx, 52, 70, 76, 77, 78, 86, 112, 114, 117, 118
Guillotin, Joseph-Ignace, 13

Guthrie, C. C., 111
Guthrie, Samuel, 33, 106
Guy de Chauliac, 104
Guy's Hospital, 17
Gwathmey, James T., x, 47, 68, 85, 113, 116
Gwathmey apparatus, 85, 86, 113
Gwathmey-Woolsey gas machine, 112
Hahn, André, 71
Hallion, 66
Halsted, William S., 41, 43, 109
Hardy, J. D., xvi
Harley, George, 49
Harrington, F. B., 87
Harvard Medical School, xxvi, 24, 25, 31, 79
Hashish, see Hemp
Hayes, S. J., 84, 109
Hayward, George, 28
Heart, 54, 87
Hebrews, 6
Hedonal, see Methylpropylcarbinol urethane
Heidbrink, J. A., 71, 85, 112, 115
Heidbrink Model T machine, 85
Heidbrink "oo" machine, 85
Heidbrink two-chamber absorber, 71
Heidbrink's first machine, 71
Heidelberg, Ophthalmological Congress, 40
Helen, 5, 103
Hemlock, 7, 8
Hemorrhage, 55
Hemp, 5, 7
Henbane, 5, 7, 8
Henderson, Velyien E., xviii, xxv, 52, 72, 115
Henderson, Yandell, xxv, 70, 112
Henry Hill Hickman Medal, 76, 80
Herb, Isabella, 51, 114
Hermann, Ludimar, 50
Hernia, 43
Herodotus, 6, 103
Hertzler, A. E., 117
Herwick, R. P., 82
Hewer, C. L., 116
Hewitt, Sir Frederic, 49, 77, 84, 109, 110
Heywood, C. F., 27
Hickman, Henry Hill, xxix, 19, 20, 21, 76, 80, 106, 175
High resistance intercoupling, 91
Hildebrandt, 42
Hillarius, 10
Hingson, R. A., 90, 118
Hirsh, Joseph, 55
Hitchcock, Fred A., 19
Hitchcock, Mary A., 19
Hobbie, Miss, 22
Hober, R., xviii
Hodges, R. M., 26
Hoff, H. E., 76
Holmes, Oliver Wendell, 30
Homer, 5
Hook, Robert, 64
Horine, Emmet F., xx
Horton, J. Warren, 91, 117
Howard-Jones, 175
Hua T'o, 7, 103

Index

Hubbell, A. O., 63
Hugh of Lucca, 7, 8, 104
Hull Botanical Laboratory, 51
Humphry Davy's "gas" machine, 17
Hunter, 47
Hunter, John, 12
Hurd, G. H., 110
Hurwitz, S. W., 113
Hustin, A., 56, 113
Hyderabad commissions, 74, 75
Hydrogen, 15
Hypnotism, 13
Hypodermic, 38, 39, 48
Hypodermic syringe, 38
Hyssop, 6
Hysteria, 15
Ice, 45
Iliad, 5
Illuminating gas, 51
Infiltration anesthesia, 42, 43
Inflatable cuff, 64, 65, 70
Ingenhouss, Johannes, 49, 105
Inhibited nervous system, 81
Inhibitory neurosis, 81
Intermittent anesthesia, 77
Intermittent flow machine, 85
International Anesthesia Research Society, 90
International College of Surgeons, 45
International Congress on Physiology, xxvi
International Medical Congress, 47, 65
International Society of Anæsthetists proposed, 175
Intestinal anesthesia, *see* Rectal anesthesia
Intravenous anesthesia, 53–63, 137–139
Intubation of the trachea, 64
Iodoform, 33
Ivy, 7, 8
Jackson, Charles A., 25, 26, 107
Jackson, Chevalier, 68
Jackson, Dennis E., 69, 70, 113, 116
Jaffe, Bernard, 26
James, N. R., 118
Jarman, Ronald, 54, 61
Jesus, 6
John, 6
Johns Hopkins Hospital, 41, 43, 87
Johnson, G. E., 89
Johnston Brothers, 108
Jones, G. W., 91, 117
Jones, Harold W., xi
Jones, Lauder, xxv
Jones, Tom, 39
Kartaševskij, 117
Keep, Nathan Colley, 32
Keith, 33
Keller, Charles M., 28
Kennedy, Catherine, xi
Kennedy, R. E., 91, 117
Ketosis, xxv
Keys, Thomas E., xix, xx, xxx
Killian, Hans, xxix
King, Edmund, 54
King's evil, 5

Kirschner, Martin, 59
Kirstein, Alfred, 68, 110
Kleiman, 6, 21, 47
Klikovich, 109
Knapp, 40
Knight, Lee Irving, 50, 112
Knight, T. A., 19
Knoefel, Peter K., xxiii, xxvi, xxx, 52, 82
Koehler, A. E., xxv
Koller, Carl, xi, xxii, 40, 109
Korff, 48, 111
Krantz, John C., Jr., 53, 117
Krawkow, N. P., 58, 111
Kropp, 61
Kuhn, Franz, 67
Kümmell, R., 112
Kummer, 42
Labat, Gaston, 114
Lafargue, 38
Lafayette, 12
Lahey, Frank, 47
Lahey Clinic, 91
Lakeside Hospital, Cleveland, 85
Landsteiner, Karl, 56
Langsdorf, 86
Larrey, Baron, 21, 45, 90, 106
Latta, 55, 106
Laughing-gas parties, 21
Lavoisier, 13
Lawrie, Lt. Col. Edward, 74, 75
Leake, Chauncey D., x, xiii-xxx, 6, 9, 21, 44, 50, 52, 81, 82, 116
Leake, Mrs. Chauncey D., xxv
Leavitt, William, 26
Lemmon, William T., 90, 117
Leopold, Prince, 35
LeRoy, 13
Lethal chamber, 44
Letheon, x, 28, 30, 177–183
Lettuce seed, 8
Levy, A. G., 76, 114
Lewis, Bransford, 42
Lewis, Dean, 49
Lewis, Ivor, 175
Lewisohn, Richard, 56, 113
Liebig, Justus von, 33, 106
Lillie, R., xviii
Linnaeus, 30
Lipoid solubility, xviii
Lister, Lord, 74
Liston, Robert, 29, 107
Liver injury, xxviii
Local anesthesia, 135-136
Local, regional and spinal anesthesia, 37-44, 62
Loevenhart, A. S., xxiii, xxiv, xxv, xxix, 82
Loewen, Storm van, 80
Long, Crawford W., xiv, 22, 23, 26, 32, 106
Louis IX, 5
Louisiana State Medical Society, 67
Lower, Richard, 54, 105
Lucas, G. H. W., 52, 72, 115
Luckhardt, Arno B., xx, xxv, 49, 50, 51, 114
Lullius, Raymundus, 9, 104

Lundy, John S., ix, x, xxi, 60, 61, 62, 78, 82, 86, 88, 116, 118
Lundy-Heidbrink kinetometer gas machine, 86
Lundy-Heidbrink model, 86
Lussem, Franz, 50
Lyman, 21
MacAlyane, Eufame, 9
McCallum, J. T. C., 60
McClendon, Adeline, 23
McCleskey, G. L., 23
MacDonald, Joseph, 90
Macewen, William, 65, 109
McGill University, 80, 81
MacIntosh, R. R., xxi
McKesson, E. I., 68, 85, 88, 111, 112
McKesson machine, 85
McMechan, Francis H., xxi, xxix, 89, 90
McMechan, Laurette van Varseveld, xxi, xxix, 89, 90
Magaw, Alice, 111
Magendie, François, 45, 71
Magill, I. W., 68, 76, 114, 117
Magnesium sulfate, 48, 58
Maine Medical School, 39
Major, Randolph, xxv, xxvi, 52
Malgaigne, Joseph-François, 32
Mandragora, xiii, 5, 6, 7, 8, 10, 11
Mandrake, *see* Mandragora
Mann, Frank, 79, 114
Mansfield, J. D., 28
Marcellus, 10
Marie Antoinette, 12
Marin, M. G., 59, 115
Mark, 6
Marsh, David, xxvii, xxx
Martin, Mrs. George, 44
Martin, S. J., 89
Massachusetts General Hospital, xiv, xx, 14, 27, 29, 87
Massachusetts Historical Society, 179
Massachusetts Institute of Technology, 91
Matas, Rudolph, 43, 65, 66, 67, 110, 111
Matthew, 6
Maxson, L. H., 117
Maydl, Karel, 65
Mayo, C. H., 50
Mayo, W. J., 50
Mayo, William Worrall, 50
Mayo Clinic, ix, xi, xii, xix, xxi, 60, 61, 86
Medical Research Council of Great Britain, 61
Meek, Walter J., xxiv, 52
Mei-Yu Chen, xxvi, 52, 116
Meigs, Charles D., 34
Meltzer, S. J., 58, 67, 68, 112
Membrane permeability, xviii
Merck and Company, xxvi, xxvii
Mering, J. von, 111
Mesmer, Franz A., 12, 13, 105
Mesmerism, 27, 29
Methylene bichloride, 44
Methylpropylcarbinol urethane, 58
Meyer, H. H., xviii

Miller, Albert H., 25, 27, 78, 83, 86, 115
Miller, William S., xxi
Miner, John R., xii
Minor surgical operations, 77
Mitchill, Samuel Latham, 15
Mock, Harry, Jr., 45
Mock, Harry E., 45
Mollière, Daniel, 46, 109
Montagna, Mazzeo della, 8
Monte Cassino *Codex*, 7
Moodie, Roy L., 39
Moore, James, 11, 105
Moreno y Mayz, 40
Morgan, Ben, 71, 86
Morpheus, 38
Morphine, xvii, xxiv, xxv, xxviii, xxix, 38, 39, 40, 71
Morphine sulfate, 48
Morse, Samuel F., 26
Morton, Elizabeth W., 25
Morton, William T. G., xiv, xx, 14, 22, 23, 24, 25, 26, 27, 28, 29, 30, 31, 35, 71, 83, 107, 177–183
Mousel, L. H., 62
Moutard-Martin, R., 109
Mravlag, Paul, xxii
Muehlberger, Clarence, xviii, xxv
Mulberry, 8
Müller, 50
Muscular rigidity, 89
Music as an aid to anesthesia, 149
Myrrh, 6
Nakagawa, Koshiro, 59, 114
Napoleon, 21
Narcylen, 114
Narkose und Anæsthesie, 115
Nasal intubation, 67
National Research Council, xxix
Nausea, 39, 82
Needle, 38, 42, 90
Neff, W. B., 116
Nembutal, *see* Barbital and barbital derivatives
Neonal, *see* Barbital and barbital derivatives
Nepenthe, 6
Nerve fibers, xvii
Nerve impulses, xvii, 72
Nerves, xiii, xviii, 11, 41, 43, 44, 72, 147
New York Academy of Medicine, 28
New York Society of Anesthetists, 47
Newton, Harlan F., 43
Nicolas of Salerno, 7, 104
Niemann, Albert, 39, 108
Nitric ether, 33
Nitrogen, 15
Nitrous oxide, xiv, 3, 14, 15, 16, 17, 18, 21, 22, 24, 25, 62, 68, 69, 71, 72, 73, 83, 84, 85, 86, 131-132
Nitrous oxide-oxygen anesthesia, 69, 73, 81, 84, 85
Noel, H., 58, 113
Nosworthy, M. D., 88, 89, 116
Novinny, 39

Index

Novocaine (procaine hydrochloride), *see*
  Procaine and procaine compounds
Nuffield, Lord, 175
Nunneley, Thomas, 49, 107
Obstetrics, 8, 32, 33, 34, 48, 69, 77, 90
Ockerblad, N. F., 115
Odom, Charles B., 44
O'Dwyer, Joseph, 65, 66
Odyssey, 5
Ohio Chemical and Manufacturing Company, 86
Ohio monovalve anesthesia machine, 86, 112
Oldenburg, 54
Olefiant gas, *see* Ethylene
Olive oil, 48
Olmsted, J. M. D., 72
Opium, xiii, 5, 7, 37, 38, 54
Oral surgery, Intravenous anesthesia in, 63
Oré, Pierre-Cyprien, 56, 57, 58, 108
Orlandi, 87
Osborne, W. A., 74, 76
Osler, Sir William, xx, 30, 177
Osler Library, xx
Ospedale di S. Matteo in Pavia, 87
Otis, 40
Overton, C. E., xviii
Oxide of azote, *see* Nitrous oxide
Oxygen, 14, 15, 19, 47, 50, 61, 62, 63, 68, 69, 71, 72, 73, 84, 85, 86, 91
Pagés, Fidel, 44, 114
Pain, xiii, xv, xvi, xviii, xix, xxviii, xxix, xxx, 3, 4, 5, 6, 12, 13, 14, 15, 18, 19, 21, 24, 26, 27, 31, 33, 36, 38, 39, 43, 44, 48
Paracelsus, 9, 104
Paraldehyde, xxx, 58, 59, 82
Paré, Ambroise, 11, 104
Parham, F. W., 67
Parrot, Miss, 25
Patroclus, 5
Payr, E., 111
Peariro, 86
Pearson, Richard, 105
Peck, Charles H., 58, 68
Pentobarbital sodium, *see* Barbital and barbital derivatives
Pentothal sodium, *see* Barbital and barbital derivatives
Peoples, S. Anderson, xxvii, xxviii, xxx
People's Hospital, New York City, 47
Pereira, 26
Peridural anesthesia, *see* Epidural anesthesia
Perlis, 59, 115
Pernice, 42
Pernocton, *see* Barbital, barbital derivatives
Pernoston, *see* Barbital, barbital derivatives
Pessel, 69
Peter Bent Brigham Hospital, 79
Peters, Charlotte H., 14
Petroleum liquid, 48
Pharmacologic factors, 80-83
Phatak, Nil, xxx
Phenobarbital, *see* Barbital and barbital derivatives

Phosphoric acid, 81
Physiologic factors, 71-80
Pien Ch'iao, 103
Pike, F. H., 111
Pirogoff, Nikolas Iwanowitch, 45, 46, 107
Plasma, 56
Plato, 30
Pliny, 6, 103
Plomley, 77
Pneumatic medicine, 15
Poggendorf, 33
Poisoning, 55, 82
Poore, Benjamin P., 178
Pope, Dr. Elijah, 22
Poppy, 5, 8, 11, 37
Porta, Giambattista della, 104
Porto, Luigi da, 10
Post, 47
Post-anesthetic care, 82
Potassium phosphate, 81
Potion of the condemned, 6
Pravaz, Charles Gabriel, 38, 107
Pravaz syringe, 38
Premedication, 48, 49, 71, 78, 82
Presbyterian Hospital (Chicago), 51
Presbyterian Hospital (New York), 66
Priestley, Joseph, xx, 14, 49, 105
Princeton University, xxiii, xxv, xxvi, 52
Prinz, 5
Procaine and procaine compounds, xxiii, 42, 44, 58, 90, 137
Propylene, 52
Pulse, 45, 87
Puncture, 44
Puységur, Count Maxime de, 13, 106
Quarterly Supplement of Anesthesia and Analgesia, 90
Quill, 54
Quincke, 41, 42, 110
Quinine alkaloid, 48
Quistorpius, J. B., 30
Radcliffe Infirmary, Oxford, England, xxi
Raginsky, 81
Rainsbotham, Francis H., 34
Ravdin, I. S., xxvii, 116
Réclus, 42
Records and statistics, 86-89, 149
Rectal anesthesia, xxix, 45-48, 142-143
Redard, 109
Refrigeration anesthesia, 44, 45, 143-144
Regional anesthesia, 41, 43
Regnault, V., 107
Reiset, J., 107
Respiration, 87
Restoration agents, 81
Reversible coagulation, xviii, 72
Revista Argentina de Anestesia y Analgesia, 117
Reynolds, Lawrence, xx
Rhinology, 40
Rice, Nathan P., 179
Richardson, Sir Benjamin Ward, xxvi, 32, 44, 50
Richter, G. H., 72

Riesman, David, 7
Riggs, John M., 24
Riggs' disease, 24
Riva-Rocci, Scipione, 87
Riva-Rocci's blood-pressure apparatus, 87
Robbins, B. H., 117
Robinson, Victor, 33
Romans, 6
Romeo and Juliet, 10, 11
Rosenberg, Paul, 67
Rothenberg, I. M., 47
Rothenberg, Solomon, 47
"Round trip" absorber, 71
Rous, Peyton, 114
Roux, 46
Rovenstine, E. A., 52, 62, 88, 89, 116
Rowbotham, E. S., 68
Royal Academy of France, 29
Royal College of Physicians and Surgeons, 80
Royal College of Surgeons of Edinburgh, 19
Royal College of Surgeons of London, 19, 31
Royal Society, 19, 21, 54, 64
Royal Society of Medicine, 76
Royal Society of South Africa, 64
Royal Victoria Hospital, Montreal, 80
Ruigh, R. L., xxvi, 52
Saez, Antonio, 45
Safety features, 146
Saglia, 40
St. George's Hospital, London, 32
St. Luke's Hospital (Cleveland), 85
Saklad, Meyer, 89
Saline solutions, 55
Sampson, Agnes, 9
Scanzoni, Friedrich W., 34
Scharpff, W., 61, 116
Scheele, Karl W., 14, 105
Scherzer, 39
Schleich, Carl Ludwig, 42, 110, 111
Schmerz, 115
Schneiderlin, 48
Schullian, Dorothy M., xi
Schuman, Henry, x, xii, xix
Schwarz, Otto Henry, 69
Schwarz, Otto Henry, Jr., 69
Scopolamine, 58
Scopolamine-morphine, 48, 142
Scrofula, 5
Scythians, 6, 103
Seattle model gas machine, 86
Seelig, M. G., 40
Seevers, M. H., 52
Seguin, 38
Semites, 6, 11
Semmler, xxvi
Sertürner, Friedrich Wilhelm, 38, 105
Severino, 45, 104
Shakespeare, 10, 11
Shannon, George E., 53, 117
Shattock, Samuel G., 56
Shields, Harry J., 43
Shock, xiii, xvii, 39, 44, 45, 55, 82
Shuman, John, xxix

Sicard, M. A., 90, 111
Sigerist, Henry, 7
Sight-feed dropper, 85
Signs of anesthesia, 77, 148
Silliman, 33
Silverman, Milton, xxx
Simpson, Sir James Y., 23, 33, 34, 35, 49, 74, 75, 107
Simpson, R. A., 89
Smith, Edgar F., xx
Smith, J. H., 25
Snow, John, 31, 32, 44, 64, 74, 77, 78, 83, 107, 108
Snow ice, 45
Society of Anæsthetists (London), 110
Sodium allyl secondary butyl thiobarbituric acid, see Barbital and barbital derivatives
Sodium amytal, see Barbital and barbital derivatives
Sodium chloride, 55, 58
Sodium citrate, 56
Sodium ethyl-methyl butyl thiobarbituric acid, see Barbital and barbital derivatives
Sodium ethylate, 44
Sodium hydrate, 69
Sodium isoamyl-ethyl-thio-barbiturate, see Barbital and barbital derivatives
Sodium phosphate, 56, 81
Somnambulism, 13, 14
Somnifen, see Barbital and barbital derivatives
Somnoform, 69
Soneryl, see Barbital and barbital derivatives
Soporific draughts, 8
Soporific sponge, 7
Sorrel, 8
Soubeiran, Eugène, 33, 106
Souchon, Edmond, 43
Souttar, H. S., 58, 113
Spear, Thomas, 26
Spessa, 39, 108
Sphygmomanometer, 87
Spinal anesthesia, 41, 42, 43, 62, 81, 90, 140-141
Sponge, 7, 8, 83
Squibb, Edward R., 107
Squire, Peter, 107
Stages of anesthesia, 77, 78, 148
Stanton, Madeline, x
Stecher, Robert M., xi
Stehle, R. L., 80, 81
Steinbüchel, von, of Graz, 48, 82
Stiles, J. A., 52, 116
Stockman, 21, 106
Stone of Memphis, 6
Stovaine, 42, 137
Striker, Cecil, 116
Stupor, 37
Sturgis, C. C., 54, 55, 56
Sturli, 56
Sudhoff, Karl, 7
Sulfuric acid, 9
Sulfuric ether, see Ether
Sun Yat Sen, xxvi
Surface tension, xviii
Susruta, 103

Index

Sutton, W. S., 45, 47
Sweet vitriol, 9
Sword, Brian C., 70, 115
Sylvester, Joshua, 35
Syme, James, 74, 75
Synapses, xvii
Syncope, 74, 76
Tait, Dudley, 42, 111
Takáts, Geza de, 42, 115
Tallmadge, G. K., 9
Tatum, Arthur J., xxiii, 60, 82
Taub, 61
Taylor, Mrs. Frances Long, 23
Taylor, Isaac E., 38, 106
Teeth, 15, 24, 25, 26, 27, 32, 63, 73, 83
Telegraph, 26
Temperature, 87
Tetanus, 89
Teter, Charles 71, 84, 85, 111
Teter gas machine, 71, 84
Theodoric, 7, 8, 83
Thomas, G. J., 91, 117
Thompson, R. C., 50, 51, 114
Thoms, 32
Thoracic surgery, 66
Timed anesthesia, 85
Touching, 4, 5
Trachea, 63, 64, 65, 66, 68
Traube, J., xviii
Treadway, Walter, xxix
Trendelenburg, Friedrich, 64, 65, 108
Trent, Josiah C., xx
Trephining, xiii, 39
Tribromethyl alcohol in amylene hydrate, xxix, 48, 59, 81
Trichlorethylene, 116, 134
Trigeminal nerve, 43
Tropacocaine, 42, 137
Truehead, 65
Tuffier, Theodore, 42, 66, 110
Tuohy, Edward B., 80, 90
Turner, J. R., 114
Twilight sleep, 48-49
United States Bureau of Mines, 91
University at Wittemberg, 9
University College Hospital, London, 32
University of Alberta, 52
University of California, 52
University of California Hospital, xxvii, 52
University of California Medical Center, xx, xxvi, xxvii
University of Chicago, 51, 82
University of London, 31
University of Maryland, 53
University of Minnesota, 80
University of Oxford, 54, 59, 175
University of Pennsylvania, xx, xxvii, 22
University of Pittsburgh, xx, 91
University of Prague, 65
University of Vienna, 12
University of Wisconsin, xx, xxiii, xxiv, xxvii, xxix, 52, 53, 76, 82, 89
Vagus, 75, 76
Valerius Cordus, xiv, 9, 104

Valverdi, 11, 104
Vehrs, G. R., 116
Velpeau, Alfred-Armand-Louis-Marie, 32, 71
Venable, James M., 22
Ventricular fibrillation, 76
Veronal, see Barbital and barbital derivatives
Vesalius, 62, 63, 64
Victoria, Queen, 35
Vienna General Hospital, 40
Vinegar, 6, 8
Vinethene, see Divinyl oxide
Vitalism, 12
Vomiting, 54, 87
Waldie, David, 33
Wancher, 47
Wangeman, C. P., 89
Warburg, O., xviii
Warm, I. S., 116
Warren, Edward, 30, 177–183
Warren, J. Mason, 180
Warren, John C., 14, 18, 22, 24, 27, 28, 29, 105
Washington, James A., 38, 106
Washington University, 25, 69
Waters, Ralph M., x, xx, xxi, xxix, xxx, 21, 53, 60, 68, 70, 76, 88, 92, 115, 116, 118
Watt, 28
Watts, James, 17, 83, 105
Webster, Daniel, 28, 30, 31
Weese, H., 61, 116
Weir, 47
Wells, Horace, xiv, xx, 23, 24, 25, 106, 175
Wells, T. Spencer, 89
West, Andrew F., xxiii
Western Reserve University, 44
White Dental Manufacturing Company, 83, 84, 108
White gas machine, 110
Wieland, H., 114
Wilks, Samuel, 17
Williams. H. W., 37
Wilson, G. W., 114
Wilson, Woodrow, xxiii
Wine, 5, 6, 54
Winterstein, H., xviii
Wisconsin General Hospital, 62
Wolff, H. G., xvi
Wood, Alexander, 38, 107
Wood, Dorothy, xxvii, 52
Wood, Paul M., xxi
Woodbridge, Philip, 91, 117
Woolsey, William C., 85
World War I, 51, 58, 77
Wren, Sir Christopher, 53, 54, 105
Würdemann, 42
Wycoff, B. S., 63
Wynter, Essex, 41
Yale University School of Medicine, xx, 60, 70, 178
Yar-Phoonk, 14
Yversen, 47
Y'Yhedo, 46
Zakheim, xxx
Zerfas, L. G., 60, 116
Zeus, 5